Fitness for Geeks

Fitness for Geeks

Real Science, Great Nutrition, and Good Health

Bruce W. Perry

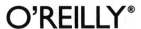

O'REILLY®

Beijing • Cambridge • Farnham • Köln • Sebastopol • Tokyo

Fitness for Geeks

by Bruce W. Perry

Copyright 2012 © Bruce Perry. All rights reserved.
Printed in United States of America.

Published by O'Reilly Media, Inc., 1005 Gravenstein Highway North, Sebastopol, CA 95472.

O'Reilly Media books may be purchased for educational, business, or sales promotional use. Online editions are also available for most titles (*my.safaribooksonline.com*). For more information, contact our corporate/institutional sales department: 800-998-9938 or *corporate@oreilly.com*.

Editor: Brian Sawyer		**Proofreader:** Rachel Head
Production Editor: Melanie Yarbrough		**Indexer:** Angela Howard
Technical Editor: Andrew "Bunnie" Huang		**Cover Designer:** Mark Paglietti
Copyeditor: Amy Thompson		**Interior Designers:** Edie Freedman & Ron Bilodeau

April 2012:   First Edition.

Revision History for the First Edition:

2012-04-12   First release

See http://oreilly.com/catalog/errata.csp?isbn=9781449399894 for release details.

OTABIND
This book uses Otabind™, a durable and flexible lay-flat binding.

ISBN: 978-1-449-39989-4

[M]

To my lovely wife, Stacy

Contents

Preface

How can we define health? Ever tried to take a stab at it? I attempt to define "fitness" and "geek" here because they appear in the title. But it seems *health* is a mélange of a lot of things—genes, lifestyle, a feeling of being safe and in charge—not all of which we can put a finger on.

We tend to grope around in defining good nutrition and health. We can be too reductionist in our view of who's healthy or whether *we* are healthy, claiming that "nutrition is 90 percent of health," or that we have achieved some perfect biomarker like total cholesterol after six tests at the doctor's office, so therefore we must be healthy. Or maybe we find out our telomeres are resilient and hanging in there, or we take a long survey on the Web, and the results pat us on the back and suggest we'll live to be one hundred. Many of these things seem like feel-good, almost delusional exercises. So much about health is mysterious, yet to be discovered, and may never be discovered. I like that aspect of it, because it leads to more experimentation. Maybe your own ideas about how to stay healthy haven't been refuted yet.

This doesn't mean that you can't aim for health, particularly if your current strategy has you waking up in the morning most days feeling pretty good. That's where my "fitness" and "geek" definitions come in.

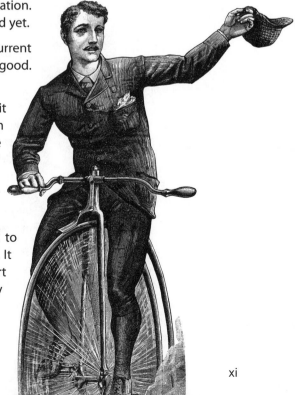

This is a book about fitness and nutrition for the independent of spirit and irrepressibly curious. The reason I have cleaved "nutrition" off from the general rubric of fitness is that, even though eating well (and the book will try to define *that* too) is part of being fit, we usually think of "fitness" as being an aspect of physical culture.

Fitness implies an underlying assumption of physical health. The *Oxford American Dictionary* defines fitness as "the condition of being physically fit and healthy." This book will discuss fitness in respect to becoming a physically stronger person and aging as well as we can. It will not advocate achieving a level of fitness, say, for a particular sport that undermines health in the process, which can actually be pretty common among all our popular extreme sports.

Mea culpa: I've done a few things in my life that some might consider extreme—like a five-hour–plus triathlon and a little mountaineering, mostly guided—but I would not claim that I was pursuing fitness during these adventures (I *was* fashioning unforgettable memories, and sometimes raising money for charity), and therein lies the difference. Since a good part of this book is about the latest and greatest gear that people are using for *self tracking*, speaking of extreme, I must pay homage here to the wonderful GoPro HD Hero helmet cams, which are tracking devices in their own right and have captured simply amazing outdoor videos for YouTube, such as that of a skier in the Alps being buried and dug out of an avalanche, and another skier launching off a cliff, unfurling a parachute, then watching an avalanche crash off the cliff behind him. Now *that's* personal tracking.

METs Anyone?

I will attempt to define fitness in terms of energy output—this book mentions *metabolic equivalent of task*, or MET, a number of times. This is a simple numerical index of the energy a person outputs during the day. So, fitness is the ability to not only have the requisite energy to get through your daily tasks, but to be intermittently capable of a high-intensity energy effort: a higher than typical MET, like lifting a heavy weight, jumping high, or running fast, relative to your age and circumstances.

We might even aspire to a more brass-tacks definition of fitness, which also comes from *Oxford-American*: the biological angle, "an organism's ability to survive and reproduce in a particular environment." You want to aspire to a level of fitness that allows you to thrive in your environment and be reasonably free of serious chronic illness. In this book's discussions of food, exercise, sleep, rest, meditation, hormesis, and other issues, I hope upon hope that readers can mine a few nuggets of information that help them "survive…in a particular environment."

The Food Angle

I like Boston Marathon winner Jack Fultz's "see food" diet—"see food and eat it" (see Chapter 7 for an interview with him)—for its simplicity. Eating in the modern world is anything but simple these days. The act of eating has been completely medicalized, and has become sociopolitically militant to boot. The vegans are hurling pies (nondairy, of course) at the meat eaters, the vegetarians are aiming online flames at the omnivores, and the raw foodists are, well, refusing to cook anything.

As you'll see in the chapter synopsis coming up, I'll provide a lot of detailed nutrition information, but it all comes down to "eat real food." Avoid processed junk and things we haven't eaten for millions of years (OK, coffee might be one exception). Yes, especially in Chapter 1, I spend a fair amount of time with the ancestral-health meme, or paradigm, that has worked its way through Western culture and among science and nutrition circles during the last few years.

The Mashed-up Ancient Angle

Humans spent hundreds of thousands of years moving around a lot outside, sleeping fairly long hours by the solar clock, and eating lots of plants and animal foods—and we carry largely the same software code inside ourselves today (human genes) as humans did back then. The closest approximations to an ancient person now are contemporary hunter-gatherers like the Maasai or the Hadzabe in East Africa, and they tend not to get our diseases.

Maybe a good part of fitness is simply getting back to our roots—not corrupting our own internal software by immobilizing ourselves in chairs, in cars, or in front of screens, moving around under the sun (making vitamin D), taking the time to sleep, and eating real food. Maybe.

Ironically enough, this is also a book about the latest technology—apps and gear that uses Global Positioning Systems, 3D accelerometers, and data connections to your own web dashboards to track personal propulsion (in running shoes and ski boots, etc.), eating, rest, and sleep. So it's a high-tech/ancient roots mashup. I certainly hope the mashup appeals and people don't find it cognitively dissonant.

A geek is someone who spends a huge amount of time analyzing the fine points of whatever interests her, ad infinitum, to a level that no one around her can possibly understand.

Annals of Experimentation

OK, now that we kind of know what fitness is, what's a *geek*?

The typical image of a geek in popular culture is the Spielbergian hero with Coke-bottle glasses who gets picked on at school, then becomes the town hero when he hacks the computers at the nearby nuclear plant that's having a meltdown. I tend to go for a broader definition, however. A geek is someone who spends a huge amount of time analyzing the fine points of whatever interests her, ad infinitum, to a level that no one around her can possibly understand. Her family members and friends are all flabbergasted and scratch their heads, until finally, with a shrug of their shoulders and a murmur of "fanatic…," they return to quotidian concerns.

When a geek focuses on fitness, that interest often manifests itself as self-experimentation. Geeks are inveterate, fearless experimenters. They want to plunge into demonstrations and proofs of conventional truths and, to this end, subject their bodies to experiments that make others squeamish, like long fasts, "hormetic" cold-river swims, guzzling pans full of leftover beet juice and admiring the red color of their pee afterward, or sometimes just going out to a beach or mountain and sprinting like wild people.

They absolutely do not automatically accept the bland marching orders of some officially anointed expert, whether it be the company dietician, a health-network M.D. they've never seen before, or the acronym-denoted bureaucracy that is determined to lecture them about how to eat and exercise.

The several people I've interviewed in the book—including two NFL pro football players, a mountaineering guide, a national expert on vitamin C, a scientist who tests the effects of fasting on mice and tumors, an MIT scientist who studies our mTOR growth pathway, and a former Israeli soldier who studied the Spartans, Greeks, and Macedonians and made up a "warrior diet"—don't necessarily fit any kind of cultural cross-section, but I think they're all fitness geeks in their own right.

I know I've always been a fitness geek. I've kept a little text log of sleep, workouts, morning heart rate, and body composition since way before the Internet became popular. I've also been educated in English and American literature and software engineering, and have spent a fair amount of time as a software programming geek. I have found many parallels between software design and fitness geekdom, such as the whole concept of antipatterns, or learning how to do something by studying how *not* to do it first. These parallels are sprinkled throughout the book—as is a little code here and there, but you don't have to be *that* kind of geek to enjoy the reading.

The "Measure First" Mantra

The final point I'll make about fitness geeks is that measuring, whether it be with the Fitbit, Zeo, Endomondo, their own software, or a simple text file, is a big part of a fitness geek's obsession (healthy obsession, I'd say). The other day, we got a mailing from the electric utility describing our home's energy usage and comparing it to that of our neighbors. We're usually right in the middle, leaning toward the most efficient and not the most gluttonous, but this time we had used way too much energy. I handed my 15-year-old daughter the graph of our energy usage and the local comparisons—"Here, you might find this interesting."

Lo and behold, I started to find yellow sticky notes all over the house, at outlets and on appliances, containing tips on how we can reduce our electricity use. Cool! The old cliché is, "What gets measured gets managed." The same is true with measuring health and fitness—the biofeedback makes a *big* difference.

How to Use This Book

This is a book that you can read from cover to cover, but you don't have to approach it linearly. You can bop in and out of it—"Hey, today I'm going to read something about macronutrients or fasting." Each chapter definitely stands on its own, so happy sampling.

This isn't a book that prescribes exactly how to eat and exercise. "If you do A, B, C, and D, you will be healthy—trust me." So many of those books come and go. I admire the determination and temerity of their authors to find the one pathway to Elysium. This book is, however, chock-full of ideas—mostly not mine originally, but certainly tested by me—of ways that you can tinker with your lifestyle and body and move into a different, healthy direction. I do appeal to some general paradigms, though, which I've mentioned—to eat real food, move around a lot, sleep copiously (things you've heard of before)—and I look at a lot of different tools that geeks have invented to help you measure and share your progress.

In terms of pursuing personal, optimal health, it's not selfish— let's shake that monkey off our backs. It's the fit person who has the energy and availability to be charitable, help others, and give more of herself.

I suppose the pursuit of optimal fitness for yourself is a lofty goal, and it's the path you take to get there that provides all the fun, stimulation, and gratification. In terms of pursuing personal, optimal health, it's not selfish—let's shake that monkey off our backs. It's the fit person who has the energy and availability to be charitable, help others, and give more of herself.

Chapter 1: *Fitness and the Human Codebase: Reboot Your Operating System*

> Too many of us are living in chairs (including the front seat of your Honda Civic or Ford Explorer), eating processed fake stuff on the run, and eschewing sleep for cable TV and social media. Isn't our internal software designed for something—Monty Python enter here—completely different? Isn't there a way we can live in the modern digital world and still feel physically vibrant? We look at cultivating respect for and seeking the wisdom of the ancients, as well as the evidence for rebooting our installed code and thus reacquainting ourselves with real food, sleep, and the great outdoors.

Chapter 2: *Fitness Apps and Tools*

> There's a lot of gear now that's designed to promote fitness, as well as for just plain time-wasting fun. *Self-tracking* is a bona fide movement among humans. Want to track your exercise (even weightlifting), analyze your chow, and view your sleep graphs for the week? There are apps and widgets for that, and more. We look at stuff like the Fitbit, Endomondo, Fitocracy, Alpine Replay, Garmin Connect, Google Earth mashups, and nutritiondata.com, among others (Zeo is covered in Chapter 9).

Chapter 3: *Macronutrients*

This is the first of two heavyweight chapters on nutrition before we turn to the "kicking up your heels" part of existence later in the book. We explore everything you always wanted to know about carbs, fats, and proteins, and then some stuff you probably didn't, like Rabbit Starvation Syndrome (the joy of living on seal fat) and the effect of fructose on your liver.

Chapter 4: *Micronutrients*

This chapter looks at everything you always wanted to know about vitamins, minerals, and phytochemicals, including some stuff that might have slipped past the school nurse during those vitamin lectures, such as "antinutrients" and what spinach might be doing to your mineral absorption, and the sorrows of vitamin deficiencies (and how easy it is to avoid them).

Chapter 5: *Food Hacks: Finding and Choosing Food*

Shouldn't you just see food and eat it? Yeah, I suppose if you were wandering through a dystopian-blasted landscape with Terminators in pursuit, but these days we can be a little more nuanced about choosing food. As in, do your wandering through weekly farmer's markets, find out what a CSA is, and get to know your local farmer (get to know him *really* well). This chapter also offers with some ideas for dealing with food shortages, price increases, and food deserts.

Chapter 6: *Food Timing: When to Eat, When to Fast*

This chapter also has a nutritional bend, but from a different angle—*not* eating for intermittent periods and the health benefits of fasting. We talk to a scientist that studies the metabolic effects of fasts, and we discuss numerous variations of fasting protocols and some of the stuff that happens with your body during fasting. We also interview the inventor of the "warrior diet," which can involve eating for only four hours per day. Hey, the Spartans did it.

Chapter 7: *The Other World: A.K.A. Outside*

This chapter looks at the absolute joy and necessity of being outside (we're programmed for it), from the point of view of walking, sprinting, hiking, body-weight exercises, running, and skiing. You learn how to do Tabata sprints, a pull-up, and your own resistance-exercise regimen on a remote beach. We talk to a former Boston Marathon winner and a mountaineer. We bring in some of our favorite tools: Endomondo, Google Earth, and Alpine Replay. And hey, I'll bet you never knew what *friluftsliv* was!

Chapter 8: Hello Gym! Navigating the Fitness Facility

You decide you gotta join the gym and get strong. Now what? We give you a rundown on the basics of resistance exercise in the gym (yeah, we figure you get the most bang for your buck by aiming to add and retain lean mass). The chapter talks about sets, reps, volume, and "repetition max," then it jumps into descriptions of about 15 different techniques, including photos and links. We talk to two NFL pro football players about the not-so-casual aspects of getting strong enough to withstand a profession as modern gladiator.

Chapter 9: Randomizing Fitness and the Importance of R & R

Ever written a `random( )` method or function in your code? Did you know that randomizing fitness, as in letting an algorithm choose a random exercise for you, might be good for you? We propose a couple of ways that you could do that (the CrossFit world has a "workout of the day" tradition), including the gainfitness.com tool. We also discuss an online tool for determining if an athlete is rested and ready to go, called RestWise. Last, but not least, is the all-important topic of sleep—and this is where you get a look at a nice piece of gear for the power sleepers of the analytic set: the Zeo Sleep Manager.

Chapter 10: Code Maintenance: Human Fueling and Supplements

Once you start going crazy on bumping up your outdoor and indoor activities, you have to start paying even more attention to nutrition. You suddenly start eating to get stronger and/or faster, not just because you're hungry. This chapter discusses some of the nuances, such as eating more of everything to add muscle, the magic hour after exercise for chowing, as well as a few supplements you might consider based on the science literature. We interview an MIT scientist about the mTOR pathway, which is the core biochemical sequence, buried just about everywhere in your body, that controls growth of both good (muscle) and bad (tumor) stuff. That's right, it's anabolic.

Chapter 11: Lifestyle Hacks for Fitness

There are so many different *potential* ways that you can hack fitness (and at least delight in the experimentation, even if they don't really work). This chapter discusses a few of them that probably do work, many falling under the rubric of hormesis, or good stress. Try cold-water swims, saunas, a nice glass of vintage grape (but not three), plus high-intensity exercise (also hormesis). "The world breaks everyone," Hemingway wrote in *A Farewell To Arms*, "and afterward many are strong at the broken places."

Acknowledgments

I always wanted to write a whole book about fitness, even before I became a geek (wait, I guess I always was a geek, they just didn't have a word for it yet—*curious dork*?). I absolutely never would have published this book, however, without the help of numerous other people.

I'll start with my family. My parents, Anne and Robert Perry, brought me up in Concord, Massachusetts (back then a land of rebels, geeks, writers, and readers), and constantly made sure that either I had a book in front of me or I was running around playing outside. No matter how hard he'd worked that day, my dad always took me outside to throw baseballs at him (note the suggestion of inaccuracy). Thereby a "fitness geek" was born. I'm grateful for everything they have done for me.

Stacy LeBaron, my wife, constantly lends her encouragement, not to mention indefatigable assistance, along with our two dear, fit children, Rachel (black belt in martial arts) and Scott (slick downhill skier in Vermont). It's tough to carve out time to write a book, and these guys are constantly covering for me so I can escape to the Vermont woods to write, not to mention inspiring new ideas with their feedback.

I'm grateful to all the busy scientists, researchers, professors, athletes, inventors, and all-around fitness geeks who took the time out of busy schedules to answer my questions, after I had "cold emailed" them out of the blue. This would have been a far lesser book without their input.

I thank my editor Brian Sawyer, who shepherded the book along from the beginning, as well as the rest of the O'Reilly team and Bob Watson, Lindsay Peterson, and Meghan Johnson, the tech reviewers, whose feedback and perspicacious efforts have made this a better book.

I'd also like to acknowledge you, the reader, and your pursuit of health for health's sake, which ends up benefitting everyone, not just yourself. Keep experimenting!

Safari® Enabled

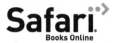 When you see a Safari® Enabled icon on the cover of your favorite technology book, that means the book is available online through the O'Reilly Network Safari Bookshelf.

Safari offers a solution that's better than eBooks. It's a virtual library that lets you easily search thousands of top tech books, cut and paste code samples, download chapters, and find quick answers when you need the most accurate, current information. Try it for free at *http://safari.oreilly.com*.

Fitness and the Human Codebase:
Reboot Your Operating System

You get up in the morning with the shades yanked down, after having collapsed under the covers at some indeterminate time past midnight (which followed several robotic hours of Facebook typing). Luckily, you'd set the coffee maker on a timer, so a quart of strong joe waits on the kitchen counter. Twelve ounces of that washes down a toasted bagel smeared with extra margarine and jelly, as you're out the door on the way to a 45-minute car commute.

It's just the beginning of a marathon bout of sitting.

The Cubicle Blues

Sound familiar? When you get to work it's an elevator ride off to the cubicle, where you refill the to-go coffee mug with joe that already tastes old, and someone's left an open box of donuts in convenient proximity. You write code until you're cross-eyed, interspersed with two meetings where you sit on your behind listening to two marketing/admin guys who love to hear themselves pontificate.

At lunchtime, you take the elevator downstairs and walk half a block to Subway, where you buy a "healthy" tuna n' cheese sub, which is almost the size of the baseball bat you used in Little League. Half of it is munched down before you get back to your cubicle and that C++ module you were supposed to finish by 5:30, which rolls around with an amazing sense of time squashed into a smaller space than you ever needed it to be.

A few times during the day, you join the crowd congregating in front of the vending machines (to which an entire work enclave has been devoted). The temptation to push a couple of buttons on this amazing invention and get *something*—chips (many varieties), a Pop-Tart, crackers and tuna salad (yup, they have those in vending machines)—is overwhelming. The lively sounds of conversation are interspersed with the ripping noise of little bags being opened.

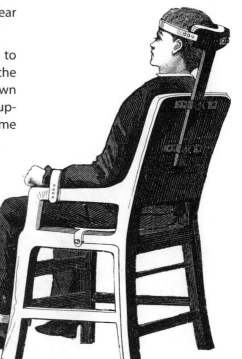

Movement, We Hardly Knew Ye

You wanted to exercise, but… it's back to the car commute and "dinner" (consisting of a Diet Pepsi and the rest of the sub while driving), when it dawns on you that you could not tell someone whether you actually walked in or physically sensed any sunlight that day. You get home, slump down onto a couch in the familiar sitting position, and, well, you feel like the bloody indefinable thing your big old cat, Hooch, who now eyes you with an inscrutable neutrality, dragged home that day.

Ditto the next day.

Free-Falling

What's wrong with this picture? Okay, so the implications of this narrative are pretty obvious. Hope I didn't lay it on too thick. You probably spent most of the day as a "chair liver."

The food you ate was "bad for you" (or simply not particularly good), and you didn't take any opportunities to move your limbs around, beyond pumping your fist in the air during an online glimpse of *ESPN SportsCenter*. You failed to stand up or walk for a reasonable period of time. The sun, bestowing life on earth, has become a stranger.

It's not your fault, you argue silently, with at least a little credibility. The work/commute schedule is crazy. You're lucky enough to have *any* job that pays pretty well.

Homing In on a Design Pattern

The messages your body undoubtedly sends you, however, roughly translated as *I feel like crap*, probably indicate that you're not really designed to live this way. In fact, a bunch of scientists, fitness experts, philosophers, economists, anthropologists, medical doctors, and overall outside-the-box thinkers have come up with the sensible hypothesis that we are *designed* for our ancestors' way of living, which was very different from the latter narrative.

We were not born to be chair livers, eating factory fare and keeping sleep hours like a vampire (unless we're in college, that is). Chapters 3, 4, 7, 8, and 9 will fill in just about all you need to know about eating right, kicking up your heels, and getting some rest. We need to find another design pattern.

… a bunch of scientists, fitness experts, philosophers, economists, anthropologists, medical doctors, and overall outside-the-box thinkers, have come up with the sensible hypothesis that we are designed according to our ancestors, who lived in a different way than the latter narrative.

DESIGN PATTERNS FOR CODE AND FITNESS

Men and women who write code for a living usually know something about design patterns. Design patterns are reusable strategies for solving common problems or tasks. The programming world borrowed this concept of design patterns from architecture—you have design strategies for buildings that always work, so why not reuse them instead of reinventing the wheel?

An example of a design pattern in object-oriented programming (OOP) is the Object Factory. OOP is a way of designing software based on the real world. If you have a website, and people join it as members, you might code a "Member" object so that you can separate that unit of Member code and have it only deal with aspects of memberships.

But you constantly need to create new Members in your code, because your website is so popular. So, the Object Factory is a piece of code whose sole purpose is to create new distinct Members. Every time your code needs to create a new Member (and store it in a database), it calls the Object Factory's getNewMember( ) method or operation. Problem solved.

Your fitness can also be based on a common design pattern—get sunlight, movement, natural food, sleep, affection, love—which we derive from our very deep past. Much of our behavior can spin off this "human design pattern."

Preinstalled Software

I tend to agree with the meme, or paradigm, that has made its way about the Web and even among the scientific journals (call it "paleo," ancestral health, the return to Eden, or whatever you want to) that we were born to move around in sunlight, eat real food, and sleep much more than our friends want us to (you know, the ones who are knocking on the door right now and trying to get you to go to that party).

As a geek, think of our situation this way. We're all born with preinstalled software, our human codebase. The genome. You know, the curlicues of DNA in our chromosomes inside the nuclei of most cells: all that ATGC code that defines what we are biologically. It is kind of cool, almost mesmerizing, how Mother Nature seems to have her own software language. Perhaps we've subconsciously invented computer programs that have the look and feel of our own internal code.

See this page at 23andMe for a nice refresher or primer on genes and genetics: www.23andme.com/gen101/genes/.

It took hundreds of thousands of years to write this software. The evolutionary process is very slow, meaning we haven't changed very much in thousands of years. We're all separated by tiny changes in our genes, such as the fact that some people can't digest lactose that well and others eat asparagus and sense a different smell in their pee (really).

"The spontaneous mutation rate for nuclear DNA is estimated at 0.5% per million years. Therefore, over the past 10,000 years there has been time for very little change in our genes, perhaps 0.005%," comments Artemis P. Simopoulos, M.D., of The Center for Genetics, Nutrition and Health, Washington, DC, USA, in a journal article from 2008.[1]

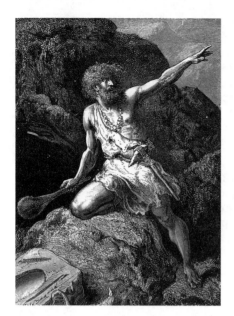

The Pre–Convenience Store Era

Our ancestors, with basically our genome, ate dead meat (as in, scavenged), wild meat that they hunted, stuff that grew, tree nuts, whatever lake or sea foods they could grab, and gobs of raw honey produced by swarms of bees made docile by the smoky fires lit beneath their nests.

Some of the time, as the weather was changing crazily around them (sound familiar?), they couldn't find any food, for days—for weeks.

Whatever, essentially, our earliest forebears could eat to remain alive, they *did* eat. It all had to be hunted and wild; they didn't have bodegas or convenience stores back then. They had to move *to* the food (no pizza deliveries or fancy caterers), and often had to chase and subdue it, if not fend off other predators who sought to reclaim their carcasses. They were outside a good chunk of the time during daylight hours.

We're so close to these ancient forebears biochemically that molecular biologists have hypothesized a link from each of us to an ultimate Mom, a primordial Eve (see the sidebar, "The Ultimate Super Mom").

Imagine that you're standing next to your grandmother in a long line. She is standing next to her mother, and then your grandmother's grandmother is the next Mom in line after that, and the string of people extends for "10,000 grandmothers," as the author Brian Fagan puts it in his book *Cro-Magnon: How the Ice Age Gave Birth to the First Modern Humans*. The 10,000th grandmother might be the ultimate Mom that all humans are related to.

THE ULTIMATE SUPER MOM: MITOCHONDRIAL OR AFRICAN EVE

Our genetic ancestors are tens of thousands of years old, and we still carry their primeval DNA in our genome. For example, genetic scientists have created deep "family trees" that are designed to trace every person in the world down the line through all the mothers and grandmas to the same woman, a kind of "super Mom" who lived roughly 150,000 years ago in East Africa.

She's called "Mitochondrial Eve" because the mitochondrial DNA (mtDNA) is where the genetic connection between ourselves and a grandmother who theoretically existed 10,000 generations ago resides.

The mitochondria are organelles within most cells, little engines that generate much of our cellular energy. They are the places, other than the cell nuclei (where most DNA is located), that also contain our genetic blueprint. A major

difference between the gene copy in the mitochondria and the copy in the nucleus of a cell is that mitochondrial DNA is inherited only from the mother—it isn't mingled together with the father's DNA.

This allows scientists to focus their analysis of genes from mother to mother as far back as they can.

The work of these molecular biologists and other scientists is a reflection of how tightly interrelated we are as humans, as well as of how close our own genes are to those of prehistoric people. "The African Eve is a fictional person, a product of molecular biology, which has used mitochondrial DNA to show that all of us, wherever we live, are ultimately of African descent," writes Brian Fagan in *Cro-Magnon: How the Ice Age Gave Birth to the First Modern Humans*.

Ancestors

The human genome goes back at least as far as about 2.5 million years, when the Lower Paleolithic era began (otherwise known as the early *Stone Age*). Actually you could trace our genes back quite a bit further, but for the sake of brevity we'll start with an upright ancestor that used tools 2.5 million years in the past called *homo habilis*.

He was followed by *homo erectus*, who trekked around his wild habitat (and often booked out of there as fast as he could) around one million years ago, and *homo sapiens* about half a million years ago. The most advanced and successful ancestor who wandered out of our original African habitat and established herself in Europe was *Cro-Magnon*, who thrived in that region beginning about 50,000 years ago. We're quite similar, anatomically and genetically, to these guys and gals.[2]

Few would disagree that a modern hunter-gatherer, or even a Cro-Magnon, is living or lived closer to our built-in design than most of us cubicle cronies!

Five Seconds to Midnight

The typical way to express the idea of us carrying the preinstalled software of those prehistoric guys and gals is that if those millions of years of human evolution could be compressed into a 24-hour clock, the last 10,000 years since the Agricultural Revolution would take place beginning at about five minutes to midnight.

The last 200 years of the Industrial Revolution began to take place at about five seconds to midnight. And the Digital Age… well, you get the metaphor. It's been an eye blink, and evolution is not fast enough to redesign us for endless couch surfing!

Designed to Get Our Butts Kicked

It's safe to say that the hunter-gatherers and us moderns are pretty similar in our genetic programming.

"Shallow" genetic changes that can dig in their heels faster are taking place all the time, according to Gregory Cochran and Henry Harpending's book *The 10,000 Year Explosion: How Civilization Accelerated Human Evolution*. These are variations on our genome; see the sidebar "Night of the Mampires: How Genes Can Affect the Way We Handle Food."

About 99 percent of our genetic history, however, has been spent interacting with our environment more like a Maasai tribeswoman, a Plains Indian, or a modern lady getting her butt kicked during an Outward Bound course, rather than the characters depicted in the TV show *Men of a Certain Age*.

The last two hundred years of the Industrial Revolution began to take place at about five seconds to midnight. And the Digital Age, well… you get the metaphor. It's been an eye blink, and evolution is not fast enough to redesign us for endless couch surfing!

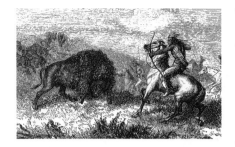

This has something to do with those eighteenth- to nineteenth-century Plains Indians being the buffest bad-asses in the world during their time.[3] They were hunters who acted like hunter-gatherers and killed, ate, made stuff out of, and revered the American bison.

Here's another evolution-related example, partly from Chapter 4 on micronutrients. We can't biosynthesize or make our own vitamin C or vitamin E, as plants can (although we *can* biosynthesize vitamin D, from the sun). We therefore evolved to get vital micronutrients like vitamins *from those photosynthesizing plants*, as well as farther up the food chain, from the animals that munched the veggies. It's part of our design; we eat plants and animals because, in turn, we need the C and E vitamins to keep our internal machinery going.

To reach the plants and animals, guess what, we had to be moving around in a cyclical pattern of hunt-gather-rest, then do-it-again. We are bipedal people, ambulatory by nature. Whether or not at any moment we could have been ripped asunder and devoured by wild beasts or stomped to death by the underestimated prehistoric bison (you can't really sugarcoat that Paleolithic life, pun intended), this scenario still represents the diet and locomotive patterns that our ancestors, and we ourselves, were and have evolved for.

NIGHT OF THE MAMPIRES: HOW GENES CAN AFFECT THE WAY WE HANDLE FOOD

Although people most likely have not developed complex genetic adaptations to a diet dominated by sugar, wheat flour, and vegetable oils, we do display code differences in our ability to handle some foods.

Many of us are *mampires*: we can consume and digest the milk from other animals.

Lactase is an enzyme that is necessary for digesting milk. According to the book *The 10,000 Year Explosion: How Civilization Accelerated Human Evolution*:

> The most dramatic examples are mutations that allow adults to digest lactose, the main sugar in milk. Hunter-gatherers, and mammals in general, stop making lactase (the enzyme that digests lactose) in childhood… But after the domestication of cattle, milk was available and potentially valuable to people of all ages, if only they could digest it. A mutation that caused continued production of lactase originated some 8,000 years ago and has spread widely among Europeans, reaching frequencies of over 95 percent in Denmark and Sweden.[4]

Humans also differ in their tolerance for salt in the diet,

according to the book:

> There is a gene whose ancestral form helps people to conserve salt. Since humans spent most of their history in hot climates, this variant was generally useful. A high frequency of this ancestral allele among African Americans probably plays a role in their increased risk of high blood pressure today. In tropical Africa, in fact, almost everyone has the ancestral version of the gene. In Eurasia, a null variant (one that does nothing at all) becomes more and more common as one moves north.[5]

So the genetic difference helps people to conserve salt in their bodies in hot climates, but it becomes a liability when you eat a lot of salt in processed foods.

Finally, the book points to evidence that some people are metabolically protected against certain blood-sugar problems:

"Researchers in Iceland have found that new variants of a gene regulating blood sugar protect against diabetes."[6] The upshot is that we're not exact replicas of hunter-gatherers; we're just very close to them.

The Cranky Anthropologist

Is it possible to live in a way that completely undermines your own software configuration? Are we corrupting our own code? Well, yeah, I guess that's where I'm leading, based on the aforementioned hypothesis of our closeness in design to our ancient forebears. Scientists call it *evolutionary discordance*.

The anthropologist Jared Diamond fumed in a famous essay from more than 20 years ago that the move to agriculture 10,000 years ago was "the worst mistake in the history of the human race" (*Discovery Magazine*, May 1987) and "a catastrophe from which we have never recovered."

Diamond emphasized the rigid class-based systems and "gross social and sexual inequalities, the disease and despotism" that agricultural systems have bred, but there were other physical and health-related downsides as well, which persist in a different nature all the way up to modern times.

> *Don't get the wrong impression from my knocks against the Ag Revolution—I love farms, particularly of the small and local variety. I just returned from one, with a juicy bag of salad materials, Macintosh apples, and blueberries. The point of this passage is that the transition from hunter-gatherer to the diet of agriculturalists had bad health consequences that are relevant today (i.e., we're still bedeviled by a high-quantity, low-nutrition diet).*

See the sidebar "A Tale of Hoe" for what the effect of the agricultural transition was on height and health in general.

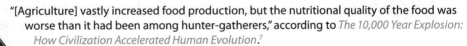

A TALE OF HOE: PROTEIN AND THUS HEIGHT "TANKED"

"[Agriculture] vastly increased food production, but the nutritional quality of the food was worse than it had been among hunter-gatherers," according to *The 10,000 Year Explosion: How Civilization Accelerated Human Evolution*.[7]

"Hunter-gatherers would rarely have suffered vitamin-deficiency diseases such as beri-beri, pellagra, rickets, or scurvy, but farmers sometimes did… it looks as if the carbohydrate fraction of their diet almost tripled, while the amount of protein tanked."[8]

Height crashed in response to this "quantity not quality diet," as did the robustness of the skeletons that paleoanthropologists have studied. The average Cro-Magnon male was between 5' 9" (176 centimeters) and 5' 10"; they were built athletically to boot.

"You can see the mismatch between the genes and the environment in the skeletal evidence. Humans who adopted agriculture shrank: Average height dropped by almost five inches."[9]

Hey, the Stone Age Was a Nasty Time

The oft-stated disclaimer is that all this hunter-gatherer talk is baloney: human longevity has never been greater than it is now, and even inside bustling, youth-oriented places like Manhattan, you can find many centenarians. In contrast, the lives of our Paleolithic ancestors were "nasty, brutish, and short," maybe averaging a third or less the length of one of those centenarians'.

A big problem with that argument, as a number of essayists have pointed out, is the concept of using an "average lifespan" to describe the health of a population of people.

As Jeff Leach pointed out in an October 2010 letter titled "Paleo Longevity Redux" in *Public Health Nutrition*:

> *The first problem with this thinking is the "average life span" math is misleading and tells us very little about the health and longevity of an individual, but rather gives us an average age of death for a given group or population. For example, a couple that lived to the ages of 76 and 71, but had one child that died at birth and another at age two ([76+ 71 + 0 + 2] / 4), would produce an average life span of 37.25. Using this methodology it is easy to see how one would come to the conclusion that this group was not very healthy.*

Along the same lines, the author of *The Black Swan*, Taleb Nassim, pointed out in an essay called "Why I Walk":

> *The argument often heard about primitive people living on average less than 30 years ignores distribution around such average—life expectancy needs to be analyzed conditionally. Plenty died early, from injuries, many lived very long—and healthy—lives. This is exactly the very same elementary "fooled by randomness" mistake, relying on the notion of "average" in the presence of variance, that makes people underestimate the risks in the stock market.*

Undoubtedly, some of those ancient lives were "nasty, brutish, and short," and inherently violent, without antibiotics, modern medicine in general, and a local police department.

In a way, the claims about brief Paleolithic lives are a red herring: the few remaining modern hunter-gatherers tend to go through their lives with only rare occurrences of the contemporary "diseases of Western civilization."

Jeff Leach concludes his essay:

> *The self-confidence that comforts us today as we review the average life span of our ancestors is misguided and tenuous when viewed through the captivating haze of modern medicine that literally props most of us up into our golden years. I doubt our ancestors would call this living. While we may live longer than our ancestors, we are in fact dying slower.*

The Modern Diet—It's Lame!

Note the "mismatch between genes and the environment" point in the "Tale of Hoe" sidebar. Things are at least as bad now in modern society as they were during the dawn of the agricultural age (at least those early farmers spent a lot of time outside doing hard-scrabble chores in sunlit gardens).

The World Health Organization estimates that lifestyle-oriented diseases will cost the global economy $30 trillion over the next 20 years (that includes smoking and alcohol abuse, as well as chowing down sugary and salt-laden snack foods).[10]

What's going on here—why do we have such a massive health crisis? Don't our experts have an incredibly deep and nuanced knowledge about how health and the body function? We've sequenced the human genome. We're even working on "nutrigenomics," or specifically tailoring nutrition and supplements to a person's genes.

I guess health isn't *exclusively* about science, medical practices, or conventional public-health recommendations, or we'd be able to apply that knowledge about how to stay healthy with greater success than we do. Couldn't we do a better job of embracing a new design pattern, one based on our own inherited operating systems?

Couldn't we do a better job of embracing a new design pattern, one based on our own inherited operating systems?

Evolutionary Discordance: It's SAD

In a 2005 article in the *American Journal of Clinical Nutrition*, the medical doctor Boyd Eaton and his colleagues pointed out how lame the diet many of us depend on—which is commonly lampooned as the Standard American Diet (SAD)—is:[11]

> *Although dairy products, cereals, refined sugars, refined vegetable oils, and alcohol make up 72.1% of the total daily energy consumed by all people in the United States, these types of foods would have contributed little or none of the energy in the typical preagricultural hominin diet.*

In a word, ouch!

Boyd Eaton also pointed out in a recent speech that "50 percent of our ancestor's diet was fruits and vegetables; now for Americans it's 13 percent, which represents a huge [decline]" in antioxidant intake (see the sidebar in Chapter 4 on those all-important antioxidants). "The skin of the fruit contains most of the antioxidants, and the smaller wilder fruits contain more antioxidants," given that you have to eat more fruit skin with the smaller, wilder varieties to fill up on fruit servings.

Taking this point to heart, I ate a lot of apples off an apple tree in Vermont this summer and early fall. The apples were smaller; I thus ate more skin and presumably antioxidants compared with larger, sweeter, store-bought apples. The apples were tarter off the tree, perhaps containing less fructose (you should watch the fructose load in your diet—see Chapter 3 on macronutrients). And hey, I had to jump and climb to get the apples, which had to be more active than cruisin' the checkout aisles!

Don't Crash Your Own Software

"As a result of the introduction of habitual physical inactivity into the pattern of daily living, the risks of at least 35 chronic health conditions have increased…"

Eaton and his colleagues have hypothesized, along with other researchers, that the "diseases of civilization," like cancer, heart disease, diabetes, and depression, could be caused by this evolutionary discordance in food intake.

In addition, some studies have pointed to the lack of physical exercise as more evidence that we are badly out of sync with our built-in codebase.

"Recent cultural changes have engineered physical activity out of the daily lives of humans," pointed out Manu Chakravarthy and Frank W. Booth in the *Journal of Applied Physiology* in 2004:[12]

As a result of the introduction of habitual physical inactivity into the pattern of daily living, the risks of at least 35 chronic health conditions have increased…we will speculate that the feast-famine cycling and physical activity-rest cycling that were related to food procurement for [hunter-gatherers] selected genes for an oscillating enzymatic regulation of food-storage and usage.

If physical activity is part of our design, why did we engineer it out of our lives? One answer is the pervasiveness of technology, which it turns out controls us, rather than the other way around. Screen life requires immobility in front of screens. In addition, we no longer have to "go get" vitamins to stay alive—they're within an arm's reach on the shelf or easily acquired without even leaving a sitting position in the car (although convenience foods often lack those very vitamins). Modern food is ubiquitous.

Ironically, our own built-in "man-page" (the software instructions for the Unix operating system) carries the imprint of our earliest low-tech ancestors, and provides many clues for maintaining fitness.

A Useful Template

Of course, most of us cannot dash out the back door and give the hunter-gatherer life the old college try.

Nor can I advocate that we all sprint out into the woods with scary face masks and beat drums, throw spears at shadows, and howl at the moon (although, now that I mention it, what a blast *that* would be). We *can* initiate a kind of mashup of modern and ancient life, though. Our preloaded software represents a useful template with which we can assess our own daily choices. We know what we're designed for; we read this book!

We've discussed nutrition a bit up to now; the rest of the book launches into the savory subjects of food, fitness, and exercise in quite a bit of detail. The movement angle of fitness is obviously very important, but to what degree?

Chair Men of the Bored

Will Ferrell leans back in the movie *Wedding Crashers* and memorably cries out, "Hey Ma—the meatloaf—we want it now—the meatloaf!" He crystallizes an evolving biological tribe we could call *Homo barcalounger*.

We've become a species of sitters, as eloquently put by a doctor in a recent online issue of the *Brooklyn Eagle*: [13]

> We move from the chair in the car to the chair in front of the computer in the office; then we go home in the chair in the car to the chair in front of a copious dinner to the chair in front of the TV. The next day the cycle repeats itself. We sit too much.

Believe it or not, scientists have coined a term for this trend: *chair living*. It has been a part of cubicle life for us geeks since the early epochs of the digital age, but many of us, along with others of the deskbound variety, have since altered our workstations to combine standing with computer work (check out the stand-up workstation called the GeekDesk at *www.geekdesk.com*).

Chair living apparently takes sedentary living to a new level.

If you're like me, you probably think of sitting as an activity that is as common as, well, standing, and that might be bad for you if you did it for 25 years in a row. It's *much* worse than that, apparently.

As James Levine, an M.D. at the Mayo Clinic in Minnesota, wrote in a November 10, 2010, journal article, "a growing body of evidence suggests that chair-living is lethal... linked to cardiovascular disease, metabolic [problems], excess weight, and shorter life span."[14]

You can read that article and weep, then, consequently, leap out of your chair. Levine goes on:

> *The human evolved over several million years to be bipedal and ambulatory. This time frame is consistent with the genetic and epigenetic design of the human physique and organ systems. Neuro-behaviorists would argue that the human brain and behavior evolved in concert. The human evolved to competitively flourish while upright with respect to providing food (agriculture and hunting), shelter (home building), and tool design (e.g., flint knives). The human evolved to feed, shelter, and invent while ambulatory. The human, simply put, was not designed to sit all day.*

The Amazin' MET

The bottom line is that you want to push up your MET for the day, because it's what we're designed for.

A very useful measure of how much we are moving throughout the day is the metabolic equivalent of task (MET), or just metabolic equivalent. It's a simple way to quantify our energy output, and it starkly underlines the differences between sitting and real movement. The MET is designed to represent the amount of energy in the form of heat we're generating, using a numeric multiple. For example, reclining in a chair is 1 MET; sleeping is 0.8.[15]

This scale moves all the way up through walking about a mile per hour on the flat (1.9), actively raking leaves (2.9), light biking or golf (5.0), to running 12-minute miles (8.5), to running faster than nine miles an hour (9.5).

We're going to be returning to METs throughout this book, particularly in the tools and exercise chapters. For example, Chapter 2 discusses a nifty little gadget called the Fitbit that you can use to measure your average MET for a day.

The bottom line is that you want to push up your MET for the day, because it's what we're designed for. We seem to be evolved for a steady oscillation of physical activity throughout the day, along with short bursts of intense, almost scary effort (yeah, exercise can be hormesis!—see Chapter 11).

Olden-days hunter-gatherers almost certainly had a higher average MET than our contemporaries.

Force Quit—Reboot

By now it should be obvious that we are built to eat Mother Nature's food, such as wild (or wild-like) meat or fish, and multicolored plants that come from organic farms and leap from the pages of *Mother Earth* magazine. We're supposed to boogie down, and we're not designed for self-imposed muscular paralysis. You might even think that this chapter belabors these points, which would amount to a harangue if not for the fact that most of these negative trends are instantly reversible.

I won't include much in this chapter about the specifics of fitness-oriented exercise and training, because so much of the book (see Chapters 2, 7, and 8) is crammed with various techniques for sprinting, resistance training, trekking (with or without weighted vests), and more for capturing all of your exercise data on a web page for various forms of analysis.

This chapter will conclude on an upward swing with the flip side of the "daily grind" we began with. It includes a couple of adjustments that bring it much closer to our installed software base—and our own pursuit of optimal fitness.

And Now for Something Completely Different

Try this: you wake up without an alarm sometime soon after sunrise, with plenty of time to spare to make it to work.

It was a good sleep; you went to bed just after nine o'clock after having a snack consisting of coconut milk blended with blueberries and a little whey powder. You're already savvy about getting enough REM sleep, but now you aim to bump up your deep sleep, or restorative NREM. You might even check out the wave chart your Zeo produced.

The first thing you do is pour a cup of black tea or coffee and go outside to this pool of sunlight you've noticed out your window.

You bask and reflect in it for a minute, perhaps followed by a few Tai Chi moves, push-ups on the lawn, or pull-ups on the jungle gym across the street from your apartment. You sip a bit more coffee and return to your living space to get ready for the commute.

Technically speaking, as you gazed up into the sky and basked in that sun, the light rays touched your retinas and were transduced by the hypothalamus and pineal gland in your brain, which has now helped set your circadian rhythms for the day.

Mindfulness

The sun you got wasn't much, not like spending the morning on the beach in the British Virgin Islands (gotta do that someday…), but it had the effect of lightening your mood, clearing your head, and kick-starting the day. You've sent the message to your body and your brain, "It's morning and I'm well rested and ready to go." (See Chapter 9 for more info on the health importance of sleep and rest.)

Every other day you stop at an intervening fitness facility to lift a few weights or do a 300-yard swim interspersed with a handful of 25-yard sprints—nothing too much, but today you're biking to the train station, where they've thoughtfully included a place to lock your rig.

The train ride into the center of the city (Boston, New York, San Francisco, Seattle, Portland, Vancouver, Montreal; Zurich, Frankfurt, Copenhagen, London, Sydney, Wellington, Tokyo, Osaka, Kyoto…) takes 35 minutes, and you stand for most of it, just because it feels better.

Geek Gear

You kind of want to rack up more activity points on this web-connected, motion-sensitive, stair-counting altitude calculator you've clipped onto your belt (yeah, it's called a Fitbit), although gear isn't strictly necessary this morning. It's just fun, in a geeky kind of obsessive way. You like quantifying and logging your exercise. This act itself seems motivating. The web charts your gear generates later are actually quite impressive. They can show your oscillating movement throughout the day, and pinpoint the days when you need more.

Gathering data is not useless when you act upon it.

The tool for adding up your daily motion mileage works with an odd "tail wagging the dog" effect; you seem to move more when you're wearing it. Further, you never really knew that ordinary movement could equate to that much mileage during the day. More than six miles sometimes, even though your walks were broken up into several smallish ones.

Plodding along on a treadmill just isn't necessary anymore. You love looking at the stats at the end of the day. Just keep moving, you say to yourself. Seek the sun.

Hard-Boiled Eggs to Go

Breakfast today was two hard-boiled eggs (eggs bought the previous weekend at a farmer's market), a piece of Swiss cheese, a bite of salmon left over from last night, and two plums plus an avocado (also purchased at the market). Yesterday, you fasted through breakfast, and that felt fine. Actually, the bit of coffee plus "intermittent fast" kept you pretty perky throughout the morning. (See Chapter 6 for more on intermittent fasting.)

You've got a little plastic bag in your backpack containing the rest of the salmon, a mixture of almonds and walnuts, an apple, and a square of 85% high-cacao chocolate. In a pinch, there's a good salad place near work. It only took a couple of weeks not to miss that bagel anymore, and especially all that crappy margarine (you go for really yellow butter now)—the sluggishness and lack of satiety it seemed to leave you with, and the way it seemed to take half the morning to digest it and the donut and scone you piled on top of it.

Hopping off the train, you walk about 30 minutes the rest of the way to work, on the sunny side of the street, even though you could have dipped into the subway or hopped on a bus.

It's morning and I'm well-rested and ready to go.

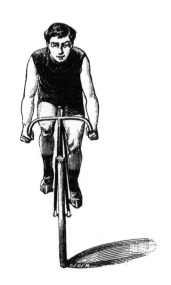

Dude, Take the Stairs

Work is on the third floor of a tall building, but you take the stairs, walking briskly past a line of people waiting at the elevator. Their auras are uniformly glum, as if someone else is pulling their strings. You have *never* taken the elevator, including that time your supervisors were standing in front of it with expectant looks, suggesting they had an axe to grind.

You take the stairs two at a time, simply because the heft in your upper leg feels good. Your heart rate gets going, but not that much; you've noticed *that* improvement over the months.

OCD About Health

The morning goes on and you switch between sitting and standing in your cubicle—standing most of the time. You have a pretty good stand-up workstation setup. Besides, the standing for hours bumps up those motion-and-mileage numbers, which no one else could possibly care about, except other users fidgeting with their tracking devices and apps and going online afterward with the data. You don't mind having an obsessive-compulsive disorder involving healthy habits. You also don't mind going without your gear for a day or two. No big deal.

About every hour or 90 minutes during the day, you head down those stairs again and back outside into the sun. When you get blocked on a sticky piece of code or logical problem, this brisk walk helps almost every time. Often, you experience casual moments outside that you always will remember and never would have experienced if you'd stayed in your cubicle all day, like that majestic hawk that hovered in the blue sky before it alighted on the ledge of a distant building.

You tried to estimate its wingspan as it hung frozen in the cerulean blue.

Hey, He Likes Me!

That handsome dude or attractive woman with the healthy glow who spoke to you out of the blue that time when you were both sitting on a bench, chilling—that hadn't happened to you in a long while; it's usually just awkward silences and departures, ships passing at night. You're going to see him/her again sometime; you're going to swap phone numbers.

You take longer walks sometimes in the city, until you find yourself drifting around with a relaxed aimlessness, kind of like Owen Wilson in the movie *Midnight in Paris*.

You have the usual "meetings" (the quotation marks question their purposefulness) in the mid-morning and afternoon. You stand during both, and it seems to have a contagious effect. Two other people stood up during the second meeting, and you could have sworn both confabs went a little faster. You're beginning to get a rep as "that healthy guy" around the office.

Knock Off Some Bench Presses

By the end of the day you've climbed about 12 floors and maybe walked a couple of miles or more (the number of miles you cover in a day, counting everything, always surprises you). A formal workout in the middle of the day is not necessary. But sometimes you duck into the company fitness facility on a rainy day and knock off some bench presses, pull-ups, and inverted push-ups. Sometimes it's just a dash on a treadmill, or some karate kicks followed by Tai Chi. It takes no more than about 30 minutes.

Your workouts almost *never* exceed that length of time. When they do, *horsing around* would be a better way to describe them than *workouts* or *training sessions*: playing catch using a winged Nerf football with your son or a friend, or gliding along a country road on a mountain bike.

It All Adds Up to Something Good

Are you getting the point here? You're able to shoulder a pretty hard job and commute, while staying healthy, mindful, and reasonably content. The days seem to flow more, instead of banging together like an extended train wreck, with you occupying the middle passenger car. Who could argue with that? You even get the monthly $50 bonus they pay at work to the employees with the fewest sick days!

The intent of the last assemblage of paragraphs wasn't to get all vainglorious and virtuous about healthy lifestyles—although it was fun to write—as much as to paint a narrative about surviving the Digital Age and emerging from your days mostly unscathed (maybe an occasional bruised ego, but it comes with the territory, right?). This chapter has introduced some basic fitness concepts that the rest of the book will cover in sometimes extensive detail:

- Living in the Digital Age, where culture, data, and networks never sleep, but still incorporating the sun, lots of walking, and outdoor experiences—living closer to the imperatives of our preloaded software (our very deep past).

- The benefits of whole, nonprocessed, real food—and even a bit of "intermittent" fasting every week.

- The advantages of incorporating ordinary exercise regimes like stair climbing, lengthy, aimless walking (no matter how cold it is!), sprints, jumps, and hill-climbing extemporaneously, when you can.

…sometimes you duck into the company fitness facility on a rainy day and knock off some bench presses, pull-ups, and inverted push-ups. Sometimes it's just a dash on a treadmill, or some karate kicks followed by Tai Chi. It takes no more than about 30 minutes.

- Using useful tracking tools and personal metrics to augment your fitness, share your progress with friends, help others work through some physical glitches or sleep issues, or for just plain time-wasting fun (when you *have* that time, that is).

- The importance of sleep and destressing; they could save your life.

- The advantages of other lifestyle tactics like freezing swims, saunas, and fasting, not to mention moderate exercise and a good drink now and then. These are examples of "hormesis," or good stress (see Chapter 11).

Unlike many faddish weight-loss and fitness schemes, the changes just described do not involve any expensive program or club fees, or drastic dietary changes (like "zero carb or fat"), except for the optional purchase of a few fun and useful gadgets or tools when you have a little extra change. In the next chapter, we look at some of these tools and apps with which you can analyze and quantify your fitness progress.

AN INTERVIEW WITH MARK SISSON

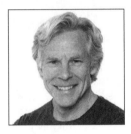

Fittingly for this chapter, we interviewed Mark Sisson of "Primal Blueprint" fame in Fall 2011. Mark is one of the pioneers of, and a powerful voice for what you might call the "live according to your design" principle.

Mark is a former elite endurance athlete, a popular blogger at *Mark's Daily Apple* (*www.marksdailyapple.com*), and he runs a health and wellness business (including conferences and vitamin supplements) under the rubric of The Primal Blueprint (*www.primalblueprint.com*).

How did you originally get into the fitness, writing, and health-supplement business?

I loved the outdoors as a kid. My childhood was one of those idyllic New England ones—staying out all day with my friends exploring the wilderness, getting into trouble, and running everywhere. Seriously, if one thing about my childhood stands out, it's the constant running. There was no real walking. We just ran around. Anyway, I got pretty good at running. I was too skinny and short to play basketball or football in school, but I excelled at cross-country. I kept running cross-country at college, where I was a biology pre-med.

I decided to forgo med school for a few years (going on 33 years now) to concentrate on running full time. I got better.

Five years of running marathons and putting in 100+ miles a week culminated in a spot in the Olympic Trials. I was at my fittest and fastest, but I was also at my sickest. That year I qualified for the Trials, I got eight respiratory infections. I had arthritis in my knees and ankles. When I wasn't running, I was hobbling around, eating whatever I could find, popping anti-inflammatories, and dreading the next training session. It sucked.

I couldn't run competitively anymore, but I could at least try to stem the damage. That was right around when triathlons started getting popular. I figured that if I couldn't run marathons competitively anymore, maybe if I spread the damage across running, biking, and swimming I could get away with it. I did, for another few years, even placing 4th in the 1982 fall Hawaii Ironman, but eventually I had to call it quits... again. That's when I got serious about nutrition and supplementation. I'd already been exploring it to enhance my performance, but now I was interested in bolstering my ailing immune system and fortifying my falling-apart-at-age-29 body. My biology background naturally led me to consider all this stuff from an evolutionary standpoint, and it just seemed to make a ton of sense. More importantly, it worked, so I decided to make a life out of it. I'd seen what chronic endurance training did to my peers, and I'd felt what it'd done to my health. I couldn't take away my past, but I felt I could help steer others away from similar mistakes.

AN INTERVIEW WITH MARK SISSON (continued)

I know your blog and the Primal Blueprint/book are very popular. Can you make a rough estimate of how many people have embraced the PB as part of their lifestyle, including overseas? It seems like the appeal would transcend culture.

It's difficult to say. I can give you the book sales figures and monthly blog visits (blog is currently over two million visits per month), both of which continue to climb steadily, but those won't necessarily tell the whole story. My most reliable marker is the number of emails I get from people with basic questions about the lifestyle. If you're asking me if riding your bike to work is Chronic Cardio (depends), if hemp seeds are Primal (sure), if intermittent fasting is right for your diabetic mother (can't say), or whether your method of cooking salmon is oxidizing the Omega-3 fatty acids, chances are you've already embraced the Primal Blueprint. I get several hundred of those emails every week, and the number has been steadily rising, including those I receive from overseas email addresses. That's my barometer—folks engaged enough to have encountered problems that need answering, typed up an email, and sent it out.

The appeal definitely transcends culture. A big help, unfortunately, has been the discrepancy between the US and other nations in degree of belief in evolution. A recent poll just came out showing that just 16% of the US believes in "secular evolutionary theory." 16%! What's scary is that figure is up from 9% in 1999.

Each element of the Primal Blueprint seems perfectly sensible to me, yet has there been any backlash?

Backlash? Some. It's not like it's being meted out by the authorities or anything, but I've noticed that the movement is getting a lot more attention in the media. I can't even remember how many articles I've read featuring some stuffy nutrition "expert" casually shrugging off the "supposed benefits" of the "caveman diet." It's the new Atkins in that it's the new whipping boy for threatened dietitians. I'm all for disagreement. I love rebuttals. I welcome them. But not when they're based on faulty premises, blatantly incorrect data, and widely held misconceptions. If detractors would come to the table with some honest arguments addressing the science, rather than making cracks about cavemen dying at 25 and asking why we still use computers, wear clothes, and drive cars, I'd be happy.

But mostly, it's just basic ignorance of all this stuff. Not ignorance in the pejorative sense, but ignorance in the "they are simply not aware of anything but the official story" sense. Old myths die hard. I have to remind myself that even though the Primal community is growing every single day, we're still a fledgling group. We're still a very vocal minority dwarfed by the millions upon millions that never even think to question what they've been told all their lives.

Do you have a favorite web-connected health or fitness gadget?

I'm with you on this one; they're fun, but usually unnecessary. I'm very much a tech guy in that my business is web-based, I blog every day, I use Twitter, but as for the health gadgets? I've never really felt the need. Actually, you know what? I do like the tech stuff that enables, rather than impedes, a more evolutionary existence. So, online forums, like my own or Paleohacks, where people can gather "with their tribe" and communicate, solve problems, get into arguments, and emerge better, more informed people. Those are cool and ultimately helpful. I'm also a big fan of F.lux, a nice app that dampens the blue light emissions from your computer screen. Blue light has repeatedly been shown to cancel melatonin production and disrupt sleep, so all those people staying up late staring into their laptop (which is basically everyone these days, right?) would probably benefit from installing it.

Fitness Tools and Apps 2

Fitness tools and apps are web-based software, hardware, or hardware/software combinations that can track and provide feedback on your fitness adventures. They are tools made in heaven for geeks, as they blend all kinds of workouts with the online and fitness worlds. Many of them are essentially wearable computers that generate reams of data and catchy, revealing web graphics. Most allow the downloading of the data so that you can do your own coding, as in GPS Exchange (GPX) XML files.

These tools often work through a cell phone app (such as Endomondo or RunKeeper), or they provide a little device or gadget that can connect with a website, as in the Fitbit Tracker. The website provides you with your own dashboard, a central place where you can view your personal stats, aggregated over the months and years, as well as digital maps of where you've been.

Quantified Self

The place to go to find out about the latest tracking devices is Quantified Self (*www.quantifiedself.com*). This web group describes itself as "a place for people interested in self-tracking to gather, share knowledge and experiences, and discover resources." It is an excellent resource for all kinds of tracking devices, posting information on the latest and greatest online web tools, beyond sports or health tracking.

For example, through Quantified Self I have found two other web tracking sites I'd like to check out in the future: FuelFrog for tracking your vehicle's fuel use, and WattVision, which can help you increase the energy efficiency of your house. The master listing of tracking tools is here: *http://quantified-self.com/guide/*.

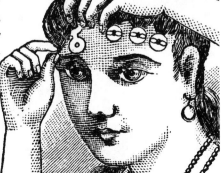

Sports and Fitness Tracking

Of course, in this book we're primarily interested in sports and fitness trackers, often using the Global Positioning System (GPS) software of your smarthone or sports watch. We've also analyzed an extra flavoring of nutrition-oriented software.

The fitness-tracking tools, a subset of which are described in this chapter, seem to have these features in common:

- They track fitness and nutrition with easy-to-record metrics and websites that automatically update colorful graphs and tables.

- They motivate the users to set goals, monitor progress, and team up and share with other users to create a self-reinforcing network—a tribe, in other words.

- In most of the cases, such as Endomondo and Garmin, the software allows the export of the data generated from fitness training (such as a GPS file), so it can be imported into another application or simply examined the way all of us geeks would read code.

For the sake of brevity, we cannot cover in detail all of the major web-based fitness tools (which include RunKeeper, Nike+, Training Peaks, and the MapMyFitness sites), but we think we've included an eclectic selection to get you started with fitness tracking apps. This chapter also describes a couple of online nutrition tools in more detail, including NutritionData and FitDay.

Who's more qualified to examine the feedback from your own body and mind than you?

Personal Metrics

These visual displays of data, on cell phones, laptops, and PCs, allow you to initiate a little investigative work on your life. For example, you may want to manage your weight, aspire to athletic goals, deal with physical issues like lowering your blood pressure (e.g., "How does my blood pressure respond to time of day or certain dietary changes?"), or simply isolate patterns and correlations in the data that you would never have pinpointed before.

> *"Hey… I'm sitting too much during the day, and not getting enough quality REM sleep."*

The personal metrics have another practical purpose, too. You can share the data with sports trainers or doctors, or you can take matters into your own hands rather than paying an expensive expert's fees. After all, who's more qualified to examine the feedback from your own body and mind than you?

Fitness tracking apps and devices can often connect and integrate each other's data. We'll get into this a bit when discussing the integration of GPS data from Endomondo or Garmin into Google Earth.

Gear ≠ Health

Fitness apps are fun and motivating, and they provide useful biofeedback, compile personal metrics in interesting ways, and are closely tied into the computer technology that you know well and love—but they are not strictly necessary for maintaining health. Our vigorous foraging ancestors did not have Fitbit or Endomondo. You can stay pretty darn healthy without fiddling with gear hanging off your belt and constantly consulting a web page.

On the other hand, many people swear by these apps for meeting new health and fitness goals, and they are, beyond a shadow of a doubt, nifty tools for analyzing personal data, playing with, and programming. They also seem to have a "tail wagging the dog" effect in terms of nudging you to accumulate more mileage and move about more.

As Chapter 1 discussed, evolution has apparently coded us for more or less continuous motion—an oscillation of movement throughout the day. Far from being a moderately harmless lazy habit, "chair living" has scientifically documented negative health effects.

Let's jump right in and examine some of these devices.

Fitbit Tracker

Fitbit is a San Francisco–based company that distributes a small motion-sensor device called the Fitbit Tracker (shown in Figure 2-1). You can clip the device to your belt, your sleeve, or wherever is handy. It has a 3D accelerometer that uses technology similar to the Nintendo Wii to analyze your motion throughout the day, compiling comprehensive statistics that you can ogle and digest later.

The device is like a pedometer on steroids. It connects with a small base station that plugs into the USB port of your computer, mainly to recharge the device, because the data can be wirelessly synced to the product's companion web pages.

The handy little Tracker has its own display that will sequentially show the steps you've taken so far for the day, your accumulated mileage, an estimate of the calories burned, and a flower icon that is meant to indicate your activity level for the last three hours (you make it grow by becoming more active).

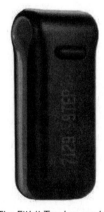

Figure 2-1. *The Fitbit Tracker captures your life in motion*

The Tracker will automatically sync its data whenever it is within 15 feet of any plugged-in base station (i.e., not just the base station plugged into your own computer).

The Dashboard

Fitbit really shines when you connect with its dashboard after logging in at *www.fitbit.com*. Figure 2-2 shows my dashboard for a day in late September. The dashboard shows how many steps you've taken (in the thousands, unless you're bedridden with a broken leg from skiing), calories burned and eaten (if you've logged them), how many miles you covered, and an Active Score, which is a numerical indication of how active you have been throughout the day.

The Active Score is a reflection of your metabolic equivalent of task (MET), which is how much energy you're expending by taking part in certain activities. Sitting all day is a MET equivalent of 1, for example. Running hard would be a MET of 9.5.[1]

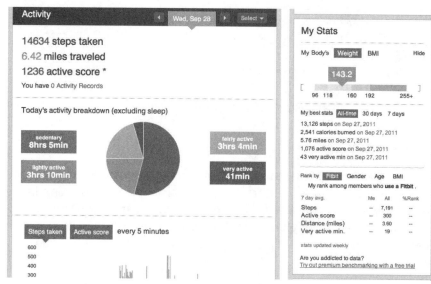

Figure 2-2. *A segment of the Fitbit dashboard*

> *The Fitbit FAQ (www.fitbit.com/faq) states that you can roughly calculate the average metabolic equivalent for the day by using this equation: METs = Active Score * .001 + 1. See the discussion in Chapter 1 on MET.*

For example, on this day, I took more than 14,000 steps (glad I wasn't counting!) and strode about 6.4 miles. My Active Score was 1236, which added up to an average MET for the day of about 2.34 (Active Score x .001 + 1). This is the equivalent MET output of someone doing light construction work.

If you're in a "generalized active state," up and down and fidgety in a healthy way, it's surprising how many miles you can amass by the end of the day. The Tracker provides a fairly accurate figure for striding (I tested it against my phone- and watch-based GPS gadgets during walks).

To provide even more precision, you can enter Fitbit's settings and specify your step and running-stride lengths.

Nifty Charts

The key advantage of the Fitbit is that it measures, with a certain degree of accuracy, your generalized pattern of activity and movement.

We seem to be designed for a steady "background noise" of movement throughout the day, rather than the "regularly scheduled workout" followed by long sedentary sits. (Think of a person hunting and gathering food.) Because it doesn't just focus on individual workouts, the Fitbit often gives you a superior reflection of your health habits compared with other tools.

For example, the "miles traveled" reported on the dashboard represents an estimate of all the mileage accumulated through the day, including walking to get the mail and climbing the stairs to fetch your raincoat. It even seems to pick up the greater effort expended when you stand rather than sitting at your workstation.

According to recent research described in a cardiology journal,[2] even people who work out most days do not benefit from this activity when they spend the rest of their time prone in front of screens (TVs, computers, video games, etc.).

If you're in a "generalized active state," up and down and fidgety in a healthy way, it's surprising how many miles you can amass by the end of the day.

Figure 2-3 shows a nice chart on the bottom left part of the dashboard indicating the activity patterns throughout the day.

All of these tools have an odd but unmistakable "tail wagging the dog" effect—they tend to increase your movement and tendency to exercise, rather than solely record and display activities.

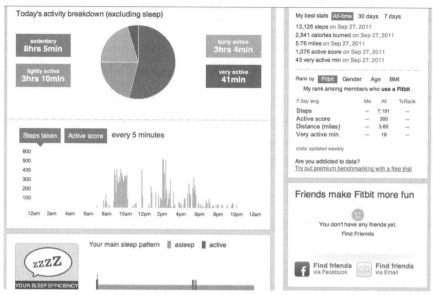

Figure 2-3. *A Fitbit chart logs your high-stepping moves*

Based on this chart, you could draw the simple conclusion that you needed to take short walks at the start and end of each day. Every step counts, and that's valid from a metabolic-health standpoint. Figure 2-3 shows the pattern of spikes (the number of steps or equivalent exercise) during my day from an easy mountain-bike ride, a walk downtown for middle-of-the-day errands, and a basketball shoot with my son at dusk.

The Fitbit does not capture non-step-related activities like biking or resistance training (beyond the general movement involved in getting on, off, and around a bike, for instance). But you can manually log these activities and thus include their caloric expenditure (the Fitbit will overwrite that segment of time with your own values for calories burned). See the sections on Endomondo and Fitocracy for discussions of capturing and logging certain sports like cycling and weightlifting.

As mentioned earlier, all of these tools have an odd but unmistakable "tail wagging the dog" effect—they tend to increase your movement and inclination to exercise, rather than solely recording and displaying your activities. You might find yourself thinking, "I'm going to walk to work today so I can bump up my Active Score. I'll try to break my time record from yesterday."

Logging with Fitbit

You can log many aspects of your lifestyle with Fitbit, thus adding to the benchmarks you set. You can also create your own variables to track (e.g., cups of coffee or beers consumed in a day). Figure 2-4 shows the tabs for food, activities (walking, biking, etc.), sleep, journal entries, and more.

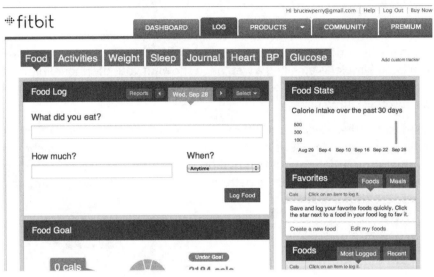

Figure 2-4. *Logging lifestyle bits in Fitbit*

The Food tab obviously allows you to keep track of calories burned and consumed, as well as a basic macronutrient ratio dealing with your percentages of carbs, protein, and fats (see Chapter 3 for more on food chemistry).

Logging all of these aspects is optional, but it gives you more ingredients for the tool's rich interface. I actually think FitDay (*www.fitday.com*) is a better tool for logging food intake, which is generally a tedious and time-consuming, if often revealing, effort. See later in this chapter for a FitDay discussion.

Fitbit will give you an analysis of your sleep patterns if you wear the tracking device around your wrist while you sleep, using the provided wrist strap. I thought it might be useful to try this once, but the idea of the device tracking me while I slept gave me the heebie-jeebies, and since I already sleep well, regard that as an optional feature. It is neat, however, to look over a chart showing the patterns of your sleep.

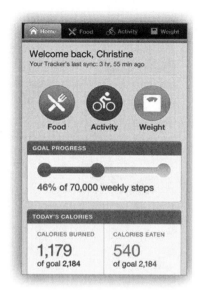

Figure 2-5. *Fitbit's screen for mobile devices*

Mobile Version

You can access Fitbit's mobile version with your smartphone browser at *m.fitbit.com*. It's not an app, but a mobile website: a manner of accessing the rich interface on a smaller screen, as shown in Figure 2-5.

Online Community

The Fitbit interface has a Community tab that gives users access to various forums where they can interact with other users. The interactive features can be as simple as emailing a web page showing your dashboard or automatically posting the data to other sites like Twitter, Facebook, WordPress, or Microsoft HealthVault.

Like most of these web-based fitness services, Fitbit also has a paid premium service that provides views of your accomplishments against a benchmark of other users, using various demographics as a filter for the data. For example, I can compare my exercise patterns against those of other men my age. Figure 2-6 shows a Fitbit bar chart from the premium service.

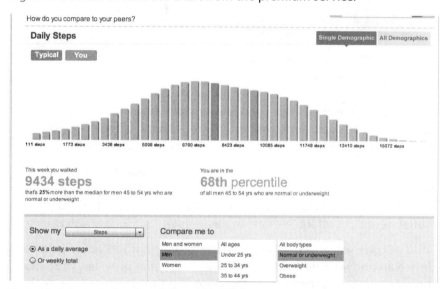

Figure 2-6. *A dynamically generated report in Fitbit*

Fitbit API

Fitbit has an application programming interface (API) for outside developers or geeks who simply want to access their own data for coding: *http://dev. fitbit.com.*

This code uses a Java API called Fitbit4J, but it also includes APIs for PHP and .NET, for instance. Developers first have to register with Fitbit (at *dev. fitbit.com*), and they receive via email authentication codes to use with their applications.

The API design is a RESTful web service that uses an open source security protocol called *oauth*. This process involves making HTTP requests for the Fitbit data, after first satisfying an authorization step by sending along the credentials the developer obtained from the Fitbit developer site.

You have a "consumer key" and a "consumer secret," both long hexadecimal numbers that look like 0f92959d8bc4483cda7bce0074d-c26bc.

There's a good tutorial on using RESTful web services with oauths at *http:// developers.sun.com/identity/reference/techart/restwebservices.html*.

One possible use for the API is grabbing your Fitbit data and mashing it up with data collected on another online fitness database, like Endomondo.

Endomondo

The Endomondo Sports Tracker is a free smartphone or Blackberry app that records your sports workouts and links the data to its website (*www.endomondo.com*).

Endomondo also sells a premium version.

On the Endomondo website, you can share your data and interact with other users. Endomondo has its headquarters in Denmark. Figure 2-7 shows what the home page looks like once you've logged in.

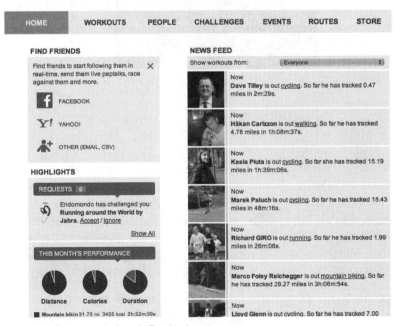

Figure 2-7. *Endomondo Sports Tracker home page*

Here's how the app works, using an example of a recent mountain-bike ride. You install the free or Pro version of the mobile app on your phone (it's available for Android, Blackberry, and the iPhone). Before you begin your workout, you fire up the app on your device and, using its interface, choose the type of sport (e.g., running, fitness walking, cycling). Then you start the timer to log your workout. Figure 2-8 shows the phone app interface.

Off I go on my mountain bike, heading for the open road with a few dips into the forest.

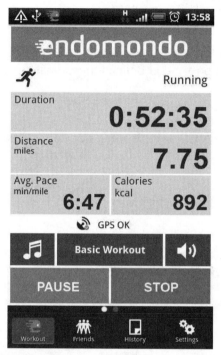

Figure 2-8. *A mobile interface for the Endomondo Sports Tracker*

Hit the "countdown" button, and a voice counts down from five or however you set it, then says "Free your endorphins!" I like that amusing feature; during the countdown, I shove the phone into a coat pocket and step into the pedals. You can configure the length of the countdown in the app's settings.

The Endomondo app uses your phone's GPS capability to track the fitness event so that it can give you dynamic mileage updates and map the workout later. As you ride along, your phone emits a pleasant voice each mile: "You've reached mile 10 in 51 minutes; last mile five minutes nineteen seconds…"

If your phone is capable of immediately uploading the training session to Endomondo's website, your friends and everyone else hooked into the site can see that you've hopped on a bike, pulled on your running shoes, or whatever, and headed out onto the trail or pavement.

The statistics, along with the audio feedback during the workout (which can include "pep talks" from your friends), are handy and fun. Figure 2-9 shows the map and statistics from my bike ride. The app uses Google Maps with interactive features to show your pace at each mile.

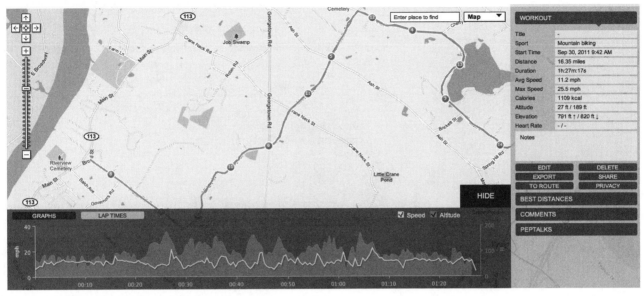

Figure 2-9. *Endomondo maps and stats*

Exporting Files from Endomondo

You can export these workouts in the GPS Exchange format (*.gpx* files) and Garmin's XML format, called TCX (*.tcx* files).

These formats represent different types of XML files that contain route, waypoint, and other GPS- and fitness-related data reflected by a mapped workout. The following site provides you with the XML schemas for several XML formats that are used by Garmin, Google Earth, and other tools (including GPX, TCX, and KML files): *http://developer.garmin.com/schemas/*.

To output an Endomondo workout as XML, click the Export button at the bottom right of the page, as shown in Figure 2-9.

What can you do with the data? Well, you can import it into another device or piece of software that supports the file type, or use XML-processing code to make additional kinds of software out of it (see the "Import Your GPS File into Google Earth" sidebar).

Here's a chunk of XML code from a *.gpx* file, for instance. This code encapsulates a couple of track points, or latitude/longitude points with an elevation and timestamp, from a mountain-bike ride:

```
<trk>
    <src>http://www.endomondo.com/</src>
    <link href="http://www.endomondo.com/workouts/ipPaf0OCq48">
        <text>endomondo</text>
    </link>
    <type>MOUNTAIN_BIKING</type>
    <trkseg>
        <trkpt lat="44.138008" lon="-72.884608">
            <time>2011-10-02T16:19:59Z</time>
        </trkpt>
        <trkpt lat="44.138008" lon="-72.884608">
            <ele>478.1</ele>
            <time>2011-10-02T16:20:03Z</time>
        </trkpt>
    </trkseg>
</trk>
```

IMPORT YOUR GPS FILE INTO GOOGLE EARTH

You can import a GPS file (such as one with a *.gpx* suffix) into Google Earth, then view the route you took within that application. Here's how to do it from Endomondo:

1. Export a *.gpx* file from within the Endomondo app (see "Exporting Files from Endomondo").

2. Launch the Google Earth application (there's a free version) and choose File→Open from within that application. I had to resave the file Endomondo exported, called *no name.gpx.xml*, to *mytrek.gpx* in the text-handling application BBEdit (notice the suffix change; I lopped off the *.xml* part) before Google Earth would recognize the file.

3. Select the file you just exported (and possibly renamed).

4. The file will open up into a Google Earth aerial view showing your route. You can use other file types as well (see *http://earth.google.com/outreach/tutorial_importgps.html#gpxfile*).

How Many Times Around the World?

Another spiffy region of the Endomondo home page is the lower-left hand corner, an ongoing aggregation of the highlights of your recorded workouts. It'll tell you how many burgers you've burned, how many times you've circumnavigated the globe, and how many trips you've taken to the moon (since I'd just began with Endomondo, I had only traversed the equator the equivalent of 0.002 times). Figure 2-10 shows this portion of the screen.

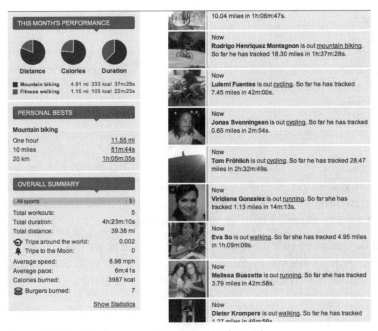

Another spiffy region of the Endomondo home page is the lower left-hand corner, an ongoing aggregation of the highlights of your recorded workouts. It'll tell you how many burgers you've burned, how many times you've circum-navigated the globe, and how many trips you've taken to the moon…

Figure 2-10. *Tracking how many burgers you've burned*

Many fitness-tracking tools take a "more is better" approach (gotta get around the earth a second time!), but, as we'll discuss in Chapter 9, over-training is not necessary to get both strong and healthy. In fact, years of overtraining can lead to ill health.

> *A common metaphor to use when representing strength training, for instance, is "digging a hole and filling it in." When you task the muscles with hard, consecutive, high-intensity training sessions, you're digging the hole deeper and deeper, but never giving your body the necessary rest to initiate the training adaptations, or the "filling in," of the hole.*

One of the strengths of Fitbit and similar tools is that you can choose to track anything, such as rest days and less intense sessions. Then you can assess how your strength gains and energy levels correspond with the number of rest days and/or easy sessions.

Fitocracy

Fitocracy (*www.fitocracy.com*) is another sports-tracking tool, as well as a community with interactive features. It has the additional benefit of providing better support than others in the areas of resistance training and body-weight exercises.

At the time I used Fitocracy, it was released as a beta version.

Along with tracking your training data, Fitocracy is built around an award system where you earn points for each exercise bout and eventually work your way up to different levels. According to its own getting started guide, "Fitocracy is a game you play to improve your fitness."

It seems to be designed to initiate friendly competition against your friends or yourself, similar to the model of computer gaming, but with a decidedly fitter result. Figure 2-11 shows a profile for a Fitocracy beginner.

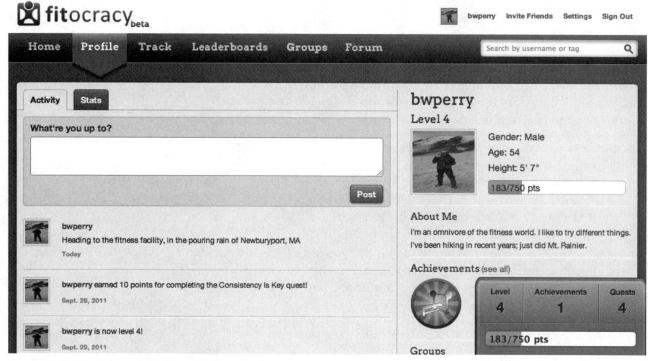

Figure 2-11. *Work your way up the fitness ladder with Fitocracy*

It is admittedly complex to input resistance-training sessions, with all the different techniques, sets, and repetitions. Fitocracy is one of the few online tools that has a rich interface for logging weightlifting, which should help the company down the line as resistance training becomes *de rigeur* for many athletes (more on this in Chapter 8).

Fitocracy's rich interface includes handy tips for describing dozens of different resistance-training routines.

Figure 2-12 shows a screen for entering a weightlifting workout that includes body-weight exercises like pull-ups and push-ups.

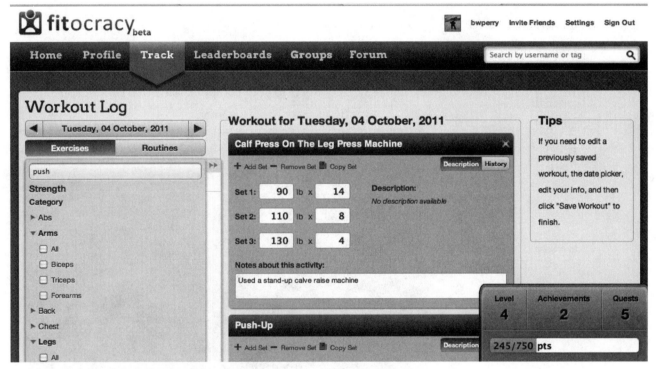

Figure 2-12. *Rich interface for logging resistance training*

You can click back and forth between training sessions on different days, as well as view a history showing when you did a particular routine before. You can log any kind of exercise activity, however, and Fitocracy autogenerates a window with suggestions, making it easy to pop up a logging window that's customized for that particular sport.

Of course, none of these sites would be complete without community features. Fitocracy has groups, a forum, a "leaderboard" showing all the point-hoarding honchos, and a feature for following other people. It doesn't seem to have a way of exporting the data yet, but it was still a beta version at the time of this writing. Fitocracy does have a mobile version, allowing you to produce a smartphone in the gym and instantly record your recent grappling with the barbells or free weights.

See Chapter 8 for a bit more on the Fitocracy mobile app, as well as on weightlifting in general.

Garmin Connect

Garmin Connect (*http://connect.garmin.com*) is the web portal you will use for any Garmin GPS tracking tool. The Garmin device (in this case a Garmin Forerunner 301) connects to your computer via a USB connection cable, as Figure 2-13 shows.

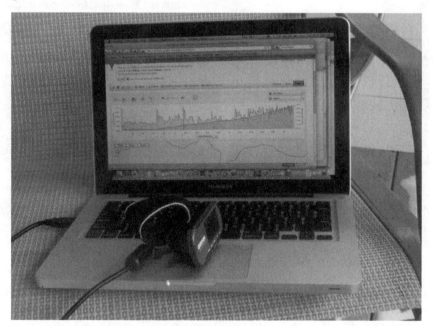

Figure 2-13. *Connecting a Garmin GPS watch to a laptop*

You have to download and install the "Communicator Plug-in" software for your PC or laptop so that your plugged-in hardware device can talk to Garmin's web-based software, which includes the dashboard showing your device's captured activities. For details, see *http://www8.garmin.com/fitness/getting_ started_communicator.jsp*.

Any one of the activities you have recorded on your Garmin watch or other device can be viewed in detail by navigating from the dashboard (at *http:// connect.garmin.com/dashboard*). If you're interested in the maps and stats for a particular workout, such as time, distance, elevation gain/loss, and pace, this data is available from the following link: *http://connect.garmin. com/activities*.

Figure 2-14 shows the stats for a hiking activity in the Alps, with all the juicy details (the screen capture does not show some additional graphics, which include separate charts describing pace and elevation over a timeline).

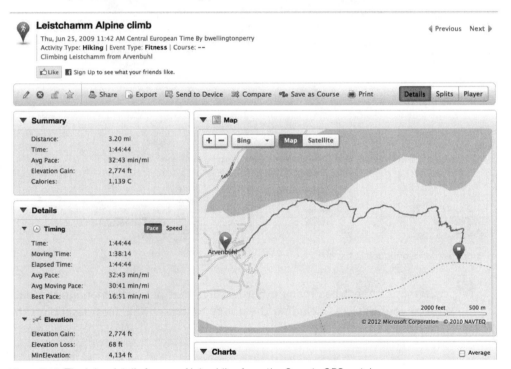

Figure 2-14. *The juicy details from an Alpine hike, from the Garmin GPS watch*

One of the niftier Garmin Connect features is the Player, which is one of the choices you can select when you are viewing the specifics of a fitness activity captured on your device. This Adobe Flash tool allows you to replay the workout from within the map embedded in your browser window. Figure 2-15 shows the Player tool.

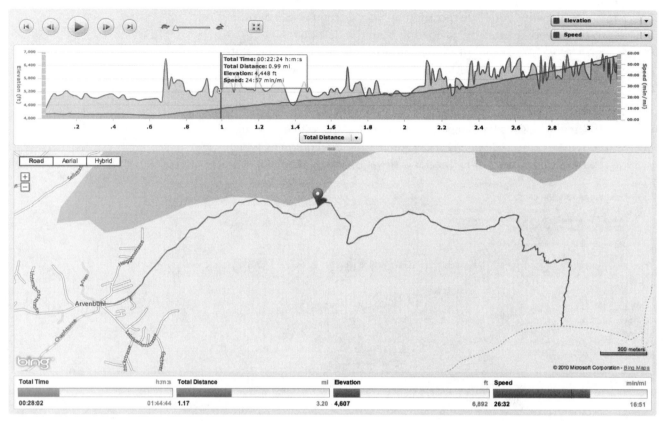

Figure 2-15. *Replaying your workout inside the map embedded in the browser*

One of the niftier Garmin Connect features is the Player, which is one of the choices you can select when you are viewing the specifics of a fitness activity captured on your device. This Adobe Flash tool allows you to replay the workout…

Garmin Connect has many other features that help you manage the data from your devices, including the ability to export XML files describing the routes.

> *Chapter 7 discusses the GPS Exchange Format(GPX), an XML language for outputting and saving routes from GPS-enabled devices.*

We'll cover a number of other sports-related apps in the fitness chapters, including GAIN Fitness (*http://gainfitness.com*) in Chapter 8 as well as the Backpacker GPS Trails pro app (*http://backpacker.com*) and Alpine Replay (*www.alpinereplay.com*) in Chapter 7.

The rest of this chapter introduces a couple of nutrition tools on the Web, as well as an example of a connected device—you use the device at home, and the data is sent to a website or to other software tools. It's called the Withings body-composition scale. Yes, you heard that correctly—your bathroom scale (this one, on steroids) can capture your data and wirelessly send it to a website.

Hmm, maybe you don't want that to happen…

NutritionData

We looked at NutritionData (*www.nutritiondata.com*) a bit in Chapter 1. This section will point out a few more interesting aspects of this tool. If you're already a NutritionData honcho, feel free to move on to the brief discussions of FitDay and the USDA Nutritional Database that follow.

For the sake of our discussion, initiate a search on mussels (the shellfish, not the ones you flex in front of a mirror): *http://nutritiondata.self.com/facts/ finfish-and-shellfish-products/4187/2*. The screen in Figure 2-16 has a graphic for "Caloric Ratio" showing the macronutrient ratio for the food.

NutritionData also gives values for "Glycemic Load" and "Inflammation." You basically want to keep the number on the left down (as in, foods that tend to spike blood-glucose levels and thus the hormone insulin and are therefore high glycemic), and increase the right hand number (reduce inflammatory foods, which in this tool means avoiding negative numbers).

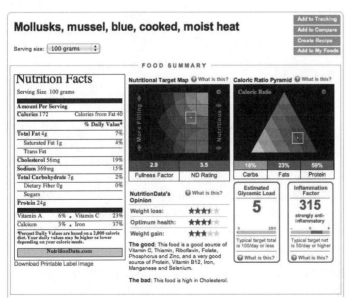

Figure 2-16. *Mussels pack a lot of protein muscle*

A macronutrient ratio represents how the food content is divided up by percent of calories into carbs, fats, and proteins. Mussels, for example, are 18 percent carbohydrates, 23 percent fats, and 59 percent protein.

This feature gives you a snapshot of the nutritional content of the food (along with the nutrition label showing about 24 grams of protein in a fairly small serving of mussels). So we know that mussels are a great source of protein, but what about fats or micronutrients?

If you scroll down to the regions representing fats, vitamins, and minerals (Figure 2–17), the data on mussels offers some pleasant surprises. This shellfish portion contains a lot of vitamin C for a protein-rich food (almost 14 grams; hey, more than enough to stop you getting scurvy!), as well as about four times as much vitamin B12 as you would need in a day.

Fats & Fatty Acids

Amounts Per Selected Serving		%DV
Total Fat	4.5 g	7%
Saturated Fat	0.9 g	4%
Monounsaturated Fat	1.0 g	
Polyunsaturated Fat	1.2 g	
Total trans fatty acids	~	
Total trans-monoenoic fatty acids	~	
Total trans-polyenoic fatty acids	~	
Total Omega-3 fatty acids	866 mg	
Total Omega-6 fatty acids	36.0 mg	

Learn more about these fatty acids and their equivalent names

More details ▾

Hydroxyproline	~

More details ▾

Vitamins

Amounts Per Selected Serving		%DV
Vitamin A	304 IU	6%
Vitamin C	13.6 mg	23%
Vitamin D	~	~
Vitamin E (Alpha Tocopherol)	~	~
Vitamin K	~	~
Thiamin	0.3 mg	20%
Riboflavin	0.4 mg	25%
Niacin	3.0 mg	15%
Vitamin B6	0.1 mg	5%
Folate	76.0 mcg	19%
Vitamin B12	24.0 mcg	400%
Pantothenic Acid	0.9 mg	9%
Choline	~	
Betaine	~	

More details ▾

Minerals

Amounts Per Selected Serving		%DV
Calcium	33.0 mg	3%
Iron	6.7 mg	37%
Magnesium	37.0 mg	9%
Phosphorus	285 mg	28%
Potassium	268 mg	8%
Sodium	369 mg	15%
Zinc	2.7 mg	18%
Copper	0.1 mg	7%
Manganese	6.8 mg	340%
Selenium	89.6 mcg	128%
Fluoride		

Figure 2-17. These mussels are stylin' from a nutrient standpoint

Mussels are also a great source of selenium, manganese, iron, and other minerals (see Chapter 4 on micronutrients). Check out the Fats & Fatty Acids box too; mussels have an Omega 3 to Omega 6 ratio of 866 mg to 36 mg, or about 24:1. This means that a small portion of mussels gives you almost a gram of Omega 3 essential fatty acids, which are generally considered a health food in moderate amounts. Our modern diet contains way too many Omega 6 fats compared to Omega 3s; see Chapter 3, for a discussion of these ratios.

NutritionData also has a self-tracking feature under the MyND section of the site. After registering, you can track and analyze the nutritional content of certain foods, as shown in Figure 2-18. Let's say you want to brag to your friends about how nutritious mussels are (thus increasing your weirdness

Mussels are a great source of selenium, manganese, iron, and other minerals.

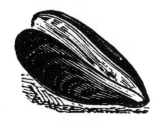

Chapter 2

quotient in their eyes). Tracking removes the need to continually search for the same food items.

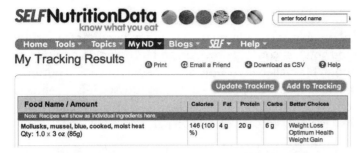

Figure 2-18. *Tracking and saving certain foods at NutritionData*

FitDay

FitDay (*www.fitday.com*) is one of the better tools around for tracking your diet and its underlying nutrition, or lack thereof. We're going to look at FitDay again in Chapters 3 and 4, but this section serves as an introduction.

FitDay is useful for the periodic tracking of a whole or partial diet to get a snapshot of its macro- and micronutrient content.

> *FitDay differs from NutritionData in this respect by analyzing numerous foods at once—an entire day's worth of eating—rather than single portions or ingredients.*

Conveniently, FitDay saves the foods you've entered before, which makes the otherwise tedious data entry go quicker the second time around. Figure 2-19 shows the table produced from a partial day's food intake. Each day you enter your food intake is saved in a calendar for later retrieval.

Food Name	Amount	Unit	Cals	Fat (g)	Carbs (g)	Prot (g)	Delete
		Total	1,100	55.8	97.7	63.9	
Almonds	0.5	oz (22 whole kernel	82	7.2	2.8	3.0	✕
Apple, raw	2	medium (2-3/4" dia	144	0.5	38.1	0.7	✕
Avocado, raw	1	avocado, California	277	25.4	14.8	3.5	✕
Cheese, natural, Cheddar or American type	1	cubic inch	69	5.6	0.2	4.2	✕
Egg, whole, cooked	1	large	83	6.1	0.6	6.1	✕
Lettuce, Boston, raw	0.5	head (5" dia)	11	0.2	1.8	1.1	✕
Turkey	5	oz, boneless, cooke	265	9.9	0.0	41.0	✕
Coffee, regular	2	coffee cup (6 fl oz)	4	0.1	0.1	0.4	✕
Strawberries, raw	4	large (1-3/8" dia)	23	0.2	5.5	0.5	✕
Orange, raw	1	medium (2-5/8" dia	62	0.2	15.4	1.2	✕
Lettuce, red leaf, raw	1	cup shredded	4	0.1	0.6	0.4	✕
Pepper, sweet, red, raw	0.5	medium (approx 2-	15	0.2	3.6	0.6	✕
Peppers, sweet, yellow, raw	0.5	pepper, large (3-3/	25	0.2	5.9	0.9	✕
Grapes, American type, slip skin, raw	10	grape	16	0.1	4.1	0.2	✕
Vinegar, balsamic	1.5	tbsp	21	0.0	4.1	0.1	✕
		Total	1,100	55.8	97.7	63.9	

Figure 2-19. *Part of a day's food intake saved in FitDay*

Conveniently, FitDay saves the foods you've entered before, which makes the otherwise tedious data entry go quicker the second time around.

This shows you exactly where all your carbs, fats, and proteins are coming from. "So what?" you might ask. Do we really have to obsess over our "macronutrient ratios"? In most cases, no. But an associated micronutrient profile can be very useful and revealing.

FitDay can drill down into a complete vitamin and mineral profile for the assemblage of food you just chowed down on and recorded, as depicted in Figure 2-20. Although bioavailability—how much of the consumed nutrient, like vitamin C or selenium, actually reached its target tissue—is a complex issue, it seems conceivable that this data will be reasonably accurate, given that you consumed the nutrients as food, not a pill.

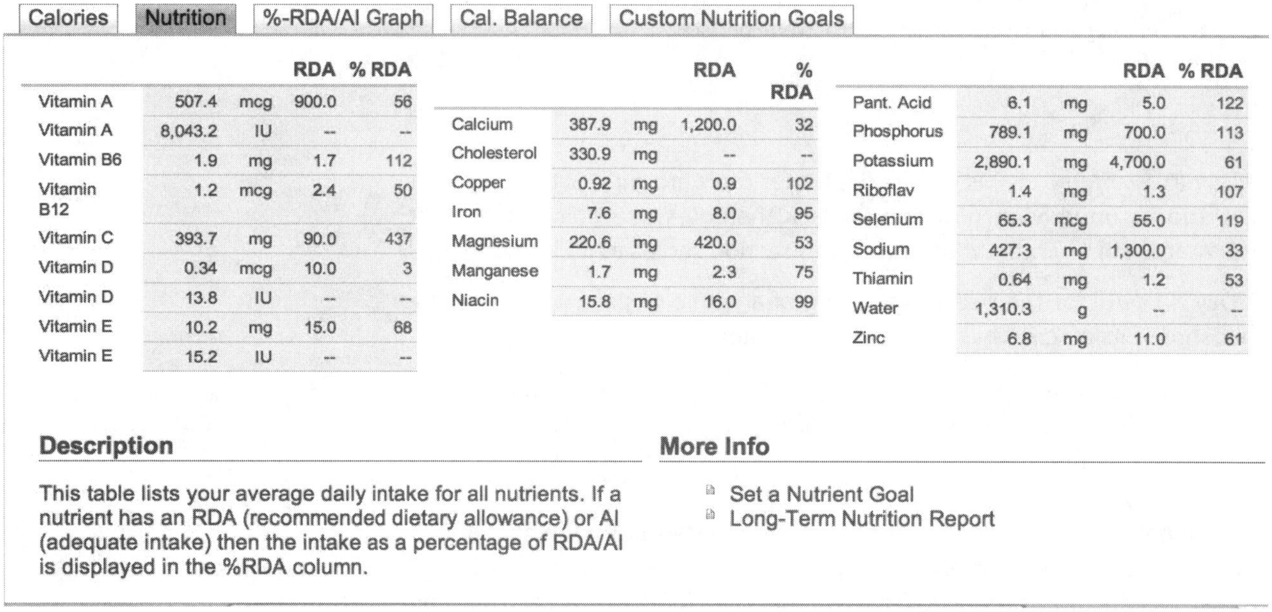

| Calories | **Nutrition** | %-RDA/AI Graph | Cal. Balance | Custom Nutrition Goals |

			RDA	% RDA
Vitamin A	507.4	mcg	900.0	56
Vitamin A	8,043.2	IU	--	--
Vitamin B6	1.9	mg	1.7	112
Vitamin B12	1.2	mcg	2.4	50
Vitamin C	393.7	mg	90.0	437
Vitamin D	0.34	mcg	10.0	3
Vitamin D	13.8	IU	--	--
Vitamin E	10.2	mg	15.0	68
Vitamin E	15.2	IU	--	--

			RDA	% RDA
Calcium	387.9	mg	1,200.0	32
Cholesterol	330.9	mg	--	--
Copper	0.92	mg	0.9	102
Iron	7.6	mg	8.0	95
Magnesium	220.6	mg	420.0	53
Manganese	1.7	mg	2.3	75
Niacin	15.8	mg	16.0	99

			RDA	% RDA
Pant. Acid	6.1	mg	5.0	122
Phosphorus	789.1	mg	700.0	113
Potassium	2,890.1	mg	4,700.0	61
Riboflav	1.4	mg	1.3	107
Selenium	65.3	mcg	55.0	119
Sodium	427.3	mg	1,300.0	33
Thiamin	0.64	mg	1.2	53
Water	1,310.3	g	--	--
Zinc	6.8	mg	11.0	61

Description

This table lists your average daily intake for all nutrients. If a nutrient has an RDA (recommended dietary allowance) or AI (adequate intake) then the intake as a percentage of RDA/AI is displayed in the %RDA column.

More Info

- Set a Nutrient Goal
- Long-Term Nutrition Report

Figure 2-20. *Micronutrient lineup in a FitDay window*

This kind of data can make a recommendation such as "maintain a potassium:sodium (P:S) ratio of at least 4:1" more concrete and thus easier to grasp. You know the foods represented in Figure 2-19 gave you a P:S ratio of 2,890 to 427, or about 6.8 to 1.

What if you just want to know what a single serving like "bagel smeared with jelly and margarine" is doing for you? No sweat, as shown in the micronutrient profile depicted in Figure 2-21.

			RDA	% RDA				RDA	% RDA				RDA	% RDA
Vitamin A	292.8	mcg	900.0	33	Calcium	31.8	mg	1,200.0	3	Pant. Acid	0.82	mg	5.0	16
Vitamin A	1,281.9	IU	--	--	Cholesterol	0.36	mg	--	--	Phosphorus	178.6	mg	700.0	26
Vitamin B6	0.15	mg	1.7	9	Copper	0.28	mg	0.9	32	Potassium	235.3	mg	4,700.0	5
Vitamin B12	0.025	mcg	2.4	1	Iron	3.9	mg	8.0	48	Riboflav	0.45	mg	1.3	34
Vitamin C	0.47	mg	90.0	1	Magnesium	53.6	mg	420.0	13	Selenium		mcg	55.0	
Vitamin D	0.0		10.0	0	Manganese	1.4	mg	2.3	60	Sodium	830.1	mg	1,300.0	64
Vitamin D	0.0		--	--	Niacin	6.3	mg	16.0	39	Thiamin	0.51	mg	1.2	42
Vitamin E	2.2	mg	15.0	15						Water	56.9	g	--	--
Vitamin E	3.3	IU	--	--						Zinc	1.3	mg	11.0	12

Description

This table lists your average daily intake for all nutrients. If a nutrient has an RDA (recommended dietary allowance) or AI (adequate intake) then the intake as a percentage of RDA/AI is displayed in the %RDA column.

More Info

- Set a Nutrient Goal
- Long-Term Nutrition Report

Figure 2-21. *The jelly-bagel sandwich tasted good, but it was hurtin' in the nutrient department*

The figures in red mean that the food is beneath the Recommended Dietary Allowance (RDA) for that nutrient (see Chapter 4). We'll give you the benefit of the doubt—you'll make up those deficits with meals later in the day.

The dressed-up wheat bagel is high in sodium and fairly deficient in nutrients, for a 614-calorie snack (300 of those calories coming from the bagel and 188 from the 1.5 tablespoons of margarine and jelly—we promised "smeared"!). When you're scarfing down that many calories, you usually want to get more bang for the buck in terms of nutrients.

The USDA National Nutrient Database

Many of the nutrition tools on the Web use the data from the USDA National Nutrient Database: *www.nal.usda.gov/fnic/foodcomp/search/*. This is a no-frills website where you can initiate searches, as shown in Figure 2-22, and/or download the entire database.

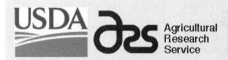

NUTRIENT DATA LABORATORY

Search the USDA National Nutrient Database for Standard Reference

Enter up to 5 keywords which best describe the food item. To further limit the search, select a specific Food Group.

Certain codes can also be searched: NDB number (the USDA 5-digit Nutrient Databank identifier); the USDA commodity code; and the URMIS number for specific cuts of meat (enter the # symbol followed without a space by the URMIS code).

Keyword(s): [_____] Help
Select Food Group: [All Food Groups ▼]
[Submit]

To view reports on foods by single nutrients, such as calcium or niacin, go to Nutrient Lists.

Use these links to access SR24 datasets or SR24 documentation.

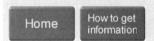

Figure 2-22. *A federal government nutrient database search*

Instead of searching this database, which is cut-and-dried, we'll show another cool way of acquiring data from this site.

Let's say you want to discover the best food sources of selenium, an important antioxidant mineral source (you'll show more than a casual interest in minerals and antioxidants after reading Chapter 4!).

Go to this URL: *www.ars.usda.gov/Services/docs.htm?docid=22114*. Scroll down to selenium, then click on the "Sorted by Nutrient Content" option.

The application automatically generates a PDF file that lists, in descending order, the best food sources of selenium (Figure 2-23). Please pass the Brazil nuts!

USDA National Nutrient Database for Standard Reference, Release 24

Selenium, Se (µg) Content of Selected Foods per Common Measure, sorted by nutrient content

NDB_No	Description	Weight (g)	Common Measure	Content per Measure
12078	Nuts, brazilnuts, dried, unblanched	28.35	1 oz (6-8 nuts)	543.5
15071	Fish, rockfish, Pacific, mixed species, cooked, dry heat	149	1 fillet	113.5
15221	Fish, tuna, yellowfin, fresh, cooked, dry heat	85	3 oz	92.0
21106	Fast foods, fish sandwich, with tartar sauce and cheese	183	1 sandwich	88.6
15037	Fish, halibut, Atlantic and Pacific, cooked, dry heat	159	1/2 fillet	88.1
05022	Chicken, broilers or fryers, giblets, cooked, simmered	145	1 cup	86.4
15128	Fish, tuna salad	205	1 cup	84.5
05172	Turkey, all classes, giblets, cooked, simmered, some giblet fat	145	1 cup	84.0
20005	Barley, pearled, raw	200	1 cup	75.4
15232	Fish, roughy, orange, cooked, dry heat	85	3 oz	75.1
20080	Wheat flour, whole-grain	120	1 cup	74.2
15111	Fish, swordfish, cooked, dry heat	106	1 piece	72.6
15121	Fish, tuna, light, canned in water, drained solids	85	3 oz	68.3
15071	Fish, rockfish, Pacific, mixed species, cooked, dry heat	85	3 oz	64.8
15119	Fish, tuna, light, canned in oil, drained solids	85.05	3 oz	64.6
15148	Crustaceans, lobster, northern, cooked, moist heat	85	3 oz	62.1
21126	Fast foods, submarine sandwich, with tuna salad	256	1 sandwich, 6" roll	60.2
15111	Fish, swordfish, cooked, dry heat	85	3 oz	58.2
15141	Crustaceans, crab, blue, canned	135	1 cup	57.9
15086	Fish, salmon, sockeye, cooked, dry heat	155	1/2 fillet	56.6
15168	Mollusks, oyster, eastern, cooked, breaded and fried	85	3 oz	56.5

Figure 2-23. *Brazil nuts are selenium-rich, and you've got the PDF for proof*

You can download an updated version of the National Nutrient Database itself (in a ZIP file), then import the numerous data files into whatever database management system you're using, such as MySQL.

Here's the link for downloading the database: *www.ars.usda.gov/Services/docs.htm?docid=22113*.

> *Release 23 of the database includes about a dozen different data files. In other words, the National Nutrient Database is relational, not one giant chunk of data.*

Pointy-Headed Searches

If you're in a very scholarly state of mind, you can search for the latest academic journal articles on PubMed (*http://pubmed.com*) or Google Scholar (*http://scholar.google.com*).

PubMed

PubMed includes "21 million citations for biomedical literature from MEDLINE, life science journals, and online books."

You can often access the entire article for free; at other times, free access is limited to the journal abstract. Figure 2-24 shows a result from searching on the Boolean expression "resistance training AND oxidative stress." Typically, the upper-righthand corner of the page containing the abstract provides any available links to the full-text version.

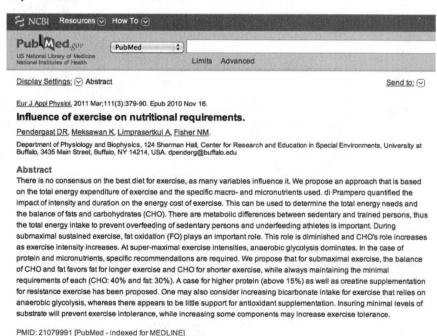

Figure 2-24. *A PubMed search result*

It's irritating, to say the least, to find an intriguing new journal article, then click on the link and discover that the publisher wants $30–$60 to read anything but the abstract. That makes it pretty hard for a student, or simply a health-conscious geek, to undertake interesting research. If you run into this problem, your college or town might have a library subscription, for instance, to an online journal-retrieval system like EBSCO that you can use for free.

Google Scholar

Google Scholar provides similar access to scholarly and academic articles on nutrition and fitness studies. Sometimes you can search on an article title to determine if the full text of the study is available, as shown in Figure 2-25.

You may want to bone up on the differences between good and bad science if you're going to become a PubMed or Google Scholar geek. This article represents a good summary: http://news.yahoo.com/difference-between-good-bad-science-read-scientific-studies.html.

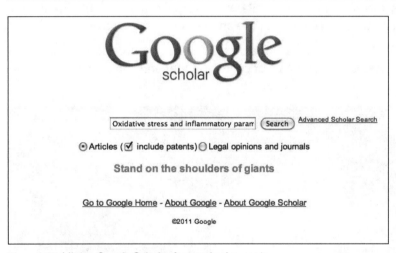

Figure 2-25. *Mining Google Scholar for cerebral nuggets*

Connected Devices

A mounting trend for geeks and techies in the sports world is the use of arrays of connected sports gear and websites. First the gadgets capture particular athletic-training events like running, biking, Nordic skiing, and hiking, then the service *broadcasts* the data to several places.

> *In many ways, this integration represents the inclusion of your fitness or health routine in "the cloud." Cloud computing in general lets you initiate more of your IT tasks, including saving and retrieving data, using devices such as smartphones and laptops that are all connected together and interrelated on the Internet.*

Many sports-gear manufacturers are taking this route, such as Garmin Connect and the Nike+ program (see *http://nikerunning.nike.com/nikeos/p/nikeplus/en_US/plus/*). We've already described Fitbit in great detail. Another device that has been integrated with Fitbit's data is the Withings body-composition scale. This is a scale that wirelessly connects to a website and uploads the data from the scale. Withings also makes a blood-pressure monitor. I guess you would call this an example of "e-health."

Figure 2-26 shows the Dashboard at *http://my.withings.com/en/*, once you have registered as a user and, of course, bought and configured the device.

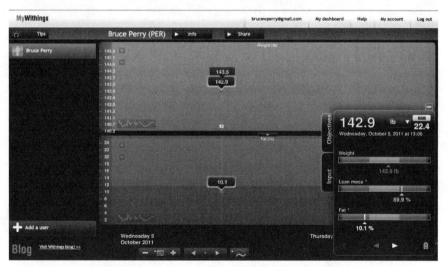

Figure 2-26. *The Withings dashboard for a body-composition analyzer*

> *To get started, you'll have to go to http://start.withings.com and download some pairing software (as in, pairing up your computer and the scale). You have to connect the scale to your computer using a USB cable. The scale then recognizes the wireless network your computer is using so it can independently connect with the Web later and wirelessly upload its data.*

What's more, Fitbit and other online communities such as Twitter, TrainingPeaks, and Google Health can also access the data from Withings and incorporate it into their own data and displays.

> *All of this is configured within a Sharing preference on the Withings dashboard—your information isn't just blindly sent out to the world.*

A body-composition scale measures not just weight, but body fat percentage. Your lean mass is the nonfatty tissue part of your body—the bones, muscles, and organs.

> *Muscles also contain fats in the membranes of cells, as well as a relatively large amount of fat that they can call upon for burning as fuel. In addition, internal organs have fats in their cell membranes, and are cushioned from body blows by adipose tissue.*

Your body fat percentage defines the part of the body that is not lean mass. It is often a more relevant detail of your physical fitness than Body Mass Index (BMI), which is skewed in people who are more muscular—they have a higher BMI, but it's reflective of more muscle than fat.

The Withings scale is pricey, at about $160. You can buy a Tanita body-composition analyzer, a device that also uses electrical impedance technology but without the web connections, for about half that amount, or you might choose to share one of these devices with your friends or teammates.

> *I suppose it's cool that you can do it, but do you really need to broadcast your weight, body composition, or blood pressure everywhere? Some might find it motivating, to know that others can track their progress; it builds in another level of accountability and motivation.*

Electrical impedance technology sends a tiny electric current through your body when you stand on the scale (don't worry, it's not dangerous!). Using an algorithm, the scale measures the feedback from this electrical current to estimate muscle vs. fat tissue. It's only a rough estimate of your body composition percentage. Numerous factors affect the results these devices spit out, including where you place the scale, how you stand on it (including whether you're in the buff or not!), and even the time of day and whether you've recently exercised. Your body composition doesn't change drastically week by week, so don't obsess over wildly fluctuating numbers. Just aim for a general trend. It's worth it to pay attention to your body composition; it's a much better reflection of health than a static weight measurement.

Your body fat percentage defines the part of the body that is not lean mass. It is often a more relevant detail of your physical fitness than Body Mass Index (BMI).

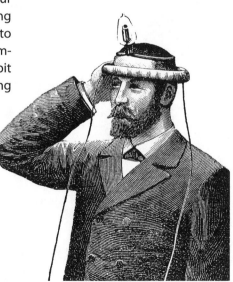

TRAINING YOUR BRAIN: LUMOSITY

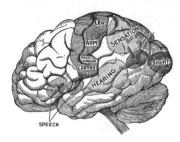

Our roundup in this chapter wouldn't be complete without a discussion of a brain-training tool. Recent neuroscience research has shown that the brain is not stuck as a static anatomical entity from birth and early development, as once thought. The brain can be strengthened and made more robust with exercise (of a cerebral nature, that is), similar to a muscle.

The fancy term for this is "neuroplasticity." According to http://en.wikipedia.org/wiki/Neuroplasticity, neuroplasticity:

> …is a nonspecific neuroscience term referring to the ability of the brain and nervous system in all species to change structurally and functionally as a result of input from the environment. Plasticity occurs on a variety of levels, ranging from cellular changes involved in learning to large-scale changes involved in cortical remapping in response to injury…

Lumosity (www.lumosity.com) is a popular online training tool that involves implementing exercises and games. The games are personalized based on the goals that you specify, e.g., improved memory, processing speed, or spatial recognition.

It's fun to use and as you progress through your customized program, the site builds a Brain Performance Index (BPI). This score is a reflection of how well you do in the games and your cognitive strength as you pump it up over time.

As the company describes it:

> Each time you play, we update your BPI to accurately reflect your current brain performance… Your Overall BPI is your average BPI across each of the five cognitive areas: attention, memory, speed, flexibility and problem solving" (www.lumosity.com/blog/bpi-brain-performance-index/).

With the "teaser" free trial, you can try out Lumosity games without the running tally of your BPI or the ability to compare it with that of other users. A fairly pricey premium version for brain games gives you these features and more. Or, you could just begin learning a new foreign language (Spanish, German, or Mandarin, anyone?).

Food Chemistry Basics:
Proteins, Fats, and Carbs

3

Most of the stuff you consume, other than the water content, is made up of *macronutrients*: substances humans require for energy, in relatively large amounts. I'm tempted to say that macronutrients are *the nutrients that you can see* (as opposed to micronutrients like vitamins or minerals), since the plate that shows the ice-cream scoop of white mashed potato laid beside a sliver of salmon clearly depicts a *carb* sitting next to a *protein* (although both foods might have a smidgeon or more of other macronutrients in them—salmon, for example, is about 40 percent *fat*).

Ta-da, the macronutrients are carbohydrates, fats, and proteins.

What do we mean by "large amounts"? That would be a total of roughly 300 to 600 grams of carbs, fat, and protein for someone who takes in from 2,000 to 3,000 calories per day (and much more for the lumberjacks and mountain guides who eat 7,000 calories per day).

You have to consume macronutrients to convert their intrinsic energy to your own fuel, as well as for the growth, replacement, and maintenance of your bodily tissues.

You could include water or fiber in the macronutrient category, but we'll focus on the top three. I'm sure you've run across protein, fats, and carbs before, even as these terms assume new meanings, propelled along by hypermarketing and branding of trendy new dietary regimes like "high protein" or "very low carb." They tend to become scientific rather than political footballs, as experts vie with one another in their health emphasis on one or another macronutrient.

Empower Yourself

This chapter goes into quite a bit of detail on these nutrients, simply because it aids your fitness efforts to understand more precisely what you're putting in your mouth. Importantly, the chapter will spend a fair amount of time on tools such as NutritionData, because they are self-empowering and no one likes making their own intellectual determinations and health choices more than a food geek.

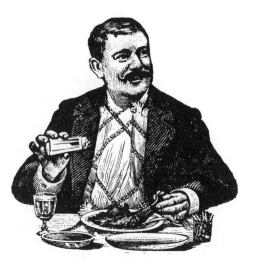

All knowledge without coercion or propaganda is a form of personal enlightenment.

The nutrition world is certainly a moving target, in terms of the debates that rage on about which of the macronutrients are healthier as foci for your diet. In my humble opinion, neither the status quo public health recommendations nor the latest inflammatory food blogs are reliable enough to slavishly follow. There's never been a better time to take the bull by the horns and do your own research.

Most geeks who are aiming for fitness have some kind of goal in mind (e.g., getting leaner, building muscle, building a baby). While we all understand that eating doesn't require a preparatory biochemical analysis (in fact, that preoccupation would probably ruin the meal before the waiter ever brought it—particularly for your dinner partners), dietary matters do entail the constant launching of complex chemical reactions in your body, as well as providing the materials for your own cells over and over again as they are regenerated by the trillions.

Therefore, understanding some of the basics behind food constituents can only be empowering. All knowledge without coercion or propaganda is a form of personal enlightenment.

In fitness terms, by eating, you're basically rebuilding yourself, and *your level of fitness starts with nutrition*.

In terms of "building ourselves," as humans, excluding water and minerals, we are composed of about 76 percent fats and 24 percent protein by calories, according to the interesting book Perfect Health Diet: Four Steps to Renewed Health, Youthful Vitality, and Long Life. *Authors Paul and Shou-Ching Jaminet, both scientists (one a physicist and the other a biochemist), argue that it makes sense to eat according to the typical proportion of fats and protein in our own bodies. Thus they conclude that we should "eat what we are," as in a majority of fats. For more explanations of their strategy, visit http:// perfecthealthdiet.com.*

Macronutrient Ratios

We'll start by discussing what a macronutrient ratio (MR) is, because this term comes up a lot in food discussions and provides a snapshot of the contents of your typical food intake.

Some people want to fine-tune their MRs, for example, in order to add lean mass (a bit more protein and calories in general), lose some extra fat (tightly connected to the previous goal), or subtract some carbs because they're not doing the "Race Across America" bike race anymore. The ratio falls into the "good to know" category; check on it once and you're good to go, unless you have to radically change your dietary components.

After discussing MRs, we'll move on to descriptions of each of the three macronutrients and what happens during digestion (because the carbs, fats, and

Chapter 3

protein that go into your mouth are reformulated—mostly ripped apart—by the time they hit your bloodstream and body cells).

The Ole 30-50-20 Maneuver

When you eat a typical meal or snack, you usually consume portions of all three macronutrients: carbs, fats, and protein. Unless you're nibbling on a stick of butter (100 percent fat *by calories*), for example, your breakfast might contain carbs and maybe a tiny bit of protein (fruit); carbs and some protein (toast); or fats, protein, and perhaps a few carbs (meat and eggs).

> *You generally don't have to obsess over your macronutrient ratio if you aim for a variety of real food: veggies, fruits, eggs, cheese, fish, meats, sweet potatoes, nuts, rice, etc. These choices should allow for settling into a sensible and healthy ratio without knowing exactly what it is. It's not as if a hawk ever flies up into the air with the aim to "bump up the fats in my macronutrient ratio." With some nudging in the right direction, it should come naturally.*

The MR is the breakdown of the percentage of calories taken up in the food by each nutrient, as in 30 percent carbs, 50 percent fats, and 20 percent protein. As the lingo goes, this would be a 30-50-20 ratio. Various essential micronutrients, such as vitamins and minerals, are in there too (hopefully!), but they are tiny by weight compared with the macros (see Chapter 4 for more information about micronutrients).

Figure 3-1 shows a FitDay (*www.fitday.com*) breakdown of what I had for breakfast this morning, about 460 calories worth of fried eggs, fruit, and cheese. Each of the fat grams is worth about 9 calories, while carbs and protein add up to about 4 calories each.

> *The term kcal or "kilogram calorie" is a more precise term in nutrition than "calorie." It means the amount of energy required to raise the temperature of a kilogram of water 1 degree Celsius. "kcal," however, has the same meaning as "calorie" in the context of this discussion.*

Food Name	Amount	Unit	Cals	Fat (g)	Carbs (g)	Prot (g)	Delete
		Total	456	33.7	23.6	18.9	
Egg, whole, cooked	2	medium	147	10.7	1.1	10.8	✖
Avocado, raw	0.5	avocado, California (l	138	12.7	7.4	1.7	✖
Coffee, regular	2	coffee cup (6 fl oz)	4	0.1	0.1	0.4	✖
Cheese, natural, Cheddar or American type	1	cubic inch	69	5.6	0.2	4.2	✖
Butter	1	pat	36	4.1	0.0	0.0	✖
Peach, raw	1	medium (2–1/2" dia)	38	0.2	9.3	0.9	✖
Blackberries, raw	2	oz	24	0.3	5.4	0.8	✖
		Total	456	33.7	23.6	18.9	

Figure 3-1. *Eggs, fruit, and cheese for breakfast*

The MR for this small meal was 19 percent carbs, 64 percent fat, and 17 percent protein, as shown in Figure 3-2. The shorthand way to describe this ratio is 19-64-17. A macronutrient ratio is generally one piece of data out of a big nutrition picture. If you really wanted to analyze your nutrition inputs, you would be better off calculating the MR for a typical week of eating, along with your calorie intake (i.e., 2,400 calories per day) and perhaps your activity levels, to put all the data into a proper context.

Hey, you can use the Fitbit tool we told you about in Chapter 2 to make this analysis.

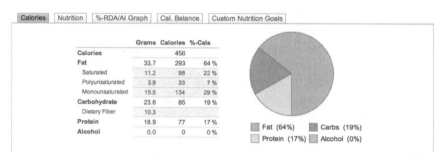

Figure 3-2. *The macronutrient ratio for a small meal, displayed on FitDay*

In this small 460-calorie meal, the ratio of fats was much higher than carbs, even though I ate less than 10 more fat grams, because fats have more than twice the calorie or energy content of carbs. They are thus considered *energy-dense* foods. The wine, beer, or other alcohol you might drink (actually containing the chemical ethanol) has about 7 calories per gram.

As you may already know, recommendations for an ideal macronutrient ratio range all over the map. Figure 3-3 shows the MRs for a number of popular diets, including the Mediterranean, Zone, DASH, South Beach, Atkins, and Ornish eating plans. They range from high-carb diets (e.g., Ornish) to low-carb, higher protein plans, which is often another way of saying high-fat diets, because the majority of calories are obtained from fat (e.g., Atkins). Figure 3-3 is derived from a 2008 article in the *American Journal of Clinical Nutrition* called "Alternatives for macronutrient intake and chronic disease."[1]

The featured eating plans differ wildly from each other; just look at Ornish (75 carbs-7 fat-8 protein) compared with Mediterranean (46 carbs-38 fat-16 protein). Each specially designed diet seems to spawn another one. I've often wondered why no one has invented the "Symmetrical Diet" or "Perfect Synchronicity" involving an exact partition of calories for all three macronutrients: 33-33-33. Not catchy enough? Or maybe I just haven't looked hard enough; it must be out there.

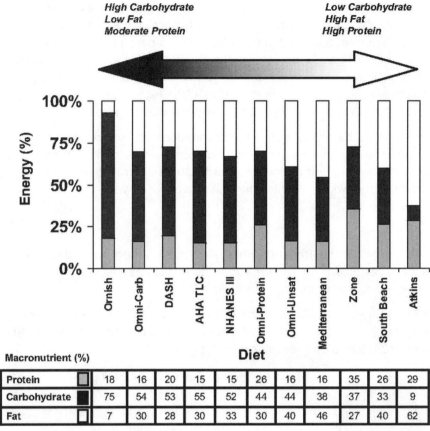

High Carbohydrate
Low Fat
Moderate Protein

Low Carbohydrate
High Fat
High Protein

Macronutrient (%)		Ornish	Omni-Carb	DASH	AHA TLC	NHANES III	Omni-Protein	Omni-Unsat	Mediterranean	Zone	South Beach	Atkins
Protein	▨	18	16	20	15	15	26	16	16	35	26	29
Carbohydrate	■	75	54	53	55	52	44	44	38	37	33	9
Fat	☐	7	30	28	30	33	30	40	46	27	40	62

Figure 3-3. *The macronutrient ratios for several popular diets (www.ajcn.org/content/88/1/1.full.pdf+html); original caption: Macronutrient profiles of popular diets, the OmniHeart and Dietary Approaches to Stop Hypertension (DASH) study diets, the American Heart Association Therapeutic Lifestyle (AHA TLC) guidelines (5), and typical US macronutrient intakes as reported in the third Health and Nutrition Examination Survey (NHANES III; 24). The eating patterns are ordered with the highest-carbohydrate diet starting on the left and the lowest on the right. The Atkins diet profile is for the life-long maintenance phase, and the South Beach diet profile is for phase 3. Small amounts of alcohol (0.2–0.8% of energy) were also present in the Ornish, Mediterranean, Atkins, Zone, and South Beach diets. Percentages may not add up to 100% because of rounding.*

If the numbers begin looking more and more like the offerings of a roulette wheel, then maybe constantly pondering and switching between them is equivalently meaningful to playing casino games with your food. Meanwhile, the Food and Nutrition Board of the Institute of Medicine, a US public health authority, has produced its own guidelines involving MRs. They are called Acceptable Macronutrient Distribution Ranges (AMDRs).

The AMDR is a "range of intake for a particular energy source that is associated with reduced risk of chronic disease while providing intakes of essential nutrients." See www.iom.edu/Global/News%20 Announcements/~/media/C5CD2DD7840544979A549EC47E56A02B. ashx for more information.

These are ranges of percentages that the Food and Nutrition Board of the Institute of Medicine recommends for each macronutrient, as follows: carbs, 45 to 65 percent for all age groups; fat, 20 to 35 percent depending on age; and protein, 10 to 35 percent. These numbers leave room for all kinds of diets, including ones dominated by carbs (65 percent), even though the accompanying comments point out that "the higher range" of carb intake leaves you open to high triglycerides and low HDL cholesterol.

For example, based on these recommendations, you could have a diet that is 65 percent carbs-20 percent fat-15 percent protein, or one that goes in a dramatically different direction: 45 carbs-30 fat-25 protein. In other words, there's a lot of wiggle room within the conventional wisdom.

RDAs

The US public health authorities also publish Recommended Dietary Allowances (RDAs) for each macronutrient (such as the RDA for carbohydrates—130 grams per day for adults).

You're probably familiar with the RDAs for vitamins and minerals. They are essentially a suggested "minimal amount for health." For example, the RDA for carbs is based on the brain's need for glucose.[2]

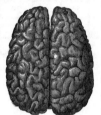

Your brain accounts for around 5 percent of your body weight, but grabs about 20 percent of your calories— mainly glucose, but also ketones, a byproduct of metabolizing fats for energy. That's a very impressive, "greedy" detail of our metabolism; if you take in 3,200 calories per day, your brain is getting about 640 calories. We'll discuss ketones at the end of the chapter.

Now we're going to move into a discussion about each of the three macronutrients.

Food molecules are like Legos. They are small molecules bonded or stuck together to make more complex ones. Starch, for example, is a big *polymer* or chain containing many *monomers*, which are glucose or sugar molecules. When you eat and digest these substances, the digestive enzymes split apart the connections between the pieces and separate them so that they can be absorbed into the body through the small intestine.

The small intestine cannot absorb whole protein, carb polymer, and fat molecules; they all have to be split up by digestive enzymes first, so the substances you are actually absorbing are glucose and other sugar monomers, amino acids (from proteins), and fatty acids (from triglycerides, the storage form of fat).

Carbs are polymers of glucose molecules. Proteins are made up of an often-complex configuration of amino acids. Fats, when you eat them in food, are composed of a glycerol molecule attached to three fatty acids in an "E" shape. These are the original Lego structures.

WHAT ABOUT COFFEE?

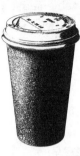

If you're like me, coffee is almost a major macronutrient for you. But can you stay fit drinking a lot of coffee? It depends what you define as *a lot*. A moderate amount—a couple of cups or a to-go mug early in the day—is probably harmless. In fact, many studies say it's good for you.

Coffee is metabolized very quickly and obviously is stimulatory for the central nervous system. Caffeine is actually considered a kind of supplement for athletes. As we discuss in Chapter 10, a strong cup of coffee or tea is a suitable supplement before a sprint, a weightlifting session, or even a longer event. Caffeine mobilizes free fatty acids and acts as a central nervous system stimulant.

People who drink coffee seem to have "reductions in the risk of several chronic diseases," according to "Coffee and Health: A Review of Recent Human Research," a 2006 article in *Critical Reviews in Food Science and Nutrition*. Coffee actually contains some micronutrients in small amounts, such as the all-important mineral magnesium.

Coffee's downsides? The obvious jitteriness you get from too much caffeine and too little kicking up of the heels.

Coffee also decreases the heart rate (in my own experience, my resting heart rate (RHR) might go from 52 to 46 or lower after a few cups of joe) and increases blood pressure—so if you've got a little hypertension, coffee might not be a great thing.

Coffee is also very addictive (with its own withdrawal symptoms—people talk about headaches, but I haven't experienced them because I haven't withdrawn yet), like that other bean, chocolate. Coffee will really mess with your sleep, and people differ in their sensitivity to it. Try drinking a big mug after 3:00 PM and see what it does to your sleep waves on a Zeo chart; you might have less REM or deep sleep, or you might simply have less sleep.

Given the number of studies they've conducted on coffee and caffeine, "the most popular drug in the world," it seems like researchers have had plenty of opportunities to find something really bad about it, and so far they haven't. As long as they don't, I'm going to continue to enjoy my morning dark roast.

See the "Coffee and Health" review article at *www.tandfonline.com/doi/full/10.1080/10408390500400009*.

We'll start our more specific introduction to food chemistry with carbs.

Carbohydrates

Carbs, or carbohydrates, seem to always be discussed as "high" or "low," but never quite in between. The latest rage is "low carb." When I was fueling long-distance races in my cardio endurance days, it was high carb with adequate protein, but keep fats low. The bodybuilders, no matter what else was happening, seemed less fat-phobic, drinking their eggs and guzzling their whole milk along with everything else they consumed.

The carbs range from the simple (sucrose or table sugar) to the complex (starch). The simplest building blocks of carbs are *monosaccharides*, single-unit molecules such as glucose, fructose, and galactose.

These molecules are rarely consumed in food as-is; they are the products of digestion that are absorbed from the small intestine into the bloodstream or liver (in the case of fructose). In other words, glucose and the others are usually connected together into *disaccharides* (two-unit sugars) or more complex food molecules called *oligosaccharides* (bigger-than-two-unit sugars resulting from the breakdown of complex polysugars). *Polysaccharides* are the most complex sugars, like starch or cellulose.

Figure 3-4 shows a sucrose molecule, which is what the table sugar you might sprinkle into your tea or coffee is made of. Sucrose is made up of a glucose molecule attached to a fructose molecule (so sucrose is actually about 50 percent fructose, which is worth keeping in mind if you want to reduce your daily fructose intake—see the sidebar titled "The Skinny on Fructose"). Every carbohydrate is made of a carbon "backbone" with hydrogen and oxygen molecules attached to it. This combination of molecules gives carbohydrates their name.

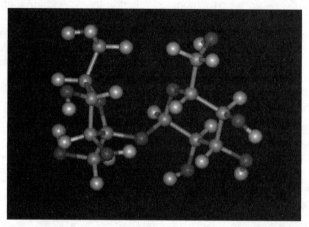

Figure 3-4. *A glucose attached to a fructose equals a sucrose (source: http://www. worldofmolecules.com/foods/); green is carbon, red is oxygen, and white is hydrogen*

Every carbohydrate is made of a carbon "backbone" with hydrogen and oxygen molecules attached to it.

When my son was finished romping about a Vermont village on Halloween, 2011, he returned with a bag full of sucrose (I'm imploring him to give a lot of it away, and/or make it last months…). When you eat candy like a 3 Musketeers bar, that mush pile of addictively tasty sucrose makes it down to the small intestine, where the sucrose molecule has to be "cleaved" into smaller parts before the sugar or monosaccharides ever make it across the intestinal barrier to the bloodstream.

Nutrients have transporters that ferry them to the great beyond across the intestinal surfaces; no sugars beyond the simple sugars or monosaccharides have these transporters.

The sucrose molecules are split apart into glucose and fructose molecules with the aid of enzymes that are present in the small intestine. The enzyme in question for the 3 Musketeers bar is sucrase (the "-ase" suffix usually signals an enzyme, just like the "-ose" suffix means a sugar). Similarly, lactose, a dissacharide milk sugar, requires lactase to be digested, and maltose has its digestive companion maltase (hey, a sensible biochemical naming strategy!).

Major Sugar Buzz

The chocolate bar, the full-sized bar that I used to like to see in my own Halloween bag, contains 40 grams of sugar.[3] This is about 160 calories that consists of 20 grams of glucose and 20 grams of fructose.

Glucose goes into the bloodstream, where it can be utilized by the brain for energy, or taken up by the muscle cells or the liver to be reassembled into *glycogen*, a special starch that animals like us store for later use (more on starch coming right up). Excess carbs can and often are stored as fat, via the sultriest term ever invented for body-fat-making processes: *de novo lipogenesis* (DNL). DNL takes place in the liver as well as in peripheral storage depots for your fats, like around your hips.

The body has to get rid of excess glucose—in a way, dispose of it—because it's toxic to cells in excess quantities. If your glycogen is already topped off (because you've eaten a lot of carbs, or you simply never use it up by moving around), so you don't have room to store more glucose in the form of starch in your body, the sugar can be oxidized (burned as fuel) by skeletal muscle cells for energy. Or, the body can store the glucose as fat in the liver or adipose tissue (other fat depots in the body).

Glucose Is Energy Fuel, but Not by the Ton

If you cannot store or burn up the glucose you've consumed, you may have the beginnings of high fasting glucose, or excess sugars dissolved in your plasma or blood. This is why the typical doc's office annual visit involves a test for fasting glucose, to determine if you're metabolically handling sugar and associated hormones (e.g., insulin and leptin) okay.

> *You can keep your blood-sugar metabolism out of the prediabetic range (measured by some medical associations or countries' standards as a persistent fasting glucose level of 100 or more) by keeping your calorie and carb consumption within bounds—i.e., in line with your total energy expenditure. Intermittent fasting helps lower your fasting glucose levels (see Chapter 6).*

The hepatic portal vein, a conduit of blood and nutrients to the liver, takes fructose, a simple sugar that is part of sucrose, to the liver to be metabolized and detoxified (see the sidebar titled "The Skinny on Fructose").

Analyzing Your Carbs

You can determine the amount of fructose in food in the following manner: search for a food like a 12-ounce can of Sprite at NutritionData (*http://nutritiondata.self.com/facts/beverages/3870/2*). This little exercise demonstrates how you can analyze food on your own, among other things. Expand the NutritionData segment on the carbohydrates in the soda-can contents, as shown in Figure 3-5.

This beverage contains about 33 grams, or 132 kcal, of sugar, and guess what? They give you a free refill. The carbs include 19,151 mg, or about 19.2 grams, of fructose and 2,399 mg (2.4 grams) of sucrose. The sucrose, however, is about 50 percent fructose, so you can determine the total fructose quantity as follows: 19151 + (2399 / 2) = 20,350 mg, or 20.3 grams.

Before you completely condemn and wipe your hands of soda, realize that a large cultivated apple also contains a notable quantity of fructose.

Carbohydrates		
Amounts Per Selected Serving		%DV
Total Carbohydrate	30.8 g	10%
Dietary Fiber	5.4 g	21%
Starch	0.1 g	
Sugars	23.2 g	
Sucrose	4617 mg	
Glucose	5419 mg	
Fructose	13157 mg	
Lactose	0.0 mg	
Maltose	0.0 mg	
Galactose	0.0 mg	
	Collapse ▲	

Figure 3-5. A 12-ounce can of soda cranks out the sugar

Apples are generally cultivated to have, among other characteristics, a large size and a sweet taste compared with the typical runty, tart apples growing in the wild. These characteristics of cultivation are usually a good thing, providing many people with fresh apples containing some antioxidants and vitamin C throughout the year. They are not a good development on the fructose front though, for reasons that are explained up ahead. Besides, eating small wild apples (admittedly hard to find for people who don't live in the countryside) provides more antioxidants. The antioxidants are in the skin, and you have to eat more of the wild apples to get the same number of calories as you would from the large store-bought apples.

...a fructose is a fructose is a fructose...

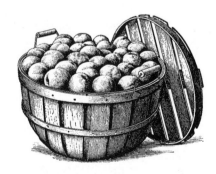

A large apple contains 4,617 mg of sucrose and 13,157 mg of fructose, according to NutritionData. Therefore, using our prior calculation, we see that it contains a total of 13,157 + (4,617 / 2) = 15,465mg, or about 15.5 grams, of fructose. This is comparable to the amount of fructose in a 12-ounce can of soda; however, the vitamin C content in an apple may help counter the negative health effects of excess fructose consumption.[4]

I don't want to dissuade people from eating apples (I eat them, particularly when I can pluck them off a tree). But the point is that a fructose is a fructose is a fructose, whether it comes from a pretty apple laid out at the store or a can of soda.

THE SKINNY ON FRUCTOSE

Many things in nature have a dose-response relationship—they might be great when experienced or imbibed in a small dose, but bad when taken in a large dose. If you were being held captive by a pirate in a small room and eating creepy-crawlies off the floor to survive, getting some fresh fruit, including its fructose content, would be a *great* life-sustaining thing.

Even once you've been released, munching on some fresh fruit once in a while would be a good idea—at the very least, it would keep you from geting scurvy (caused by a severe vitamin C deficiency).

Apparently, though, consuming *lots* of fructose—the simple sugar or monosaccharide found in plants but more typically consumed in the form of table sugar or high-fructose corn syrup (HFCS)—can be very unhealthy, in fact toxic. In regular doses as low as 50, 70, to 100 grams[5,6] per day,

fructose can induce insulin resistance (a precursor to other problems such as diabetes and obesity), chronic inflammation, weight gain around the abdomen, a fatty liver, excess uric acid, and other problems.[7] Fructose appears similar in terms of its negative effect on the liver to booze or ethanol, its fermentation byproduct.[8]

Basically, seek to eliminate the consumption of fructose- or HFCS-containing sodas and numerous other processed foods, and you avoid munching on commercial apples or watermelon all throughout the day (although vitamin C does seem to diminish the not-so-good fructose effects). Lemons, for example, are a great source of vitamin C and low in fructose. Just keep in mind that it's a dose-response relationship (everything in moderation).

Exercise also seems to help offset some of the bad metabolic aspects of fructose.[9]

When you drink cow's milk, part of what you consume is lactose, which is a sugar that is made of one part glucose and one part galactose.

One cup of whole milk contains about 13 grams of sugar, all of that in the form of 12,836 mg (or 12.8 grams) of lactose. The whole milk has a macronutrient ratio of 30-49-21, meaning that it is 49 percent fats. About 70 percent of its calories come from fat and protein (see http://nutritiondata.self.com/facts/dairy-and-egg-products/69/2).

The lack of lactase, an enzyme that splits apart lactose into its digestible constituents of glucose and galactose in the small intestine, is commonly known as lactose intolerance. People with this common form of indigestion don't get along with regular milk, often replacing it with soy milk.

The book The 10,000 Year Explosion *by Gregory Cochran and Henry Harpending poses the theory that the human genetic mutation that allowed people to maintain lactase production after weaning, giving them the ability to digest the milk of other animals (not just their mom's), was an important factor in the spread of Indo-European languages. They posited that drinking the milk made the people who originated these languages stronger nutritionally and allowed them to spread their influence. You really have to give this book points for originality!*

Maltose is a disaccharide composed of two glucose molecules bonded together. When barley is malted during the brewing of beer, this process breaks down the barley starch into maltose. Yeast will later use this sugar to fuel its lifecycle, producing alcohol and carbon dioxide as byproducts.[10]

Polysaccharides, or Starches

Polysaccharides are many sugars bonded together, sometimes consisting of thousands of glucose monomers. In other words, they are big complex Lego structures of glucose and other molecules. This is why they are commonly referred to as *complex carbohydrates*.

A complex carb is ultimately a big interconnected blob of sugar. When digested, it's split apart into many glucose monomers and released relatively quickly into the bloodstream, at least in terms of its effect on your metabolism. Some complex carbs or starches, like potatoes and white bread, have a higher glycemic index—an old measure of the effect of foods on glucose and insulin spikes in the blood—than table sugar. A complex carb like brown rice does not contain any fructose, however, which is a good thing if you're looking for more carbs but no more fructose. Fiber-containing complex carbs such as squash have an added advantage in that they beneficially feed the microbiota in your colon after their incomplete digestion in the small intestine.

Polysaccharides include the starches we eat, such as a banana or a baked potato; glycogen, the animal starch we store in our muscles and liver (as well as a few other less substantial stores); and cellulose, which we cannot digest but often are implored to chew down as fiber.

Ruminant animals or herbivores like grazing cows, sheep, goats, bison, moose, and elk have specially designed stomachs that use microorganisms to ferment cellulose, whether it be grass or sticks or twigs or weeds, into a digestible substance, which is eventually absorbed by their systems as short-chain fatty acids. So, while they are herbivores or plant eaters, they have a high-fat diet!

We can digest starch because we have the enzyme amylase in our saliva, as well as in the pancreatic juices that help break the starch down in our small intestines. Amylase helps break up starch into maltose, the double-glucose sugar, and maltase takes care of the rest of the job so the glucose can be absorbed into the bloodstream.[11]

Protein

Protein is a critical structural and functional component of the human body, and commonly represents anywhere from 10 to 30 percent of a person's daily caloric intake. If you have a 2,400-calorie diet and 25 percent of it comes from protein, you're getting 600 calories, or 150 grams, of that macronutrient.

The ability of the body to properly metabolize protein foods *diminishes at an intake of about 35 percent of calories*, which is why you are not advised to go crazy on protein intake and try to get the majority of your calories from it. A potentially fatal condition known as "rabbit starvation syndrome" can occur with a diet dominated by lean protein and deprived of fats and carbs.

Early American explorers and pioneers discovered that dependence in the wilderness on meat that didn't contain enough fat, like rabbits, caused nausea, diarrhea, and sometimes death.[12]

Vilhjalmur Stefansson, the famous Arctic explorer from Canada (he ended up his exciting life as Director of Polar Studies at Dartmouth in Hanover, New Hampshire), also commented on the ill effects and futility of trying to survive on skinny animals in the far north with the Inuit. He spent a few years living with the Inuit on Arctic expeditions about 100 years ago, and his writings and self-experiments cast light on the Inuit's, and our own, ability to live almost exclusively for months on meat and fat. His book *My Life with the Eskimos* can be found at *http://www.amzn.to/My-Life-Eskimo*.

> *Where did the Inuit derive their vitamins, such as C, on this seal- and whale-meat diet? "Fediuk [analyzed] the vitamin C content of 100-gram (3.55-ounce) samples of foods eaten by Inuit women living in the Canadian Arctic: Raw caribou liver supplied almost 24 milligrams, seal brain close to 15 milligrams, and raw kelp more than 28 milligrams."[13]*

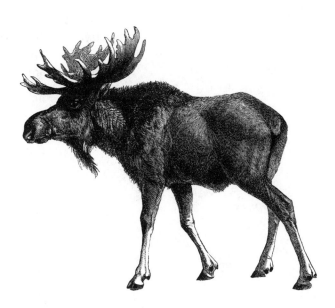

Proteins Do Important Stuff

The body requires protein in big and small ways. Human genes are essentially recipes for creating proteins. Skeletal muscle incorporates proteins called myosin and actin; bones are about one-fifth composed of the protein collagen, which dominates connective tissue such as ligaments and tendons. Organ tissue, the gut, skin, hair (keratin), and blood vessels also contain structural proteins.

Proteins are also functional; they do important stuff. Examples of the functional proteins are hormones that are made of protein (including glucagon, insulin, and growth hormone), immune system cells such as antibodies, enzymes (the catalysts for the body's chemical reactions, and used in digestion itself), as well as red and white blood cells. Figure 3-6 shows a hemoglobin molecule, a protein complex in red blood cells that carries oxygen throughout the body.

Proteins are like Lego structures, but this time the Lego pieces are *amino acids*, the protein's building blocks. The body can build thousands of different proteins using numerous combinations of these almost two dozen ingredients.

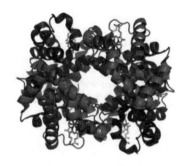

Figure 3-6. *A hemoglobin molecule contains protein in blue and red, and iron in green* (*source: http://en.wikipedia.org/wiki/ Hemoglobin*)

The body synthesizes from 500 to 1,000 pounds of protein, depending on the person's size, during a lifetime![14]

Here is some nomenclature involving proteins: 10 or more amino acids stuck together form a *polypeptide* (and two are a dipeptide and three a tripeptide). A polypeptide with more than 50 amino acids is called a *protein*, which can be composed of as many as 10,000 amino acids.[15]

Proteins have to be broken down into their constituent amino acids to be digested. This happens first in the stomach and then in the small intestine, employing a number of enzymes, including peptidases, proteases, and trypsin.[16] The protein building blocks, the amino acids, make their way to the liver (where some are actually metabolized for energy), then into the bloodstream, where the cells take them up to help make more proteins.[17]

FROM A PROGRAMMER, THE HACKER'S DIET

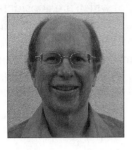

We interviewed John Walker, who wrote *The Hacker's Diet*, founded Autodesk, Inc., and coauthored the AutoCAD software. He lives in Switzerland, and we conducted our email interview in November 2011.

When did you write the 'The Hacker's Diet' book?

The book was written in 1989–1990. It circulated as samizdat PostScript and PDF files until 1994, when the first web edition was released. There have been two subsequent web editions in 1994 and 2005, all with essentially the same content but improved formatting and navigation as HTML/XHTML has evolved. An EPUB edition was released in 2011.

I gather you've approached the issue of losing weight using an engineer's perspective. What is the crux of the strategy?

To lose weight, eat fewer calories than you burn; to gain weight, eat more calories than you burn.

The slope of a moving average trend line of daily weights provides an accurate measure of calorie balance.

A pound of fat is equivalent to around 3,500 calories, so if you have a 500-calorie-per-day deficit, you'll lose about a pound a week.

What is the importance of tracking, metrics, and tools in your system? What other concepts are used that a developer might be familiar with (e.g., design patterns)?

In my view the flaw in most diet plans is that they are "open loop"—they prescribe a regimen of food and exercise, but provide no means to adapt to the differences among individuals and changes in circumstances. In *The Hacker's Diet*, feedback is integral to the concept, as illustrated by the figure at the start of this chapter: *www.fourmilab.ch/hackdiet/e4/losingweight.html*.

Daily tracking and plotting of the trend both eliminates much of the psychological rollercoaster of weight loss and management, and also allows one to adapt when circumstances change long before a problem gets out

of hand, even if you don't understand the cause of the change. For example: *www.fourmilab.ch/fourmilog/archives/2006-07/000726.html*.

The main concepts used in the system and the tools are:

- Exponentially smoothed moving averages as a means of low-pass filtering out of day-to-day noise in weight measurements (largely due to water retention).

- A linear regression fit to the smoothed trend line to determine its slope, from which calorie balance and rate of weight loss or gain can be calculated.

- A feedback system which adjusts meal plans based upon the measured calorie balance to achieve the desired rate of weight loss and permanent maintenance of weight when the goal is achieved.

I've written a bit in this book on ancestral health and "Paleo." Do you think these concepts have a place in a health regimen?

I have been experimenting with my own flavor of Paleo since December 2010 and have, so far, been very impressed with the results, particularly in blood pressure and cholesterol levels. I believe that both the evolutionary and biochemical arguments for Paleo are credible, and that people concerned with health and longevity should seriously consider it.

That said, while some people report weight loss after switching to Paleo, you certainly don't need to adopt Paleo to lose weight—as long as you manage your calorie balance, it doesn't matter what you eat. It may (and almost certainly will) be easier to lose weight if you eat a well-balanced diet of healthy food, but the main reason to do so is better health, not weight management in itself.

Do you have any favorite tools or gadgets?

I'm a software guy, so I'm not particularly into gadgets and gizmos. I am a great believer in Donald Knuth's practice of "Literate Programming," and use his CWEB/CTANGLE tools for C/C++ programming and Nuweb for development in Perl and other languages. The entire source code for my 2007 online set of tools for *The Hacker's Diet* is published in Literate Programming form: *www.fourmilab.ch/hackdiet/online/download/1.0/hdiet.pdf*.

Essential Amino Acids

Proteins are composed of any of 20 amino acids, 10 of which are considered essential because they have to be obtained in your diet. The body cannot synthesize its necessary proteins if these 10 amino acids do not show up in adequate amounts in your diet: isoleucine, leucine, lysine, methionine, phenylalanine, threonine, tryptophan, and valine, as well as arginine (for infants) and histidine (for infants) (from *Human Anatomy & Physiology*, by Elaine Marieb and Katja Hoehn).

> *Exercise Physiology, by William McArdle et al., lists only eight amino acids as "essential," and points out that infants cannot synthesize histidine and children have "a reduced capability for synthesizing arginine."*

The rest of the 20 amino acids are: alanine, asparagine, aspartic acid, cysteine, glycine, glutamic acid, glutamine, proline, serine, and tyrosine.

Eating Protein

When you eat protein-containing foods such as meats, fish, eggs, cheese, nuts, and plant foods, as we mentioned, proteases and other enzymes split up the big block of Legos into their separate amino acids, which can then be absorbed in the small intestine and released to the liver and bloodstream.

The body can do a number of things with these amino acids, depending on your physical needs:

- The cells can take them up and use them as raw ingredients for proteins.

- The liver can make glucose out of them for energy purposes, in a process called *gluconeogenesis.*

- They can also be stored, after conversion by the liver to glucose or lipids, as glycogen (i.e., muscle fuel) or fat.

> *Yes, both excess carbs and excess protein in the diet can be stored as excess fat.*

Proteins that are already in the cells (not coming in as part of your food) are constantly being degraded or split up into their constituent amino acids and resynthesized into new proteins the body needs. It's a very complicated and ingenious metabolic process by which the liver finds so many different uses for proteins and amino acids, but one of the important elements of the sequence is that when the liver has to metabolize amino acids (in order to make glucose out of them, for example), the organ breaks down the amino acids into ammonia, which is converted to urea and excreted out via the kidneys in the urine.

> *Ammonia is toxic when it builds up in the blood, which makes the excretion of urea throughout the day so important. The rate at which this conversion takes place in the liver is limited, which is why the body cannot tolerate unlimited amounts of protein, as in "rabbit starvation syndrome."[18]*

Cells can take up the amino acids for their own use, such as new protein synthesis by muscle cells.

> *An iPhone and Android app exists for amino acid aficionados, appropriately called Amino Acid Reference.*

If you aim for optimal health, you need to get all of the essential amino acids in high enough quantities from your diet. Meat and fish eaters have an easier time of it than vegetarians, for instance, because these meat constituents are generally complete proteins—they have all of the essential amino acids in greater than trace amounts. Eggs are a great source of essential amino acids for vegetarians (eat copious amounts of pastured eggs), as is the occasional whey protein shake (see Chapter 10 for more details on sports nutrition).

FERMENTED SOY AS A SMALL PROTEIN SOURCE

Ever tried tempeh, miso, or natto? If you're Asian, Indonesian, or a vegetarian/vegan, your answer will probably be "Yes." These are fermented soy products: the first originated in Indonesia, and the last two are well-known Japanese foods. They are part of a long lineage of traditional Eastern foods that consist of soy-based protein that is fermented; this removes most of soy's nasty antinutrients, which prevent the absorption of minerals and protein (see the "Antinutrients" section in Chapter 4). Natto's a really good source of vitamin K. These are also decent soy-based protein sources, albeit in small amounts.

You get the protein, without the meat fats, if you so desire. I've been adding tempeh to my salads, and liking it. It has the consistency of a softer cheese, and tastes a bit like bland meat. It'll soak up sauces and dressing if you add it to salads or soups (miso is often made into a soup, such as at Japanese and Thai restaurants).

So how does tempeh look, for example, as a protein source? It's a complete source of protein, about 5 grams in a 28-gram serving. Tempeh is actually a high-fat food when you come right down to it, having a macronutrient ratio of 20 percent carbs-47 percent fat-33 percent protein (now that you're an expert on MRs!). Four ounces, or about 112 grams, of tempeh contains a lot of Omega 6 fat and has a poor n-6:n-3 ratio of more than 10 to 1. It's a decent source of vitamins and minerals.[19]

Natto has a similar profile, but is more nutritious in terms of vitamins/minerals and has an almost equal amount of protein compared with tempeh, with the same problem of an unfavorable Omega 6 to 3 ratio (in the form that must be converted, unfortunately at a low rate, to the long chain versions that our bodies really need).[20]

To show you how to analyze food for its protein quality, we'll do a quick check of lamb, salmon, and bananas with NutritionData. This searchable web database for nutrition information has a good section on its result pages for protein. Figure 3-7 shows the page for a small slab of cooked lamb, which the site gives a good protein score (anything over 100 is a complete protein).

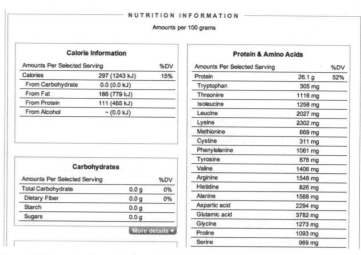

NUTRITION INFORMATION

Amounts per 100 grams

Calorie Information

Amounts Per Selected Serving		%DV
Calories	297 (1243 kJ)	15%
From Carbohydrate	0.0 (0.0 kJ)	
From Fat	186 (779 kJ)	
From Protein	111 (465 kJ)	
From Alcohol	~ (0.0 kJ)	

Carbohydrates

Amounts Per Selected Serving		%DV
Total Carbohydrate	0.0 g	0%
Dietary Fiber	0.0 g	0%
Starch	0.0 g	
Sugars	0.0 g	

More details ▾

Protein & Amino Acids

Amounts Per Selected Serving		%DV
Protein	26.1 g	52%
Tryptophan	305 mg	
Threonine	1116 mg	
Isoleucine	1258 mg	
Leucine	2027 mg	
Lysine	2302 mg	
Methionine	669 mg	
Cystine	311 mg	
Phenylalanine	1061 mg	
Tyrosine	876 mg	
Valine	1406 mg	
Arginine	1548 mg	
Histidine	826 mg	
Alanine	1568 mg	
Aspartic acid	2294 mg	
Glutamic acid	3782 mg	
Glycine	1273 mg	
Proline	1093 mg	
Serine	969 mg	

Figure 3-7. *Lamb gets a good protein score*

Many of the amino acids are in lamb in a quantity in excess of a gram, and the four ounce piece of meat has 26 grams of protein, a bit less than a quarter of what a training athlete would need in a day. *Salmon is also an excellent source of amino acids*, as Figure 3-8 shows. A six ounce filet has about 40 grams of protein, with more than 3 grams of the important muscle-building amino acid *leucine*. It also has more than 300 mg of *tryptophan*, an important biochemical precursor in the synthesis of the neurotransmitter serotonin, as well as the hormone melatonin.

> *Tryptophan in food may help make you sleepy before bedtime, because serotonin has a calming effect, and melatonin is a hormone that plays a role in sleep regulation.*

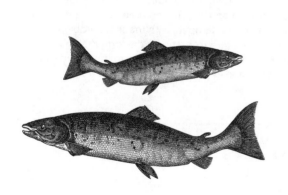

NUTRITION INFORMATION

Amounts per 1/2 filet (154g)

Calorie Information

Amounts Per Selected Serving		%DV
Calories	356 (1491 kJ)	18%
From Carbohydrate	0.8 (3.3 kJ)	
From Fat	186 (779 kJ)	
From Protein	169 (708 kJ)	
From Alcohol	~ (0.0 kJ)	

Carbohydrates

Amounts Per Selected Serving		%DV
Total Carbohydrate	0.0 g	0%
Dietary Fiber	0.0 g	0%
Starch	0.0 g	
Sugars	0.0 g	

Protein & Amino Acids

Amounts Per Selected Serving		%DV
Protein	39.6 g	79%
Tryptophan	444 mg	
Threonine	1736 mg	
Isoleucine	1825 mg	
Leucine	3218 mg	
Lysine	3637 mg	
Methionine	1172 mg	
Cystine	425 mg	
Phenylalanine	1546 mg	
Tyrosine	1337 mg	
Valine	2041 mg	
Arginine	2370 mg	
Histidine	1166 mg	
Alanine	2395 mg	
Aspartic acid	4057 mg	
Glutamic acid	5911 mg	
Glycine	1900 mg	

Figure 3-8. *A salmon filet cleans up with essential amino acids*

The absorption during digestion of amino acids is quite slow—anywhere from 3 to around 10 grams per hour (that's only 12 to 40 calories per hour), depending on how much you weigh and whether the protein has a fast (whey protein) or slower (raw eggs) absorption rate—compared with fats (about 14 grams per hour) and carbs (60 to 100 grams per hour, in terms of a glucose drink). So, if you eat 40 grams of protein, your body may take about eight hours to absorb and utilize the amino acids.[21]

Just for the sake of comparison, let's check out the amino acid content of a starch: bananas. A banana actually contains all the amino acids, but in very small amounts: less than 100 mg each (a large banana, after all, provides just 1.5 grams of protein). As shown in Figure 3-9, though, the banana scores more than 30 grams of carbs, including over 6 grams of glucose and fructose, and even a little maltose.

Calorie Information

Amounts Per Selected Serving		%DV
Calories	121 (507 kJ)	6%
From Carbohydrate	112 (469 kJ)	
From Fat	3.8 (15.9 kJ)	
From Protein	5.0 (20.9 kJ)	
From Alcohol	0.0 (0.0 kJ)	

Carbohydrates

Amounts Per Selected Serving		%DV
Total Carbohydrate	31.1 g	10%
Dietary Fiber	3.5 g	14%
Starch	7.3 g	
Sugars	16.6 g	
Sucrose	3250 mg	
Glucose	6772 mg	
Fructose	6596 mg	
Lactose	0.0 mg	
Maltose	13.6 mg	
Galactose	0.0 mg	

Collapse ▲

Fats & Fatty Acids

Amounts Per Selected Serving		%DV
Total Fat	0.4 g	1%
Saturated Fat	0.2 g	1%
Monounsaturated Fat	0.0 g	
Polyunsaturated Fat	0.1 g	
Total trans fatty acids	~	
Total trans-monoenoic fatty acids	~	
Total trans-polyenoic fatty acids	~	
Total Omega-3 fatty acids	36.7 mg	

Protein & Amino Acids

Amounts Per Selected Serving		%DV
Protein	1.5 g	3%
Tryptophan	12.2 mg	
Threonine	38.1 mg	
Isoleucine	38.1 mg	
Leucine	92.5 mg	
Lysine	68.0 mg	
Methionine	10.9 mg	
Cystine	12.2 mg	
Phenylalanine	66.6 mg	
Tyrosine	12.2 mg	
Valine	63.9 mg	
Arginine	66.6 mg	
Histidine	105 mg	
Alanine	54.4 mg	
Aspartic acid	169 mg	
Glutamic acid	207 mg	
Glycine	51.7 mg	
Proline	38.1 mg	
Serine	54.4 mg	
Hydroxyproline	~	

Collapse ▲

Vitamins

Amounts Per Selected Serving		%DV
Vitamin A	87.0 IU	2%
Vitamin C	11.8 mg	20%
Vitamin D	~	~
Vitamin E (Alpha Tocopherol)	0.1 mg	1%
Vitamin K	0.7 mcg	1%
Thiamin	0.0 mg	3%
Riboflavin	0.1 mg	6%
Niacin	0.9 mg	5%
Vitamin B6	0.5 mg	25%
Folate	27.2 mcg	7%

Figure 3-9. *A large banana chalks up the carbs on NutritionData*

A medium-sized sweet potato has 1/10th the glucose and fructose of a large banana. A banana is a good source of potassium, however, so that's the trade-off.

Fats

Fats, or *fatty acids*, are an important macronutrient both for food intake and as a source of energy when you are *not* eating and generating energy from your own stored tissue. Fats are also important because they contain fat-soluble vitamins such as A, D, E, and K, as well as other nutrients.

> *I use the mnemonic device "a deck of cards" to remember the vitamins in fats: ADEK, or "a deck." Not bad, huh?*

Many fat-containing foods also contain protein and/or carbs; in fact, it's quite common to get all three macronutrients in your food.

We get our fats from a variety of foods, including dairy (e.g., butter, whole milk, cheese), veggies like avocados and olives, meat, fish, nuts, coconut oil, nut butters, and oils (olive, peanut, coconut, etc.). Later in the chapter, we'll take a closer look at the fat content of certain foods using our trusty NutritionData tool.

The form in which fats are both stored and eaten is called a *triglyceride*. This is an E-shaped molecule with a glycerol backbone attached to three fatty acids, as Figure 3-10 depicts.

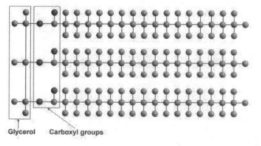

Figure 3-10. *A triglyceride molecule (source: http://www.reducetriglcerides.com/reader_triglyceride_molecules.htm)*

> *The body also contains fats in the form of phospholipids in cell membranes, cholesterol (which is crucial for synthesizing steroid hormones and making vitamin D in the skin), and other less substantial forms, but the vast majority of fat is stored in lipocytes, or fat cells, in the body's fat depots such as adipose tissue and muscles.*

Each one of the three fatty acids in a triglyceride is a hydrocarbon chain (often just described as a chain of carbon atoms) that is liberated at digestion and eventually released to the bloodstream. In other words, after you consume an animal or a plant fat (veggies also contain fats!), the simplified version is this: an enzyme called *pancreatic lipase* splits up the triglyceride into separate molecules, including the three fatty acids, so that they can be absorbed in the small intestine (a triglyceride cannot be absorbed in its present bulky state).

When the body stores fats, they are reassembled into triglycerides, and when you metabolize fats for energy, they are split up (yet again, just as in digestion) and are transported by proteins in the form of free fatty acids (FFAs) in the blood. Somewhat similar to the other macronutrients, the FFAs are the Lego pieces that can be fit together into the triglyceride structures, along with the glycerol molecule. Figure 3-11 shows an FFA called lauric acid, a shorter-chain fat with 12 carbons in its chain.

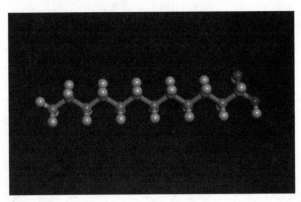

Figure 3-11. *Coconut milk and human breast milk contain lauric acid (source: http://www. worldofmolecules.com)*

The body can store fats in a waterless environment, and therefore they are a more efficient, lightweight storage medium for a human's onboard energy. We each store about 100,000 calories' worth of fat. Carbohydrates have an affinity for water, on the other hand, and therefore weigh more, including the water, as stored glycogen. It would take about 67 pounds of stored glycogen to represent the equivalent energy of 10 pounds of stored fat![22] This must be one of the reasons that we only store about 1,200 to 2,000 calories' worth of glycogen, our own starch.

Free fatty acids have common names like lauric or stearic acid, along with a numbered symbolic notation, such as 12:0. This means that lauric acid, a saturated fat, has 12 carbon atoms and 0 double bonds along its chain. Before your eyes glaze over with this reminder of geeky Mr. Taylor's Chem 101 class back in Wichita Falls, realize that the length of a fatty acid chain is always even, and represents a good geek detail for understanding fat nutrition. We promise!

SatFats vs. PolyFats

A saturated fat (satFat, my abbreviation) is a molecule that has a straight, noncurvy orientation (without the "kinks" or double bonds of the other fats). This orientation allows the satFats to fit together snugly and remain solid at room temperature (like cheese, or butter, before they get moldy and rancid!).

On the other hand, a *polyunsaturated* fat (polyFat) has more than one double bond along its carbon chain (which is where the *poly* prefix comes from). This creates a bend, or kink, in the molecule. That structural aspect keeps polyFats liquid at room temperature.

A polyunsaturated fat that is much discussed for its health benefits, an Omega 3, is called eicosapentaenoic acid (EPA).

Forget it, don't even try to pronounce it.

EPA has a notation that looks like 20:5, n-3, indicating that this fatty acid has 20 carbon atoms and 5 double bonds, and that the first double bond is located three carbons in from the Omega end of the chain (i.e., at the end of the "toes" of the E-shaped structure, rather than at the location where the fatty acid chains connect with the glycerol molecule).

Only a food chemist really wants to practice memorizing these complicated notations. You can impress your friends, however, by calmly explaining to them the difference between saturated and polyunsaturated fat; one's kinky!

A *monounsaturated* fat (monoFat), like the oleic acid in olive oil, has only one double bond in the molecule.

Eating Fat

To sum up, the various fats in your food arrive in the form of saturated, monounsaturated, or polyunsaturated fats, and often a mixture of all three of these substances.

Olive oil, which you can use in your homemade salad dressing, contains the following types of fats: monoFats (about 75 percent); satFats (about 14 percent), and polyFats (about 11 percent).[23] Olive oil's principal monounsaturated fatty acid is an 18-carbon chain fat called *oleic acid*.

Olive oil is a liquid at room temperature. The higher the number of double bonds in the fat's chemistry, the more likely it will be a liquid at room temperature. Animal fats tend to contain more monounsaturated (one double bond) and saturated fats, and thus tend to be solid at room temp. Vegetable oils, true to their name, are only usually liquid at room temp and contain more polyunsaturated fats.[24]

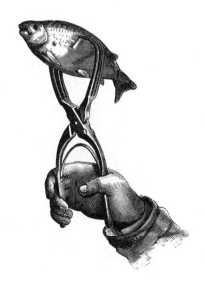

The health advice for eating fat can be summed up this way: eat a reasonable amount of monounsaturated fats, as in olive oils, avocados, and macadamia nuts, as well as fish and many meats, and try to even out the ratio between Omega 6 fats and Omega 3s (subsets of the polyFat; see the "Omega 6 vs. Omega 3 Fat Ratio" section).

Saturated fats have recently had the air let out of their tires as the demon of your diet (see the "Saturated Fat Has Some of the Air Let Out of Its Tires" sidebar on related scientific studies and opinions), so we don't have to be so phobic about them. They might even have anti-inflammatory effects for some people, particularly if you've replaced a lot of simple carbs or sugars with them.

Coconut milk is fine, as are high-quality cheeses and grass-fed meats, and the satFats you get in the small chunks of the 100-percent high-cacao chocolate I eat (addictively) are acceptable and healthy additions to the diet.

Figure 3-12 shows all the other fats (some in trace amounts) that olive oil contains, from the handy NutritionData tool. A teaspoon of olive oil is 100 percent fat by calories, with 5 grams totaling about 45 calories (9 calories per gram, because it's a fat!).

This is how you can find out the fat content of your food: do a search at NutritionData, then scroll down to the boxed area reserved for Fats & Fatty Acids. This shows that a teaspoon of olive oil also contains almost half a gram (439 mg) of linoleic acid, or Omega 6 fats, a subset of polyFats. There's the oleic acid: "18:1 undifferentiated"—more than three grams of it.

I told you those fat notations could get pretty geeky!

Rather than just a teaspoon of oil, let's analyze the fat content of typical fare for an American Friday night: a large pizza slice with pepperoni. The dish sounds delectable, but, like all of life's vicissitudes, that dinner's nutritional profile is likely to be a mixture of joy and regret.

Fats & Fatty Acids		
Amounts Per Selected Serving		%DV
Total Fat	4.5g	7%
Saturated Fat	0.6g	3%
4:00	0.0mg	
6:00	0.0mg	
8:00	0.0mg	
10:00	0.0mg	
12:00	0.0mg	
13:00	~	
14:00	0.0mg	
15:00	~	
16:00	508mg	
17:00	1.0mg	
18:00	87.9mg	
19:00	~	
20:00	18.6mg	
22:00	5.8mg	
24:00:00	0.0mg	
Monounsaturated Fat	3.3g	
14:01	0.0mg	
15:01	~	
16:1 undifferentiated	56.5mg	
16:1 c	~	
16:1 t	~	
17:01	5.6mg	
18:1 undifferentiated	3207mg	
18:1 c	~	
18:1 t	~	
20:01	14.0mg	
22:1 undifferentiated	0.0mg	
22:1 c	~	
22:1 t	~	
24:1 c	~	
Polyunsaturated Fat	0.5g	
16:2 undifferentiated	~	
18:2 undifferentiated	439mg	
18:2 n-6 c,c	~	
18:2 c,t	~	
18:2 t,c	~	
18:2 t,t	~	
18:2 i	~	
18:2 t not further defined	~	
18:03	34.2mg	
18:3 n-3, c,c,c	~	
18:3 n-6, c,c,c	~	
18:4 undifferentiated	0.0mg	
20:2 n-6 c,c	~	
20:3 undifferentiated	~	

Figure 3-12. *For olive oil, mostly monounsaturated fat, Omega 6, and palmitic acid, a saturated fatty acid*

HOW DOES THE "PALEO" DIET MEASURE UP?

There's been an explosion of Romantic Primitivism in Western culture. It must have something to do with how moribund the so-called benefits of modern civilization have become (you can only spend so much time in cubicles staring at screens with cell phones plastered to your ear).

Just look at how popular escapist journeys into the backcountry or the outback and Burning Man have become. Every region now boasts multiple weekend races where the participants are required to mimic the opening scene of the film *Gladiator*, beating their bare chests, shaking toy spears, and sprinting off with war cries into the woods. The nutrition counterpart of this Spartan movement is the Paleolithic, or Paleo, diet, which is making a comeback after about 50,000 years.

The Paleo diet is a delicious combination of meats, fish, veggies (e.g., tubers like sweet potatoes), fruits (mostly of the berry kind), nuts, and "offal" (not awful!), as in bone marrow and liver pate. I had a bison heart recently from the Full Circle Bison Ranch in southern Oregon; it was delicious and nutritious (marinated in balsamic vinegar and spices, then baked for a while on a low temperature). Many people, like myself, add dairy to Paleo, as in whole milk, cheese, and eggs (the real Paleo diet most likely included bird's eggs, but certainly no cheese or cow's or goat's milk).

The Paleo diet has measured up quite well lately in the few studies that have compared it with other dietary regimens, according to a 2010 journal wrap-up.[25] Here are a few quotes from the article:

A randomized controlled trial of 29 patients with ischemic heart disease and either glucose intolerance or [Type 2 Diabetes Mellitus] (T2DM) were randomized to 12 weeks of a Paleolithic (i.e., lean meat, fish, fruit, vegetables, root vegetables, eggs, and nuts) or a Mediterranean-like Consensus diet based on whole grains, low-fat dairy products, vegetables, fruits, fish, oils, and margarines. The Paleolithic group showed an improved glucose control and a greater decrease in waist circumference when compared with the Consensus group.

Fifteen patients with T2DM were randomized to either a Paleolithic diet or a diabetes diet and then crossed over after 3 months. Patients were on each diet for 3 months. Compared with the diabetes diet, the Paleolithic diet produced lower mean levels of hemoglobin A1c, triacylglycerol, diastolic blood pressure (BP), weight, body mass index (BMI), as well as waist circumference and higher mean serum high-density lipoprotein levels.

Whether the Paleolithic diet will become a suitable prescriptive alternative remains to be determined by more extensive studies on a larger number of participants.

Lively discussions of the Paleo diet and its practitioners can be found on *www.paleohacks.com* and other websites.

It wouldn't be fair if we didn't indicate the whole lineup of macronutrients, including protein and carbs. Figure 3-13 from NutritionData shows the Fats & Fatty Acids results for a 14-inch pizza slice with pepperoni topping.

The pizza slice includes 12.1 grams of fats, or 109 calories, which happens to be 37 percent of the total 298 kcal.

This is pretty high in calories for just one pizza slice. Multiple slices would obviously be a very energy-dense meal. Better be climbing a mountain the next morning, or better yet, back off from the slices and eat some blueberries.

Fats & Fatty Acids

Amounts Per Selected Serving		%DV
Total Fat	12.1 g	19%
Saturated Fat	5.3 g	26%
Monounsaturated Fat	3.7 g	
Polyunsaturated Fat	2.2 g	
Total trans fatty acids	~	
Total trans-monoenoic fatty acids	~	
Total trans-polyenoic fatty acids	~	
Total Omega-3 fatty acids	188 mg	
Total Omega-6 fatty acids	1749 mg	

Learn more about these fatty acids and their equivalent names

More details ▾

Figure 3-13. *The fatty acid lineup for a slice o' pepperoni*

The macronutrient ratio, the whole shebang, for the pizza slice is 46 percent carbs-37 percent fats-17 percent protein. You can assume that the vast majority of the carbs (and thus up to half of all the calories) came from the refined flour of the pizza crust. See the "Now for Something Completely Different on the Crust Front" sidebar for a recipe involving an alternative crust.

NOW FOR SOMETHING COMPLETELY DIFFERENT ON THE CRUST FRONT

What follows is a recipe for pizza crust for when you want a break from the grains, wheat, and refined flour, but you still want to pile the fixings onto your pizza slices (recipe courtesy of *www.girlgoneprimal.com*).

1 large head of cauliflower

2 cups cheese (mozzarella, cheddar, or a combo of both)

2 eggs

Optional herbs (thyme, fennel, oregano, basil & parsley all work wonderfully)

Method:

Preheat oven to 200 degrees Celsius. Line pan or pizza stone with baking paper.

Rice the cauliflower by putting florets into a food processor and buzzing until finely processed (but not mushy). Place cauliflower into a microwave-safe bowl and zap for 6-8 minutes. You should end up with about two cups of riced cauliflower.

Mix in cheese and eggs until smooth. Spread evenly over baking paper in a round shape. Sprinkle with herbs. Place in oven until golden on top and starting to crisp around the edges (around 15 minutes in my oven).

Remove from oven and add desired toppings. I used sliced tomato, sliced capsicum, mozzarella and parmesan cheese, mushrooms, and some meat (I only had salami). I choose to sprinkle cheese on the base, with the toppings rather than placing it between the base and the toppings (as directed in the original recipe). The cheese in the base helps keep the topping in place and connected to the base.

Place completed pizza back in the oven until the cheese melts and toppings are cooked to your preference. Cut and serve while hot. Also delicious reheated.

You can see that the pizza slice contains all three fatty-acid classifications. About 44 percent of the fats come from saturated fats (we can reasonably assume a lot of that comes from the cheese, since mozzarella cheese, for example, is about 58 percent saturated fat).

The saturated fat isn't necessarily bad (five grams or so, almost matched by a similar amount of monounsaturated fat) from a health standpoint, compared with the refined carbohydrate represented by the pizza crust.

Oh no, here it comes again, some glum preachy advice about not eating too much pizza! I'm imitating my son here, who's heard enough from me about nutrition. He calls me, with a derisive tone, "Mr. Healthy Guy."

The crust might contribute to the fat gains brought on by excessive energy-dense foods. Just ease up on it, do yourself a favor.

SATURATED FAT HAS SOME OF THE AIR LET OUT OF ITS TIRES

When I was a young tyke soccer player, I used to eat bacon and eggs for breakfast. Then, the night before a game, my mother would make me a steak, and I used to eat the fat because it tasted good. Then I used to go out onto the field and run everyone's butts off (and occasionally get my own tail kicked)—in other words, the ingredients for that training table seemed to work. I guess we're supposed to conclude that I was dying of heart disease, then? Too much saturated fat in the eggs and steak?

Many of us have grown up with public-health guidelines that say to avoid saturated fats at all costs. Eat it, get a heart attack. Yet, it's very easy these days to find dissenting or at least moderating opinions, including among health and nutrition experts.

At the very least, you need fats to absorb fat-soluble vitamins: A, D, E, and K ("a deck of cards—ADEK"). And fats, including saturated, can be anti-inflammatory for some people, particularly if they replace more inflammatory foods.

The American Journal of Clinical Nutrition published a study in March 2010 that cast doubt on whether the consumption of saturated fats is a serious risk factor for cardiovascular disease. Led by Dr. Ronald Krause of the Children's Hospital Oakland Research Institute, Oakland, CA, the meta-analysis reviewed the results of 21 studies.

The review concluded that "there is insufficient evidence… that dietary saturated fat is associated with an increased risk of CHD, stroke, or CVD [cardiovascular disease]." The full review is available at *www.ajcn.org/content/91/3/535.full*.

In a related opinion piece published in the same journal online in January 2010, the authors wrote:

The evidence that supports a reduction in saturated fat intake must be evaluated in the context of replacement by other macronutrients. Clinical trials that replaced saturated fat with polyunsaturated fat have generally shown a reduction in CVD events, although several studies showed no effects.

An independent association of saturated fat intake with CVD risk has not been consistently shown in prospective epidemiologic studies, although some have provided evidence of an increased risk in young individuals and in women. Replacement of saturated fat by polyunsaturated or monounsaturated fat lowers both LDL and HDL cholesterol.

However, replacement with a higher carbohydrate intake, particularly refined carbohydrate, can exacerbate the atherogenic dyslipidemia associated with insulin resistance and obesity that includes increased triglycerides, small LDL particles, and reduced HDL cholesterol.

In summary, although substitution of dietary polyunsaturated fat for saturated fat has been shown to lower CVD risk, there are few epidemiologic or clinical trial data to support a benefit of replacing saturated fat with carbohydrate.

See the related *Scientific American* article at *www.scientificamerican.com/article.cfm?id=carbs-against-cardio* and the opinion article itself at: *www.ajcn.org/content/91/3/502.full*.

Omega 6 vs. Omega 3 Fat Ratio

Apparently, another piece of dietary-fat data to pay attention to is the ratio of Omega 6 to Omega 3 essential fatty acids. Here, with the pizza slice, it is 1,749 mg to 188 mg, or about nine to one in favor of Omega 6. So what are Omega 3 and 6 fats, and why should you care about them?

Omega 3 and 6 fats are subsets of the polyunsaturated fats. They, in turn, are super-categories for a number of different Omega 3s and 6s, each with their own technical names. The two groups of fats are often referred to by the position of the first double bond in their molecules: n-3 and n-6.

The first revealed essential fatty acids were called vitamin F until scientists decided, "Hey, they're not really vitamins, they're macronutrients—fats."

Both n-3s and n-6s play a number of important roles in the body, including the provision of the raw ingredients for the biochemicals of the immune system called *prostaglandins*.[26] Both fatty acids are used in the body's cell membranes, and n-3s are particularly important for the developing brains of youngsters and babies, as well as the aging brains of us old coots.

We have to eat these essential Omegas because the body does not have the wherewithal to synthesize their long-chain versions, such as EPA (the unpronounceable one) and DHA (another n-3 fat), as well as arachidonic acid, an n-6. Two food chemicals in our diets that are raw materials or precursors for these essential fatty acids are the shorter-chain fats linoleic acid, an n-6 fat, and alpha-linolenic acid (ALA), an n-3, or Omega 3 fat.

Bump up those n-3s

A biochemical the body needs called arachidonic acid is synthesized from linoleic acid (the n-6) using enzymes. Linoleic acid competes for the same enzymes that help make EPA and DHA (the two downstream n-3s our bodies require) from ALA.

Too much n-6 in the diet, for example, will tend to ramp *down* the production of the important EPA/DHA Omega3 nutrients, because they compete for the same enzymes. And thus the Omega 3s don't make their way into cell membranes, brain matter, and other places where they do good work.

The western SAD diet contains too high a proportion of Omega 6 fats. It is easier to get n-6 fats than n-3s, particularly if you consume a lot of polyunsaturated vegetable oils like corn, soy, or safflower oil (as in, things that are cooked in those oils), which are rich n-6 sources.

A number of otherwise healthy foods, like eggs (15 to 1 ratio of n-6 to n-3; a pastured egg will have higher amounts of n-3s though), avocados (15 to 1; but you don't want to stop eating avocados and lose all that healthy monounsaturated fat), almonds (2,000 to 1, more than three grams n-6; but a very good source of vitamins, minerals, and phytochemicals), and walnuts (4 to 1, with most of the n-3 in the form of ALA), have unfavorable n-6 to n-3 ratios.

Nutrition is often a trade-off between benefits, drawbacks, and uncertainties involving the synergies of certain foods with others on the same plate. This is why it's sensible to vary the types of food you eat, so you can attenuate or "hack out" any mistakes or imperfections in food choices. E.g., you don't have to stop eating nuts like almonds or macadamias, but make sure that you are getting good sources of n-3s.

Our genes are selected for closer to 1:1

Scientists have posed a theory that humans are genetically programmed for an Omega 6 to Omega 3 ratio of closer to 1:1. This is based on the different composition of foods that our wild-eating Paleolithic forebears chowed down on (like seafood), as well as what they *didn't* eat, like Burger King french fries and salad dressing made out of soy oil.

> *The french fries have an n-6 to n-3 ratio of about 30 to 1, but at least equally bad are the six grams of the Franken-lipid trans fatty acids, which you should never eat.[27]*

"Studies on the evolutionary aspects of diet indicate that major changes have taken place in our diet, particularly in the type and amount of essential fatty acids and in the antioxidant content of foods," writes Dr. Artemis P. Simopoulos in the *Asia Pacific Journal of Clinical Nutrition*. "It has been estimated that the present Western diet is 'deficient' in Omega-3 fatty acids with a ratio of Omega 6 to Omega 3 of 15-20/1, instead of 1/1 as is the case with wild animals and presumably human beings."

> *An Omega 6 called conjugated linoleic acid, or CLA, appears to be pretty good for us. You can find it in grass-fed beef and pastured or free-range eggs, for example. See www.eatwild.com/healthbenefits. htm and any CLA search on Google Scholar, such as http://scholar. google.com/scholar?q=conjugated+linoleic+acid&hl=en&btnG=Sear ch&as_sdt=1%2C46&as_sdtp=on.*

Omega 6 fats tend to be more inflammatory when overconsumed, and Omega 3 fats are anti-inflammatory in nature. So how do you help correct your own ratio so it falls more on the Omega 3 side? *Eat rich sources of Omega 3 fats (including EPA/DHA) like seafood and shellfish* every few days: salmon, arctic char, herring, sardines, tuna, mussels, mackerel, oysters, halibut, crab, and shrimp.

Legitimately pastured eggs and meats are richer sources of Omega 3 than their industrially produced counterparts, but some of these foods can also be somewhat high in Omega 6 fats (e.g., even grass-fed beef has an n-6 to n-3 ratio of 4 or 5 to 1).

You can get lots of servings of small but significant amounts of n-3 fats such as ALA from fresh veggies like broccoli (92 mg and a 4 to 1 ratio of n-3 to n-6). Even fruits like bananas and blueberries have small amounts of ALA. The conversion rate by the body of ALA to EPA and DHA (the building of a shorter-chain n-3 into a longer-chain one), however, is quite low: in men, as low as 8 percent of ALA is converted to EPA and 4 percent to DHA.

Nutrition is often a trade-off between benefits, drawbacks, and uncertainties involving the synergies of certain foods with others on the same plate.

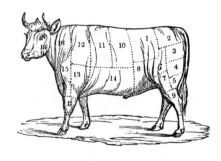

Chapter 3

This means that if you eat eight grams of ALA, it converts into far less than a gram of EPA or DHA, the forms your body really needs. The conversion rate is higher in women, according to the Linus Pauling Institute's description.[28]

> *A tablespoon of caviar, or fish roe, wouldn't you know it, is good for you, if not your wallet. It's a good source of minerals and vitamin B12 and has more than a gram of Omega 3 fatty acids, with about an 80 to 1 ratio of n-3 to n-6 essential fatty acids. So if you run into a Russian fellow who wants to gift you his caviar container for that extra ticket to the Knicks game...[29]*

It also helps to cut back on foods and oils that are rich in Omega 6, because as we mentioned, they are ubiquitous in the Western diet. Here's a tiny but telling example: a small portion of wheat crackers, like the amount that I used to routinely eat (14 of them) contains almost a gram of Omega 6 because they're cooked in a vegetable oil like soy oil; they have an n-6 to n-3 ratio of about 19 to 1.[30]

You have to watch out for nuts, too, and their Omega 6 content. A small portion of macadamia nuts, however, has healthy monounsaturated fats and a 5 or 6 to 1 n-6 to n-3 ratio—not too bad a trade-off.

The foods richest in Omega 6, according to NutritionData, are various vegetable oils (sunflower, safflower, grapeseed, soy), various types of mayonnaise (hold the mayo!), sunflower seeds, and fast-food sauces such as "creamy ranch" and "spicy buffalo."

Health Hack: Testing for Omega 3

You can actually test the Omega 3 content of your body fat, as another health hack. The tests examine the fat content of the cell membranes of red blood cells for its percentage of EPA and DHA. These cells turn over in the body every three to four months, so the tests are designed to determine your recent n-6 and n-3 consumption. There are commercial testers such as OmegaQuant or GeneSmart, or you could just ask your doctor to order the test.

Although potentially interesting, this is a very minor element of biomarker testing (I'll probably indulge in this test one day anyway). It would be pretty meaningless unless you'd taken care of the major fitness issues first, like body weight, cutting back on refined sugar, inflammation, and a solid exercise program. Most of the time, just upping your fish intake and backing off of industrial vegetable oils will give you the most bang for your buck in this arena.

Ketones

We'll conclude with a brief discussion of ketones, or ketone bodies, simply because they are elements of nutrition (particularly lower-carb approaches) and fasting that many people are curious, or simply bewildered, about these days. Ketones are also involved in fat metabolism.

The body has three nutrient pools that it calls upon to fuel itself: fats, carbs, and proteins, roughly in that order of magnitude. The heart and skeletal muscles don't at all mind using fat for metabolic fuel; these are the free fatty acids that are liberated from our fat stores (triglycerides) or provided by the fats on our plate. At rest, our brains are usually hogging most of our glucose (they use up to 20 percent of our total energy).

The mitochondria—the little power plants inside our cells, such as the skeletal muscle and heart muscle cells—can readily metabolize stored or dietary fat to produce our body's energy. When resting, such as when we are sitting in a chair or sleeping, about 70 percent of our metabolic energy comes from burning fat. We appear to be *designed* for fat burning, given that fat represents the vast majority of our stored energy and is what we're mostly burning when we're not eating (in the "absorptive state") or in a high-speed cycle or road race.

> *Our fat-metabolic machinery apparently cannot keep up with the high oxygen requirements of speedy endurance exercise (such as when hammering along at heart rates of 140 beats per minute or more)—otherwise, racers wouldn't need "GUs" and PowerBars (basically concentrated sources of glucose) to keep them from bonking during marathons and triathlons. See Chapter 10 for the skinny on sports nutrition.*

When you're taking part in an intermittent fast or are otherwise low on carbs (i.e., fasts of less than a day, very low-carb diets, and particularly during starvation), the liver reaches a fork in the road along its metabolic pathway for generating energy from fats. A chemical in the metabolic pathway called acetyl-COA builds up in the absence of another chemical that would usually be present in enough quantity if more carbs were around.[31]

The liver then generates another fuel source called *ketones*, out of the acetyl-COA. The ketones enter the energy mix along with the fatty acids and the glucose made from the amino acids harvested from muscles (*gluconeogenesis*).

Ketones are an ancient biochemical among living things, a common energy substrate (babies are apparently born metabolizing a lot of ketones to keep things going, as their proportionately huge brains use 60 percent or more of their fuel). Ketones actually provide more calories per gram than glucose (about 4.76 calories per gram compared with glucose's 4 per gram).[32]

At rest, our brains are usually hogging most of our glucose.

The heart and brain can utilize ketones for energy, and as at least one scientific study indicated, the heart uses energy more efficiently on them.[33]

A number of researchers and doctors have theorized that our bodies have evolved this ketone-utilizing pathway to preserve muscle and continue to fuel the brain during extreme swings of food availability and scarcity (if ketones are being burned, less muscle, which is necessary for moving your body around and surviving, has to be squandered making glucose out of amino acids).[34]

"Fats are metabolized to ketone bodies, which replace glucose as a major fuel for the brain," explained Dr. Thomas Seyfried, a professor at Boston College who has implemented studies of ketogenic diets, and who was interviewed for Chapter 6, our fasting chapter. "Ketone body metabolism reduces inflammation and enhances [the] metabolic efficiency of most cells."

The next time I pick up some kind of virus, you can bet that I'm going to try to fast it out of me—have a lengthy tea fast, for example. Not that getting sick is the only reason to fast. My body will start burning ketones at a certain point for energy, and as long as the fast is working, this is not a development I'm particularly going to mind.

Micronutrients:
Vitamins, Minerals, and Phytochemicals

4

Tiny components can have huge effects. Even if you're not a weather scientist who embraces Chaos Theory (the flutter of a butterfly's wings in Mexico changes weather patterns in America), you know a computer chip the size of a fingertip can contain millions of invisible gates, and the loss of that chip means that the seven-million-pixel Photoshop montage you've been working on for that DVD cover just vanished forever.

The Nutrient That Roared

A seemingly innocuous glitch can bring down software programs comprising hundreds of thousands of code lines. Ever heard of that impossible-to-find "divide by zero" bug? Just because something is small doesn't mean that its influence isn't *giant*. Such is the case with the micronutrients in our diet.

"Vitamins schmitamins," you might say.

All you have to know is that the continuous deprivation of really tiny amounts of vitamins B1 (thiamine) and B3 (niacin) can give you nasty, potentially fatal diseases called beriberi and pellagra, respectively. These diseases have been very common throughout human history.[1] And these vitamins are recommended only in the *micrograms* per day.[2]

If your dinner was a beach, the B vitamins would be a palmful of sand.

Apples vs. Twinkies

What about vitamin C, which has been urged upon you ever since that apple banged around in active competition with the Twinkie inside your lunchbox?

According to a 2004 study that tested thousands of Americans for their health status, up to 3 in 10 Americans have either a deficient (about 7 percent of them) or marginal vitamin C status, meaning that if the C starvation continues, they could be a few months away from real scurvy symptoms[3] (see the sidebar "Vitamin C: Helps Keep Your Tissues and Fat-Burning Capabilities Intact").

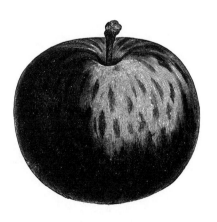

Full-blown scurvy is a potentially fatal and ghastly disease, involving bleeding from ruptured blood vessels, as well as the overall disintegration of collagen, the fibrous, bodily connective tissue found in tendons, ligaments, cartilage, skin, bone, muscles, and veins. Vitamin C must be present for the synthesis of collagen, which is why you literally fall apart without it!

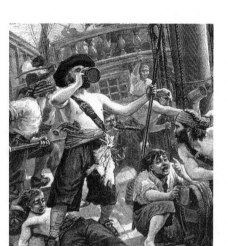

British sailors keeled over with scurvy, but the cats on the ships survived.

Now that I've mentioned it, a medium-sized apple contains about 8.4 mg of vitamin C (you need on average about 6 mg of vitamin C per day to avoid death!), so you need to go quite a bit farther than the apple to reach the RDA of 90 mg for men and 75 mg for women.

It's a Snap to Keep Yourself Topped Up

The good news is that it's generally very easy for the vast majority of people to get enough micronutrients via their diet alone (if you make the effort to educate yourself on food composition), or through a combination of food and supplements.

You have to derive micronutrients from your diet and/or supplements, because the body cannot make most of them itself. In fact, we've evolved a love affair with plants due to that age-old drawback of not being able to synthesize life-giving chemicals like vitamin C or E as plants can (see the sidebars on vitamin C and antioxidants).

You might recall this story: the British sailors keeled over with scurvy, but the cats on the ships survived, because they could synthesize their own vitamin C (thus the "Limeys" began eating fruit like vitamin C–containing lemons and limes to survive sea voyages).

What's Ahead?

People have a small but crucial requirement for vitamins or minerals in their food. An upcoming section explains the daily requirements for micronutrients, which the Food and Nutrition Board of the U.S. National Academy of Sciences establishes and calls Recommended Dietary Allowances, or RDAs.

Sometimes a doctor, or a friend, or the local guru who seems to have read every Asian philosopher and can walk anywhere barefoot, scratches his chin and says something like, "Maybe you should take more magnesium. . ."

Because it's generally to your advantage to be able to distinguish magnesium from vitamin C (for beginners, one's a mineral and the other is a vitamin), this chapter will also provide brief descriptions of many of the key vitamins and minerals.

Along the way, the chapter gives you tips on reading a vitamin Supplement Facts label, as well as sensible reasons to aim for some of the "super foods" like the tiny but mighty phytochemicals.

The end of the chapter has a guide to a few of the online tools you can play with for analyzing your nutrient intake. After all, knowledge is power, especially self-knowledge. Your nutrient profile might begin as a sad story, but it's going to end in triumph.

Let's get some definitions out of the way first.

What Are Micronutrients?

A *micronutrient* is a tiny constituent of food or a biochemical that plays a vital role in basic physiology, such as a vitamin, a mineral, or a phytochemical—that is, a chemical made by plants, such as beta-carotene, lycopene (in tomatoes), or resveratrol (in grapes).

Macronutrients (discussed in Chapter 3) are the dietary components used for fuel and making things, and are thereby used up in the process: protein, carbohydrates, and fats. Micronutrients are used for chemical reactions (vitamins can be cofactors for enzymes) and/or stored in the body as part of its structure or chemistry (e.g., calcium and phosphorus in bone), or as antioxidant defenses (vitamins C, E, and the mineral selenium).

Micronutrients are often measured in milligrams or micrograms. There are about 28 grams in one ounce; a single U.S. dollar bill weighs about 1 gram. A milligram (mg) is one thousandth of a gram. A microgram (mcg) is about one millionth of a gram.

Sodium chloride (salt), for example, is a "macromineral" that people eating Western diets typically get more than enough of from processed foods. A macromineral is usually required in the diet at a quantity of at least 100 mg or more per day, but all of our descriptions will mention specific RDAs along the way.

To picture a milligram, imagine one grain of salt out of a saltshaker. Some of the trace or "microminerals" we list in this chapter, like iodine or selenium, along with B vitamins, for example, are only recommended in a few mg per day, or in some cases, a few *micrograms*.

Figuring Out Your Daily Micronutrient Requirements

As in the user-testing and bug-tracking tools of the software world, you have to have some kind of metric to determine whether you're getting enough of a micronutrient or not. You may know you're getting 50 mg of vitamin C per day, but then what? Is that too much, not enough, or adequate for your age or gender?

In the U.S., the Food and Nutrition Board of the National Academy of Sciences has set the daily requirements for vitamins and minerals. They call them Recommended Dietary Allowances (RDAs), and they are usually

A micronutrient is a tiny constituent of food or a biochemical that plays a vital role in basic physiology, such as a vitamin, a mineral, or a phytochemical—that is, a chemical made by plants.

expressed in milligrams or micrograms. The RDAs are the amounts of the chemicals that will keep you out of deficiency for that vitamin or mineral (meaning, they are not *maximum* intakes by any means). They are part of a larger rubric called Dietary Reference Intakes, or DRIs (see the end of this section for an explanation of the "dietary alphabet soup").

Some of the vitamin recommendations are in International Units (IU), such as for vitamins A and D.

> *To convert from IUs to micrograms, for vitamin D: 1 IU = 0.025 mcg (so 40 IU vitamin D = 1 mcg). For vitamin A: 1 microgram = 3.33 IUs.*

An RDA is pretty easy to understand: for example, 90 mg of vitamin C for male adults and 75 mg per day for female adults.

The RDAs are not generally hard to meet by eating whole foods such as fruits and vegetables, but that hasn't prevented the vast majority of Americans—more than 90 percent of us—from falling short of the requirements, according to Dr. Jeffrey Blumberg, the director of the Antioxidants Research Laboratory at Tufts' Jean Mayer USDA Human Nutrition Research Center on Aging.

A multivitamin is "insurance" against being deficient in vitamins and minerals, he said, but not a substitute for healthy foods. Eating healthfully versus taking supplements is a "false dichotomy."

The vast majority of people need to do both, but you shouldn't view supplements as taking the place of fresh plant foods, which, unlike your multivitamin-mineral (MVM) supplement, contain dozens of important phytochemicals like beta-carotene, lycopene, flavonoids, and epicatechin (in green tea).

> *Some newer supplements are jammed with a lot of "super ingredients," but these products are unregulated and may be fraught with uncertainty. You might as well graze the farmer's markets and stands for fresh sources of flavonoids and other phytochemicals, because these appear to be roughly the types of nutrient sources that humans have sought throughout our evolution.*

We probably evolved to graze on plant foods and thus inherit their protective antioxidant and anti-inflammatory defenses (see the sidebar "Antioxidants: Cultivate Your Inner Nerf"). "We lost the ability a long time ago, when we became human, to synthesize these compounds [internally] ourselves," Blumberg said.

Graze the farmer's markets and stands for fresh sources of flavonoids and other vphytochemicals.

That's all you really have to know about RDAs; they are not a *maximum* amount for your intake, but rather the minimum amount required to keep you from becoming deficient (the upper limit is abbreviated as TUL). For what it's worth, the overall DRI is explained here: *http://www.ars.usda.gov/News/docs.htm?docid=10870*.

According to this site, the DRI's are actually a set of four reference values (of which RDAs are one).

> *"Recommended Dietary Allowance (RDA) is the average daily dietary intake of a nutrient that is sufficient to meet the requirement of nearly all (97-98%) healthy persons.*
>
> *Adequate Intake (AI) for a nutrient is [...] only established when an RDA cannot be determined. Therefore a nutrient either has an RDA or an AI. The AI is based on observed intakes of the nutrient by a group of healthy persons.*
>
> *Tolerable Upper Intake Level (TUL) is the highest daily intake of a nutrient that is likely to pose no risks of toxicity for almost all individuals. As intake above the UL increases, risk increases.*
>
> *Estimated Average Requirement (EAR) is the amount of a nutrient that is estimated to meet the requirement of half of all healthy individuals in the population.*

ANTIOXIDANTS: CULTIVATE YOUR INNER NERF

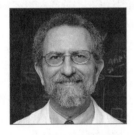

There's an easy way to help soak up oxidative stress in the body, the rust and decay that is behind aging and many chronic diseases (oxidation causes a bitten apple to turn brown on the shelf, and iron to rust): eat lots of the tiny phytochemicals that turn on a protein in the cell's nucleus called Nrf-2 (it's pronounced "nerf2").

"Our major focus is looking at polyphenols like the flavanoids as antioxidants and anti-inflammatories; dark chocolate, green tea, and tree nuts for example: almonds, walnuts, pistachios. Their skins are extremely rich in these compounds," explained Dr. Jeff Blumberg, the director of the Antioxidants Research Laboratory at Tufts' Jean Mayer USDA Human Nutrition Research Center on Aging. "One of the principal roles of these [compounds] are as phytoalexins—defense agents against insects, molds, ultraviolet light, any environmental toxicant—and [humans] may well have evolved to use those compounds for similar kinds of purposes."

Similar to our inability to synthesize vitamin C for use in our cells, we may have evolved to graze on plants to borrow their internal defenses against pathogens.

It turns out, however, that polyphenols are "lousy antioxidants," Blumberg said. "Very good in vitro as antioxidants,"

but we don't absorb them in high enough quantities to deal with the higher concentrations of free radicals in the blood and tissue. "To mop up all of the [reactive oxygen species, another name for free radicals], you need a big mop. The concentration of vitamin C, glutathione, and nitric acid are thousands of times higher" than the flavanoids.

Polyphenols "are still very good anti-inflammatories," which goes hand in hand with oxidative stress. "If you provoke oxidative stress you can provoke inflammation. They are both intimately involved in the pathogenesis of diseases, like cancer, heart disease, as well as neurodegenerative diseases like Parkinson's and Alzeimer's. Free radicals can cause damage to DNA, protein, enzymes; the damaged molecules stimulate the immune system to take care of them," which gives rise to the inflammation.

By eating lots of fruits and veggies, you can turn on an anti-inflammatory pathway called "nerf2" after a protein in the cell's nucleus: Nrf-2. "One of the primary pathways—the way these compounds work in very small concentrations in the cell are through cell-signaling transduction pathways," Blumberg explained.

"We have complex pathways that ultimately end up turning on or turning off our genes; we do this every day, and our diet plays a big influence on this, particularly the phytochemicals.

ANTIOXIDANTS: CULTIVATE YOUR INNER NERF (continued)

Nrf-2 turns on the antioxidant response element on the genome, in your genes; it [thereby] upregulates antioxidant enzymes such as superoxide dismutase and glutathione peroxidase. It can turn down some of the inflammatory genes—cytokines and interleukins that stimulate the immune system when you don't want it to be stimulated; and this all happens at the genome level because of what you eat.

You don't need too many of these compounds like you need a [a certain number of milligrams of vitamin C], all you need to do is turn on this one pathway, a few molecules will do it. It's a huge amplification system.

There are a number of polyphenols which have been demonstrated (all with in vitro studies, of course) to modulate Nrf-2, including curcumin (turmeric), sulphoraphane (broccoli), epicatechin (green tea), procyanidins (berry fruit), and caffeic acid phenethyl ester (honeybee propolis)."

You can turn on your own protective pathways by aiming for more antioxidant-containing ingredients in your diet.

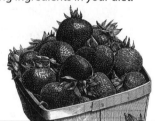

Aim for Farms and Markets

Taking a multivitamin/mineral supplement is about half (or less) of the picture of micronutrients. The other half is the fun part: eating for health.

I try to aim for foods from local farms and farmer's markets (see Chapter 5, for more on finding and choosing food). I seek to get most of my vitamins and minerals from healthy foods. By targeting healthy foods, I mean piling on the veggies (carrots, lettuce, yellow/red/orange bell peppers, broccoli, asparagus, etc.) and fruits (lots of berries, fresh apples, oranges, bananas, lemons), as well as eating pastured dairy (butter, cheese, milk), coconut milk, grass-fed meats, fish (including shellfish), a fairly neutral grain like brown rice (grains can be problematic), as well as some nuts, seeds, and plant oils like a little olive and coconut oil.

The tools we discuss at the end of this chapter will help you determine whether your vitamin and mineral consumption is adequate or not. The *degrading* of nutrients in kept food is an issue, too. Oxidative damage (think juice in paper cartons, or old refrigerated veggies that have changed in color) can degrade a food item's nutritional content, and supplements whose expiration dates have passed will no longer have the potency indicated on the bottle.

Use common sense: a ready-to-drink carton of OJ may quickly lose its vitamin C content in the refrigerator (using glass containers and drinking it fresh from frozen are better), according to Professor Carol Johnston at Arizona State University. Gnarly-looking veggies orphaned in the back of the food drawer have probably also lost a lot of their antioxidant and vitamin power. Check the expiration date of any multivitamin/mineral supplements (MVMs).

For most of us, life involves a marathon of over-programming and scheduling that keeps us sitting down most of the time and snatching random food items here and there on the run. As a result, some of us might benefit from a multivitamin/mineral supplement, but a healthy dose of skepticism in regard to the quality and efficacy of these products is in order.

The *bioavailability* of these artificially manufactured nutrients is a highly significant variable as well, according to a 2006 executive summary in the *American Journal of Clinical Nutrition*.[4] Here's their take on this issue:

> *Key factors determining the bioavailability of micronutrients are the chemical form in which the nutrient is presented to the intestinal absorptive surface, the presence of other competing chemicals in the intestinal lumen, the concentration of food constituents (such as phytates and other chelating agents) that bind to the nutrient and make it unavailable for absorption, intestinal transit time, and enzyme activity.*

> *A nutrient may affect not only the absorption of other nutrients, but also the transport, tissue uptake, function and metabolism of other nutrients.*

> *The following URL, a search of Google Scholar, provides much food for thought on the matter of nutrition in a pill: http://scholar.google.com/scholar?q=efficacy+of+multivitamin+mineral+products&hl=en&btnG=Search&as_sdt=1%2C46&as_sdtp=on.*

We can probably benefit from a measure of insurance. You might mix and match a supplement (e.g., D3, calcium, magnesium) with healthy foods from local farms in season. If you are a nutrition power user, and I'm guessing many of the readers are, you could actually test yourself for vitamin and mineral insufficiencies before committing to certain MVMs and nutrient intakes.

I recently spent the better part of three days climbing Mt. Rainier, a 14,411 ft. active volcano near Seattle, Washington. Nothing grows up there. All water comes from melted snow. The food the guides cooked in the mess tent was outstanding in taste (veggie burritos loaded with avocados and tomatoes, gorpy oatmeal, and mounds of cheesy eggs and bacon), but I couldn't have lived on it 100 percent of the time, in terms of micronutrient intake. Obviously, if I were spending weeks on a mountaineering trek in similar environs, I would consider bringing a vitamin and mineral supplement to buoy up my nutrition.

Not only is the research mixed or inconclusive on whether MVMs actually prevent chronic diseases,[5] but there are undoubtedly huge differences in quality among the thousands. of available MVM-related products.

READING AN MVM SUPPLEMENT FACTS LABEL

Every MVM supplement comes with a Supplement Facts label. If it doesn't, you'd better give it the heave-ho. You should read the label before you take any of the substances (whatever form they're in: pill or liquid or chewable), especially before handing some of them to a child or other family member.

Figure 4-1 shows one of these Supplement Facts labels. The first column specifies the micronutrient, like vitamin E or calcium (this supplement happens to include only one mineral; it's a special vitamin and phytochemical combination).

The next column is the Amount Per Serving. This is the micronutrient amount you're going to get if you ingest the recommended serving, in this case, two wafers.

The amounts are in mg, mcg, and IUs. This can be confusing, as different nutrients use different units of measure: for instance, vitamins A, D, and E are labeled in IUs; vitamin C in mg; and folic acid in mcg.

The more you learn about micronutrients, the greater comfort you will have rattling off the IUs vs. the mcgs, however, since each of the vitamins and minerals are almost always paired with the same unit of measurement whenever you come across them. You'll get used to them.

The next column, % Daily Value, puts this information into better perspective. This number represents the percentage of the vitamin or mineral you will ingest in one serving, relative to the public health recommendations for a daily amount of the nutrient.

For example, 100 percent means you're getting some amount akin to the RDA for that micronutrient; 400 percent states that a serving contains four times the recommended minimum amount.

The cross-shaped glyph signifies that public health bodies (such as the Food and Nutrition Board in the U.S.) have not established a recommended amount for that substance. It might be a "super food" such carotenoids or blueberry extract that the government has not yet come up with a standard for.

Supplement Facts
Serving Size 2 Wafers
Servings Per Container 30

	Amount Per Serving	% Daily Value
Calories	10	
Total Carbohydrate	3 g	1%*
Vitamin A (as beta-carotene)	5,000 IU	100%
Vitamin C (as ascorbic acid)	60 mg	100%
Vitamin D3 (as cholecalciferol)	1,000 IU	250%
Vitamin E (as d-alpha-tocopheryl succinate)	30 IU	100%
Thiamin (as thiamin mononitrate)	1.5 mg	100%
Riboflavin	1.7 mg	100%
Niacin (as niacinamide)	20 mg	100%
Vitamin B6 (as pyridoxine HCl)	2 mg	100%
Folate (as folic acid)	400 mcg	100%
Vitamin B12 (as cyanocobalamin)	6 mcg	100%
Biotin	300 mcg	100%
Pantothenic acid (as D-calcium pantothenate)	10 mg	100%
Calcium (as calcium citrate)	50 mg	5%
Choline (as choline dihydrogen citrate)	20 mg	†
DHA concentrate	50 mg	†
Proprietary fruit and veggie blend	300 mg	†
Carotenoids concentrate		
Apricot, carrot, mango, melon, peach, summer squash, tomato, cantaloupe, plum and watermelon		
Cruciferous/Organosulfides concentrate		
Asparagus, beet greens, broccoli, garlic, Brussels sprouts, cauliflower, kale, leek, onion and radish		
Flavonoids concentrate		
Black currant, blueberry, cranberry, tangerine, celery, grapefruit, lemon/lime and orange		
Fruit enzyme concentrate		
Papaya and pineapple		
Isoflavone concentrate		
Soybean		
Lutein concentrate		
Spinach and kale		
Phenolics concentrate		
Apple, cherry, grape, pear, raspberry and strawberry		
Super foods blend		
alfalfa, artichoke, peas and red beet		

* Daily Values are based on a 2,000 calorie per day diet.
† Daily Value not established.

Figure 4-1. *Vitamin Supplement Facts label*

Cooking Alters Micronutrient Content

If you don't take an MVM supplement or your use of them is sporadic and strategic, remember that various forms of cooking have a significant effect on the nutritive value of veggies, fruits, and meats.

For example, if you cook (and drain the boiling water from) a stalk of broccoli, with the assumption that you will be ingesting fantastic amounts of vitamin C and B12, keep in mind that the boiling itself may reduce the vitamin content by 75 percent and 50 percent, respectively.[6]

> *A study showed varying effects of boiling on veggies such as broccoli and asparagus.[7] For asparagus, boiling actually raised its "[free] radical scavenging activity," or RSA (a measure of antioxidant activity), by 10 percent, and 15 percent of the original vitamin C content of the veggie was left in the cooking water. Broccoli retained only 83 percent of its RSA after boiling, and the cooking water had a high antioxidant value as well.*

There are many solutions to this conundrum. If you're cooking a stew, then make sure you consume the broth with the stew contents, because this liquid will likely contain some of the nutrients.

If you boil veggies on occasion, you can be hardcore like me: take the leftover boiling water and use it as a base or an ingredient for a smoothie. The study referenced by the last note pointed out that a stalk of boiled broccoli, for instance, leaves about 28 mg of its vitamin C in the cooking water (the water alone containing about a fifth of a good day's worth of C for the average person). For sure, the water tastes a little weird at first, but be creative, as in the upcoming sidebar.

You can also impress your friends and appall your guests by simply guzzling the leftover water out of the pan.

As we saw in Chapter 2, there are many handy tools for helping determine the nutritional content, or lack thereof, of your diet. We'll take another look at some of these, and introduce a few new ones, in "Getting Micronutrient Information Online: Web Tools," at the end of this chapter. The "FitDay on Vending-Machine Fare" section gives the lowdown on some of the "food-like substances" some of us geeks like to eat.

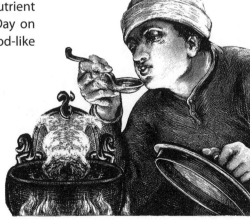

CAPTURING THE COOKED VEGGIE'S NUTRITION IN A SMOOTHIE

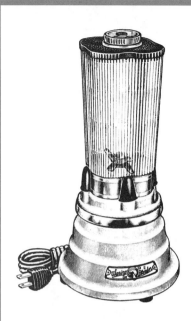

Here's a recipe for a smoothie that will help recapture some of the vitamins and minerals lost when boiling a vegetable (for you steamers out there—and I'm one of them—that cooking style also reduces veggie nutrition). Mix the following ingredients in a blender:

1 grated carrot

½ a lemon (more vitamin C)—you could substitute an orange or the like, but lemons have less fructose

About 4–8 ounces coconut milk (healthy fats, calcium)

1 scoop of whey protein mix (branched-chain amino acids)

A handful of raspberries (phytochemicals and taste)

½ teaspoon of local honey (a bit of sweetness)

1 tablespoon Greek-style plain yogurt (consistency, calcium)

Pour in water from boiling asparagus and broccoli, or any other veggie. Mix well. I tried this at home, and it was delicious. Then I ate the warm veggies with a nice pat of pastured butter and a piece of chicken from Gaylord Farm in Vermont that I had in the freezer. *Voilà!*

Grade School Nurse Fondly Recalled

If you're like me, you pretty much slept, or teased Gilda McGillicuddy in the seat next to you, when the elementary school nurse bopped in for a lecture on "The Importance of Vitamins." The following sections contain a wealth of knowledge about vitamins and minerals, and I've designed it to be a digestible and concise package. You can even skip over it to the online tools section at the chapter's end and just return to this section for later reference.

The Linus Pauling Institute's Micronutrient Information Center at Oregon State University is one of the best places around for finding out more detailed biochemical information about these substances: *http://lpi.oregonstate.edu/infocenter/*. Whenever possible, each nutrient has a reference back to the LPI pages.

Vitamins

Vitamins are organic molecules (the ones containing carbon atoms) that are cofactors or helper molecules for enzymes that play vital roles in the body. Back in the early part of the last century, the term "vitamin" was formed from "vital amines," when it was thought that all vitamins were amine molecules.

Vitamins aren't used for energy themselves, but they are crucial for many of the internal chemical reactions by which our body's machinery can utilize protein, carbs, and fat for fuel.

Food scientists don't consider a nutrient a vitamin unless it's essential for our metabolism or other vital systems, and must be obtained via the diet. Monkeys, apes, humans, and some birds, for example, have lost the ability to synthesize vitamin C. We can biosynthesize vitamin D from exposure to ultraviolet (UV) light from the sun, however, and some bacteria in our guts can synthesize vitamin K, a fat-soluble vitamin.

Enzymes are biochemicals (usually proteins) that catalyze or initiate chemical reactions but are not used up by those reactions. Enzymes commonly end with the suffix "ase," as in *lactase*, the enzyme that allows people to digest milk sugar or lactose, or the enzyme in saliva that disassembles starch into smaller sugars, *amylase*.

We don't use up vitamins for energy, as we do carbohydrates or protein in food, but they take part in numerous essential chemical reactions, or simply are hormones themselves, like the active form of vitamin D.

Even though vitamin D might get all the splashy headlines these days, the eight B-complex vitamins and vitamins A, C, E, and K also play crucial roles in the basic physiological processes that keep us alive.

Fat-Soluble Vitamins

A subset of vitamins can be stored in body fat and are thus described as "fat-soluble." This characteristic has two main ramifications. First, to properly absorb these vitamins in supplement form, it helps to consume them with a little dietary fat (e.g., a blob of Greek-style yogurt). Furthermore, eating healthy fats, like a pastured egg, an avocado, or coconut milk, will help you derive more fat-soluble vitamins, because the fats you are digesting contain the nutrients.

Second, since fat-soluble vitamins can be stored, you can potentially overload your body with fat-soluble vitamin supplements. Although it's difficult to do, you could, for example, take in too much vitamin A in cod liver oil and potentially accumulate toxic levels of this vitamin.

> *An upcoming section is devoted to vitamin-A toxicity, or hypervitaminosis A. For an article that goes into more scientific detail, see http://lpi.oregonstate.edu/infocenter/vitamins/vitaminA/.*

This is the reason why you shouldn't start taking mega doses of vitamin A (or *any* supplement, for that matter) without reading the supplement labels and checking the RDA for adults and kids first (see the sidebar earlier in this chapter on reading the Supplement Facts label).

The fat-soluble vitamins are vitamins A, D, E, and K.

> *I made up my own mnemonic device for remembering them: "a deck of cards," ADEK. It's a start, right?*

Vitamin A

This vitamin is available in the diet in two forms:

- Retinol, or *preformed vitamin A* ("true" vitamin A) from animal sources like eggs, pastured butter, fish, meats, and cod liver oil.

- Pro-vitamin A carotenoid, the vegetable- and fruit-based beta-carotene (found in orange and other brightly colored foods like carrots, cantaloupes, peaches, sweet potatoes, and leafy veggies), which the body can convert into retinol, albeit at a low conversion ratio.[8]

There is an international conversion factor for foods and supplements called the *retinol activity equivalents* (RAEs), described in the upcoming "Retinol Activity Equivalents for Vitamin A" sidebar. For example, 12 units of beta-carotene are about the equivalent of 1 unit of vitamin A or retinol.[9]

Beta-carotene is also an effective antioxidant.

You could theoretically (given the cooking method and your individual ability to incorporate food; i.e., no potential digestive problems, age, etc.) acquire all the vitamin A you need for a day from a medium-sized carrot, a baked sweet potato, and a salad ingredient of spinach. In fact, that would probably give you more than you need (unless you're an athlete putting in mega miles).

The body converts retinol from these various forms of vitamin A into retinoic acid, which is the molecule responsible for vitamin A's biological effects.

For example, retinoic acid affects gene transcription, and thereby affects how certain bodily proteins are synthesized (some tissues have retinoic acid receptors, or RARs).[10]

Vitamin A is essential for the health of your retinas, particularly for night vision. If you bump up your vitamin–A containing veggie intake after a period of deficiency, you might notice the night-vision difference right away. As you're driving at night, can you read the small print on those luminescent street signs?

Vitamin A has a crucial anti-infective role in the immune system. Retinol is required in the body for the normal functioning of epithelial cells, the "first line of defense" that line the airways and digestive tract, for instance. The body needs vitamin A to develop white blood cells such as lymphocytes, which are central to our immune system.[11]

"Vitamin A appears to facilitate the mobilization of iron from storage sites [in the body] to the developing red blood cell for incorporation into hemoglobin, the oxygen carrier in red blood cells," according to the online Linus Pauling Institute (LPI) article at *http://lpi.oregonstate.edu/infocenter/vitamins/vitaminA/index.html#function*.

Vitamin A is essential for the health of your retinas, particularly for night vision. If you bump up your vitamin–A containing veggie intake after a period of deficiency, you might notice the night-vision difference right away.

RETINOL ACTIVITY EQUIVALENTS (RAEs) FOR VITAMIN A

Not all vitamin A is created equal. If you ingest beta-carotene, which the body can convert to vitamin A or retinol in small amounts, you can use the following equation to estimate the equivalent consumption of retinol (retinol is the "pure" vitamin A form found in foods like liver, eggs, fish oil, milk, and cheese):

```
RAE Vitamin A = mcg retinol + (mcg beta-carotene equivalents/12)
```

Mcg stands for micrograms. If you eat a medium-sized carrot that has 0.0 mcg of retinol and 5,054 mcg of beta-carotene (according to NutritionData), that veggie represents an RAE of about 421 mcg. The U.S. Recommended Dietary Allowance is 900 mcg RAE for males over 14 and 700 mcg RAE for females over 14, rising to 770 mcg RAE for a pregnant woman and 1,300 mcg RAE for a lactating mom.

The RDA for kids is 300 mcg RAE for ages 1–3, 400 mcg RAE for ages 4–8, and 600 mcg RAE for ages 9–13. So you can see that with one measly carrot, people are well on their way to meeting their dietary requirements for vitamin A. That's where the sweet potato and spinach come in.[12]

Vitamin A toxicity

Since vitamin A is a fat-soluble vitamin, it is possible to take too much pre-formed vitamin A (you *do not get* vitamin A toxicity, or hypervitaminosis A, from eating a lot of carotenoids, as found in carrots, bell peppers, sweet potatoes, and mangos, for instance).

Although fairly rare, hypervitaminosis A has serious symptoms, such as liver abnormalities, reduced bone density, and cerebral edema (what occurs with the onset of the severe form of high-altitude sickness). Most people fully recover by simply stopping the overdosing of A.

Check the tolerable upper limit (TUL) for vitamin A before you start imbibing a lot of preformed vitamin A in the form of supplements or cod liver oil, for example.[13]

Vitamin A amounts are specified in IUs. To convert IUs to micrograms: 1 IU of A equals 0.3 micrograms.

I did a search on cod liver oil at *www.nutritiondata.com*. Figure 4-2 shows what I found. Look at that retinol amount for just one tablespoon: 4,051 micrograms. The TULs specify that adults shouldn't take more than 10,000 IU or 3,000 mcg of retinol per day, and kids aged four to eight should take no more than 3,000 IU or 900 mcg.[14]

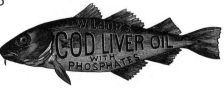

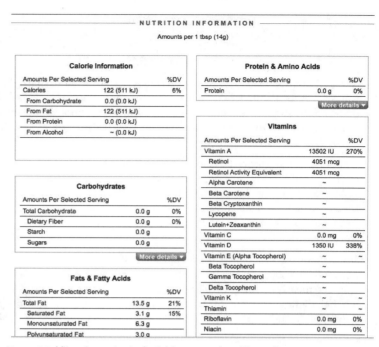

NUTRITION INFORMATION

Amounts per 1 tbsp (14g)

Calorie Information

Amounts Per Selected Serving		%DV
Calories	122 (511 kJ)	6%
From Carbohydrate	0.0 (0.0 kJ)	
From Fat	122 (511 kJ)	
From Protein	0.0 (0.0 kJ)	
From Alcohol	~ (0.0 kJ)	

Carbohydrates

Amounts Per Selected Serving		%DV
Total Carbohydrate	0.0 g	0%
Dietary Fiber	0.0 g	0%
Starch	0.0 g	
Sugars	0.0 g	

More details ▾

Fats & Fatty Acids

Amounts Per Selected Serving		%DV
Total Fat	13.5 g	21%
Saturated Fat	3.1 g	15%
Monounsaturated Fat	6.3 g	
Polyunsaturated Fat	3.0 g	

Protein & Amino Acids

Amounts Per Selected Serving		%DV
Protein	0.0 g	0%

More details ▾

Vitamins

Amounts Per Selected Serving		%DV
Vitamin A	13502 IU	270%
Retinol	4051 mcg	
Retinol Activity Equivalent	4051 mcg	
Alpha Carotene	~	
Beta Carotene	~	
Beta Cryptoxanthin	~	
Lycopene	~	
Lutein+Zeaxanthin	~	
Vitamin C	0.0 mg	0%
Vitamin D	1350 IU	338%
Vitamin E (Alpha Tocopherol)	~	~
Beta Tocopherol	~	
Gamma Tocopherol	~	
Delta Tocopherol	~	
Vitamin K	~	~
Thiamin	~	
Riboflavin	0.0 mg	0%
Niacin	0.0 mg	0%

Figure 4-2. *Vitamin content of a tablespoon of cod liver oil*

Again, it is quite easy to get enough vitamin A by eating whole foods such as vegetables that contain carotenoids, salmon (an RAE of 229 mcg), and two scrambled eggs (an RAE exceeding 600 mcg).

Vitamin D

If ever a vitamin could be deemed "sexy," it would be vitamin D.

The hype surrounding vitamin D seems to be spreading: a very tanned checkout girl, who looked like she'd recently broken Owen Wilson's and Matthew McConaughey's hearts (at the same time), recently told me she'd spent the weekend "getting her vitamin D" (and she probably *did* get her D that way).

Everywhere you look, another "media story based on a study" touts the vitamin's multifarious benefits.

The hype seems to have at least a partial basis in fact.

Photosynthesis has generated vitamin D in life forms on earth for millions of years, and it is a remarkable biosynthetic mechanism by which we can create a vital chemical for our bodies from sunlight.

We're like plants, basking in the sun for reasons much more important than an excuse to wear Ray-Bans.

The human genome has hundreds of sites known as vitamin D receptors (VDRs), indicating that the active form of vitamin D can bind with these sites and affect gene expression (meaning some "health-positive" genes can be turned on, and/or genes that have negative effects can be switched off).[15]

We geeks are often indoor creatures

Along with sunblock, which will screen out the ultraviolet (UV) rays that help produce vitamin D, modern life—specifically, Facebook, Twitter, Netflix, cubicle life, and every other excuse to sit in a glorified box in front of a screen—has driven us indoors, where we were never really designed to spend a lot of time in the first place.

Back in my own software engineering days, I tried to walk in the sun as much as possible during the workday. I walked half an hour or more every morning from the train along Cambridge, MA's sunny sidewalks (yeah, the sun comes out in New England, sometimes). I went outside several times a day to find splotches of sun in Kendall Square. Right now I'm headed off to sit on a rock in the sun and swim in a Vermont waterway called the Mad River. Of course, I take some D supplements too. I *do* spend the winter in New England, a region and time of year not usually known for sunshine.

Your vitamin D status is a relevant marker of health. A Massachusetts General Hospital study found that among 290 patients entering the hospital with a variety of ailments, about 57 percent of them were vitamin D–deficient, with blood levels of 15 ng/ml (nanograms per milliliter) or less.[16]

A September 2009 study of more than 3,000 older folks in the U.S. found that "compared [with] those [who had] optimal vitamin D status, those with low vitamin D levels were three times more likely to die from heart disease and 2.5 times more likely to die from any cause."[17]

The biosynthetic process

Here's how we naturally produce our own vitamin D. The skin generates *cholecalciferol*, the inactive form of vitamin D, when cholesterol molecules in epidermal cells are exposed to ultraviolet radiation.[18]

The liver converts this biochemical to *calcidiol*, or 25-hydroxyvitamin D, abbreviated 25(OH)D—a prehormone and the form of vitamin D that blood tests detect (see the "Testing for D" section). A prehormone is a substance that other tissues in the body convert into an *active* hormone, a signaling chemical that binds with receptors and launches chemical reactions in the body.

It's good to know all this stuff because you're probably going to be testing for vitamin D, and the doctors will be casually tossing around terms like "25(OH)D." Besides, you can also impress tanned checkout girls (or guys) with your advanced vitamin-D know-how!

Photosynthesis has generated vitamin D in life forms on earth for millions of years, and it is a remarkable biosynthetic mechanism by which we can create a vital chemical for our bodies from sunlight.

It's a dessert topping—it's a hormone!

An enzyme in the kidneys called 25(OH)D-1α-hydroxylase further modifies this chemical calcidiol to *calcitriol*, or 1,25-dihydroxyvitamin D. This is a secosteroid hormone that is responsible for most of vitamin D's physiological effects. A *secosteroid* hormone is similar to a steroid hormone like testosterone and estrogen, but has a slightly different molecular structure.

This hormone binds with hundreds of sites throughout the body that have vitamin D receptors, and thereby affects how many of our genes are expressed.

Vitamin D is an essential molecule for bone health, but it has also been associated with promoting insulin sensitivity (where your cells are able to admit glucose and amino acids in response to the presence of insulin in the bloodstream), preventing the cell proliferation associated with certain cancers such as those of the prostate, breast, and colon, as well as helping prevent high blood pressure.[19]

Sources of Vitamin D

Along with exposure to the sun, you can also build up your vitamin D with food and supplements.

Some foods are fortified with vitamin D3 (like milk, about 115 to 124 IU per 8 ounces[20]), or contain moderate vitamin D3 levels without fortification (grass-fed or free range eggs and salmon). A can of sardines has about 250 IU of vitamin D3, but that's not enough for a day.

The sun might still be the best way to get vitamin D, for the same reason we drink water through our mouths instead of running off to inject it intravenously—because that's the way we're designed. It's also impossible to develop vitamin D toxicity from the sun, unless you're also taking too high a dose in supplemental form. My guess is that surfers and lifeguards who aren't covered by a wetsuit and sunblock all the time have pretty healthy D levels.

> *A recent study of some people in East Africa who live pastoral or hunter-gatherer lifestyles, the Maasai and the Hadzabe, noted that their mean 25(OH)D levels fell into the mid to high-40s range. The Maasai's mean levels were "48 ng/ml (119 nmol/L) and ranged from 23 to 67 ng/ml," and the Hadzabe's were "44 ng/ml and ranged from 28 to 68 ng/ml." A "deficient" level, according to U.S. standards, is beneath 32 ng/ml (see http://blog.vitamindcouncil.org/2012/01/25/new-study-vitamin-d-levels-of-the-maasai-and-hadzabe-of-africa/).*

But what about those of us who live in the northern latitude—not near the equator, in Australia, or in the U.S. sunbelt—or have a darker skin color, which makes it more difficult compared with lighter-skinned people to make D from the sun (especially in northern regions)?

> *Obesity also makes photosynthesized vitamin D less bioavailable. See http://hjira.com/acjn/72-3-690.full.pdf.*

Supplements

Vitamin D3 supplements are cheap (about $30 per year for a daily 2,000 IU dose, the last time I looked) and readily available. The National Institutes of Health (NIH) has recommended that adults, kids, teens, and pregnant women take 600 IU per day, the minimum amount necessary for bone health. As for blood levels, "levels ≥50 nmol/L (≥20 ng/ml) are sufficient for most people," according to an NIH fact sheet.[21]

> *In terms of vitamin D, 40 IU equals 1 microgram (mcg). So if you take a 4,000 IU dose daily, you're getting about 100 mcg.*

However, the Vitamin D Council, an advocacy group, recommends that both adults and kids should attain a D serum level of about 50 ng/ml (125 nmol/l).

There is obviously some disagreement between the recommended levels of the federal government and the Council, which suggests that the public-health recommendations move too slowly to track the latest D research findings. In other words, the active form of vitamin D affects much more, physiologically, than calcium and bone health.

You could take the conservative approach and consider the U.S. government's recommended dose, then test to determine if the supplement's effects are adequate. Also see this page for the Vitamin D Council's recommended amounts and its rationale: *www.vitamindcouncil.org/about-vitamin-d/how-to-get-your-vitamin-d/vitamin-d-supplementation*.

If you're vitamin D–deficient, there seems to be some evidence that remedying that condition will aid an athlete's or a weekend warrior's sports performance. See the "Better D Status Boosts Sports Performance" sidebar.

Supplement thoughtfully

To reach the higher levels in your blood tests, in almost all instances, you would have to take more supplemental D3 than the NIH's recommended 600 IU per day, although how the body responds to vitamin D3 supplements varies from one person to the next. Some adults may attain healthy levels with 600 to 2000 IU per day; for others, it may take 4,000 IU or more per day.

Fat-soluble vitamins can be stored in human adipose tissue, so toxicity is possible when thoughtlessly supplementing with vitamins A and D, for instance, especially for kids. Their low body weights make them more vulnerable to toxicity when their dosages are recklessly scaled upward. An adult dose of 5,000 IU per day will not have the same effect on a kid who weighs 50 pounds.

The federal government puts the TUL for D3 at 4,000 IU per day for males and females of age 9 and above, "while symptoms of toxicity are unlikely at daily intakes below 10,000 IU/day."[22]

Other D3 researchers have noted that the TUL could be much higher than that, since about 30 minutes of full-body, high-noon sun exposure will generate up to 20,000 IU naturally.

"Excessive sun exposure does not result in vitamin D toxicity, because the sustained heat on the skin is thought to photodegrade previtamin D3 and vitamin D3 as it is formed," according to a National Institutes of Health Dietary Fact sheet on vitamin D. For more information, see *http://ods.od.nih. gov/factsheets/vitamind/#h8*.

Testing for D

Testing your D3 levels involves asking your doctor to have it included in a blood workup during a typical routine checkup or using one of several private testing services.

The result will be in the form of a number representing your blood level of 25-hydroxyvitamin D. In the U.S., this will most likely represent a 25-hydroxyvitamin D (sometimes shortened to "25 (OH) D") level in nanograms per milliliter (ng/ml), a figure like "48 ng."

Other countries, like the United Kingdom, may provide this number in nanomoles per liter (nmol/L), resulting in a number that is about 2.5 times higher (48 ng is 120 nmol/L).

According to the NIH, levels greater than 20 ng/ml are "generally considered adequate for bone and overall health in healthy individuals,"[23] but other researchers or advocates, such as the Vitamin D Council, advocate a higher number—50 ng/ml or more.

Science Daily reported on a February 2011 study that found much higher daily doses of vitamin D were required to protect most adults from cancer. "We found that daily intakes of vitamin D by adults in the range of 4000–8000 IU are needed to maintain blood levels of vitamin D metabolites in the range needed to reduce by about half the risk of several diseases—breast cancer, colon cancer, multiple sclerosis, and type 1 diabetes," according to a doctor at the UC San Diego Moores Cancer Center.[24]

Again, you have to test yourself periodically if you're going to boost your supplementation of vitamin D3.

Vitamin E

Vitamin E is one of the body's primary antioxidants. Since it's stored in body fat, vitamin E helps prevent the destruction by free radicals of the fats in cell membranes. Fats are a major component of cell membranes, so vitamin E has a key role in cell biology. Vitamin E also helps combat the oxidation by free radicals (the bad guys, when they're not being used to destroy invading germs) of low-density lipoproteins or LDLs.

LDLs are protein-fat-cholesterol complexes that travel through the bloodstream.

Vitamin C helps regenerate the antioxidant capacity of vitamin E—an example of two vitamins working synergistically and why you should aim to keep up to speed on all vitamins.

The liver secretes a form of vitamin E called alpha-tocopherol.[25]

Naturally sourced vitamin E is called d-alpha-tocopherol; the synthetically produced form is dl-alpha-tocopherol.[26]

The RDA for adults from adolescence on is 15 mg. One ounce of almonds, about 23 nuts, gives you 7.4 mg, which is almost half of the vitamin an adult needs to reach the RDA. Avocados (providing 4.5 mg, about a third of the RDA), olive oil, Swiss chard, spinach (cooked and raw), asparagus, and sunflower seeds are also very good sources of vitamin E.

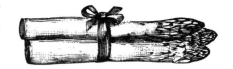

Avocados, olive oil, Swiss chard, spinach, asparagus, and sunflower seeds are also very good sources of vitamin E.

E and C supplements

Some studies have cast doubt on the efficacy of supplementing with vitamin E, as well as C for that matter, according to the National Institutes of Health in the U.S.[27] On the other hand, supplementing up to the RDA for these vitamins in most cases can't hurt. For a vitamin C–related supplement discussion, see the "Vitamin C: Helps Keep Your Tissues and Fat-Burning Capabilities Intact" sidebar.

Vitamin K

Vitamin K, another fat-soluble vitamin, plays an important role in blood clotting (the "K" comes from the German word "koagulation"), bone health, and preventing or reducing the calcification of arteries.

There are two naturally occurring forms, broadly referred to as *K1* (phylloquinone) and *K2* (menaquinone). The easiest way to think of vitamin K is that it puts calcium where it belongs (the bones) and removes it from where it doesn't belong (the arteries).

Plants manufacture K1, which is the vitamin K that newborn infants are given (I found it jarring—as the "husband witness," milling around somewhat ineffectually—when immediately upon both of my children's births, they were jabbed in the leg with a vitamin K1 shot, even before being wrapped in a blanket). The usual healthy suspects—parsley, spinach, leafy green lettuce, kale, broccoli, and olive oil—are good sources of vitamin K1.

Some bacteria in the large intestine generate K2, one of the few instances where a vitamin can be synthesized in the body (see below for the food sources of this nutrient).

Why should you even think about foods and supplements containing K2, if the gut flora can synthesize it? Because antibiotics can kill the bacteria in your gut that produce it, and it's a fairly important and underestimated vitamin that calls for insurance measures to make sure you're getting enough.

The bacteria make a range of K2 designated as MK-*n* (MK-4 in meats or supplements; MK-8 or 9 in cheese), where "n" stands for a 5-carbon unit on the side of the molecule, according to the Linus Pauling Institute's page on K2: *http://lpi.oregonstate.edu/infocenter/vitamins/vitaminK/*.

For example, menaquinone-4 (MK-4) means the molecule has four 5-carbon units.

Grass-fed cheese appears to be a good source of K2, according to Mark Sisson's *Mark's Daily Apple* page: *www.marksdailyapple.com/cheese-unhealthy/*.

Cheddar cheese, Swiss cheese, eggs, and chicken contain MK-4 in higher amounts than other foods.[28]

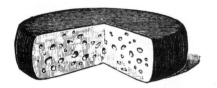

These comments on vitamin K2 contained in cheese and Natto (a fermented soy food popular in Japan that is a very good source of minerals and protein), from a 2004 Dutch study published in the *The Journal of Nutrition*, are eye-openers:

> *Cheese has not been established as a dietary risk factor for cardiovascular disease in epidemiological studies, despite its high levels of saturated fat and salt. We hypothesize that menaquinones in cheese (MK-8 and MK-9) could exert a beneficial effect in the cardiovascular system and that the high cheese consumption in France and the Mediterranean countries may possibly account for lower prevalences of [heart disease].{...}*
>
> *In healthy Japanese subjects who consumed fermented soybean (Natto) high in menaquinone (especially MK-7), serum concentrations of MK-7 and carboxylated osteocalcin were significantly increased.[29]*

K2 activates a protein called *osteocalcin* that builds or remodels bones by binding calcium to a mineral matrix. In fact, K2 works together with vitamin D and calcium to keep your skeleton healthy and strong. The active form of vitamin D, calcitriol, plays a role in the synthesis of osteocalcin.

Another vitamin K–dependent protein called *matrix Gla protein* (MGP) helps prevent the calcification or hardening of soft tissue and cartilage. Runners and cyclists, keep that one in mind as you consider vitamin K2 supplementation.

Water-Soluble Vitamins

The water-soluble vitamins do not have to be eaten with fat to be absorbed, and it's harder to overdose on these vitamins, as the body can flush them out via the urine. This doesn't make these substances—the eight B-complex vitamins and vitamin C—any more innocuous or less important than the fat-soluble ones, though. Some of the most infamous nutrient-related diseases are caused by deficiencies in C (scurvy), thiamine (beriberi), and niacin (pellagra).

B vitamins

This group of eight vitamins—B1 (thiamine), B2 (riboflavin), B3 (niacin), B5 (pantothenic acid), B6, B7 (Biotin), B9 (folic acid), and B12—has a wide variety of vital roles in the body. The MVM supplements will refer to the whole group of them as a *B-complex vitamin*.

Your first question might be: what about all those missing Bs (B4, B8, B10, etc.)? The short answer is that scientists decided that they weren't "vitamins" anymore, for reasons such as the body's ability to synthesize them.

Thiamine (B1) was one of the first vitamins ever discovered, in the late nineteenth century. "The story of thiamine is the story of beriberi, the disease caused by thiamine deficiency."[30]

In the early 1880s, for example, a Japanese naval physician named Kanehiro Takkaki found that adding meat, fish, and vegetables to the white-rice seaman's staple helped to cure a disease that had cut a swath through sailors, many of whom had languished on a low-level diet of polished white rice.

> When you remove the brown skin on rice, usually accomplished by milling machines, to make "polished white rice," even the tiny amounts of thiamine present in brown rice are lost. Beriberi, the horrible disease that has been common in populations that depend on rice in their diets, is broken down into "dry," "wet," and "cerebral" beriberi (see http://lpioregonstate.edu/infocenter/vitamins/thiamin/).

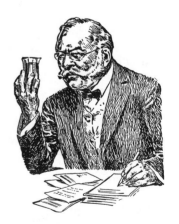

Thiamine plays a number of crucial roles as a coenzyme (an essential assistant for an enzyme) in basic metabolic processes.[31]

Transketolase, for example, is a key enzyme for synthesizing DNA and RNA, among other biochemicals. Its presence in diminishing amounts in red blood cells is taken for a possible sign of thiamine deficiency.

The RDA of thiamine is only 1.2 mg for an adult male and 1.1 mg for females. Three scrambled eggs provide just 0.1 mg, the same amount you get from a cup of plain yogurt, about 4 ounces of cooked brown rice, or one slice of beef liver. Thiamine tends to be in lots of foods in tiny amounts.

B2 (riboflavin) is involved in the metabolism of food (carbs, protein, and fats), as well as in the formation of other B vitamins such as niacin into their corresponding coenzymes.

B2 is an integral part of a coenzyme that assists glutathione, for example, one of the body's major built-in antioxidants.[32]

Similar to B1, the riboflavin RDA is 1.3 mg for adult males and 1.1 mg for females 19 and older. An apple (0.1 mg), a small Atlantic salmon filet (0.7 mg), and a hard-boiled egg (0.3 mg) get you most of the way there, according to NutritionData.

Niacin (B3) is also known as nicotinic acid, but it has no relation to the nicotine in cigarettes.[33]

Severe deficiency in B3 vitamins can cause *pellagra*, a disease whose name may be derived from the Italian words for "rough skin."

Pellagra is considered the disease of the four Ds: dermatitis, diarrhea, dementia, and death. As explained in Frances R. Frankenburg's book Vitamin Discoveries and Disasters, *once the Europeans imported maize, or corn, from North America, pellagra began to spread in Europe. Maize is a cheap source of calories, but not of good nutrition; the niacin (B3) is bound and not absorbed unless the corn is soaked in limewater or another alkaline solution—a process called nixtamalization—as is done to make Mexican tortillas. The preColumbian and preHispanic populations of the Americas did not have the same problems, because they knew how to mix corn with other foods.*

The liver can also synthesize B3 from the amino acid tryptophan (an amino acid is a building block for proteins), but it takes a lot of tryptophan (60 mg) to make 1 mg of B3. As an amino acid, tryptophan is a component of good protein sources like turkey, salmon, eggs, and whey protein. For example, half a filet of salmon will give you about 450 mg of tryptophan (along with many other amino acids).

The RDA for niacin is 16 mg per day for an adult male, and 14 mg for a female. That tasty filet of salmon will give you about 14 mg of niacin alone: other good sources include a 6-ounce serving of chicken breast (almost 20 mg), turkey (a little less than chicken), half a can of tuna (about 5 mg), and an avocado (about 3 mg).

Vitamin B5, or *pantothenic acid,* is essential for all forms of life, due to its conversion to coenzyme A (CoA).[34] CoA is a cog in a central metabolic pathway of biology called the Krebs or citric acid cycle, by which cells generate energy from food sources.

The adequate intake (AI) for pantothenic acid, since it doesn't have an RDA, is 5 mg per day for adults. You can get vitamin B5 pretty easily from foods: a

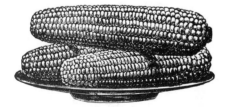

Maize is a cheap source of calories, but not of good nutrition.

small piece of wild Atlantic salmon has 3 mg, half a chicken breast has about 1 mg, and a California avocado has 2 mg.

Vitamin B6 is a coenzyme for glycogen phosphorylase, an enzyme involved in the cleaving of glucose from glycogen (the way the body stores starch in the muscles).

Glycogen is a long chain of glucose molecules. When your muscles need energy (you're standing up now, right?), the muscle cells look to acquire it from glycogen, which is like their own food pantry.

The muscles also have their own stored fats, from which they derive a substantial amount of their fuel. Interestingly, the fats inside muscles store more energy in calories than the total amount of glycogen that your body stores.

The chain of glucose molecules that make up glycogen has to be broken up into the separate pieces of glucose so that cells can use the latter for energy (see Chapter 3).

Coenzymes are like an enzyme's essential assistant; they bind with the enzyme and are a part of the chemical reactions that enzymes initiate.

B6 is also a coenzyme in the production of glucose or fuel from protein, a pivotal metabolic process called *gluconeogenesis*. Reactions that are dependent on B6 are also involved in the nervous system, such as generating serotonin from the amino acid tryptophan, and synthesizing the neurotransmitters dopamine and norepinephrine.[35]

Vitamin B7 (biotin) is also an enzyme cofactor.[36] Remember that scene from *Rocky* when Rocky Balboa chugged the raw eggs before heading off on another Philadelphia jaunt? Well, think twice. Raw egg whites contain a chemical called avidin that binds to biotin, prevents its absorption, and can lead to biotin deficiency.[37]

The AI for biotin or B7 is 30 mcg per day for an adult.

Folates are the form of *vitamin B9* found in food, while *folic acid* is the synthetic form found in supplements and fortified foods.

The U.S. government has required breads, cereals, flours, corn meals, pastas, rice, and other grain products to be fortified with folic acid since 1996, because people eat these foods in large amounts, and the grains are poor natural B9 sources. The RDAs for B9 are based on a term called *dietary folate equivalent* (DFE).

According to the NIH fact sheet for folate, "DFE accounts for the easier absorption of folate in supplements and fortified foods compared with folic acid found naturally in foods, which is absorbed only about half as well. One DFE = 1 microgram food folate, which = 0.6 microgram folic acid from supplements and fortified foods."[38] So, the DFEs are 600 mcg per day for

In biochemistry, the niacin coenzymes NAD and NADP play central roles in the metabolism of macronutrients (carbs, protein, and fats), as well as in the reactions involving the synthesis of molecules such as cholesterol and fatty acids.

pregnant women, 500 mcg for lactating women, and 400 mcg per day for adult men and other women.

Broccoli, asparagus, and spinach are good sources of folates, along with the fortified breads and other foods. For example, only eight spears of boiled asparagus will give you about 180 mcg of B9, and a pretty big spinach salad or two hard-boiled eggs provides about the same. Two tablespoons of salt-less peanut butter only give you about 24 mcg of B9.

> *Which is better for B vitamins, a grass-fed or non-grass-fed beef steak? A quick search on NutritionData shows that a similar gram-weight of grass-fed steak has more niacin, folates, B6, and pantothenic acid, sometimes by a magnitude of two or three, than the other steak (http://nutritiondata.self.com/facts/beef-products/10525/2). The exception is B12: both are good B12 sources, and the conventional steak provides almost all you need.*

Vitamin B12 is a cofactor for several enzymes. These include molecules that help synthesize DNA and build hemoglobin, which carries oxygen in the blood throughout the body. This is why B12 deficiencies can lead to anemia, an inadequate number of red blood cells.

Vitamin B12 is mostly found in animal products like fish (including good sources like shellfish), beef, turkey, and chicken, as well as dairy products like eggs, milk, and cheese. Plant foods do not contain B12, so vegetarians have to obtain it by eating dairy products or with supplements. Two pastured eggs, hard-boiled, and a cup of whole milk will get you all the way there.

The RDAs for B12 are 2.4 mcg for adults, and a bit more for pregnant or lactating moms.[39]

Vitamin C

Also called *ascorbic acid*, this vitamin from fresh fruits and veggies is pivotal for many reasons, which is why you were harangued so much as a child to eat your apples and drink your OJ. For one, it is essential for synthesizing the protein-containing structural component of ligaments, bones, tendons, and blood vessels called collagen (see the accompanying sidebar on vitamin C).

The body also uses vitamin C "as a cofactor for catecholamine biosynthesis, in particular the conversion of dopamine to [the neurotransmitter] norepineph-rine," according to an article in the *American Journal of Clinical Nutrition*.[40]

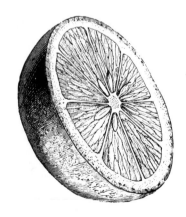

Vitamin C is a powerful aqueous-based antioxidant. It helps mop up the reactive oxygen species in the watery parts of cells. It also helps recharge vitamin E after that vitamin has neutralized oxidative stress in the fatty parts of cells, such as their membranes.

Vitamin C deficiency is infamous for causing scurvy, a potentially fatal disease that beset British sailors in the 17th and 18th centuries, and it still rears its ugly head in the modern world.

VITAMIN C: HELPS KEEP YOUR TISSUES AND FAT-BURNING CAPABILITIES INTACT

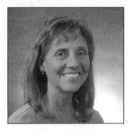

"I love vitamin C, it's so interesting, and totally unappreciated," Carol Johnston, a Ph.D., nutrition professor, and vitamin C researcher at Arizona State University in Phoenix, confided one afternoon in late September 2011. "Vitamin D gets all the press right now, but here we have a major vitamin C issue going on."

She was talking about some National Health and Nutrition Examination Survey (NHANES) data from 2004 that showed 31 percent of Americans to be either *scorbutic* (with vitamin C blood levels indicating scurvy) or with "marginal vitamin C status" (meaning that "your body tissues are not operating optimally because there is too little of vitamin C there for optimal pathways and metabolism").

She had me convinced; vitamin C is perhaps "the new vitamin D," in terms of the attention we should be paying it.

Vitamin C must be present to produce collagen, the super-strong connective tissue protein in tendons, cartilage, bone, and blood vessels. However, collagen has an important immune system role as well, according to Johnston. "We have defense collagens, little toll-like receptors on immune cells that actually recognize pathogens," Johnston explained. People who are deficient in vitamin C (up to a third of Americans) have a "marginalized ability to stay infection free."

Vitamin C is also a cofactor for making carnitine, a pivotal protein that shuttles fatty acids into the cells mitochondria to be burned for energy. "Some of the fatigue associated with early marginal C status could be related to carnitine [depletion]," Johnston said, because your metabolic system for using fats for energy is compromised.

The fatigue "could [also] be related to norepinephrin," she said. "No one's really looked at that" from a scientific research standpoint. Vitamin C is necessary for the production of norepinephrine, which the adrenal glands release as part of the fight or flight response. It's also a neurotransmitter that affects how the heart contracts.

The typical adult stores about 1,500 mg of vitamin C in her body, according to Johnston, mostly in the liver and adrenal glands.

What about *bioavailability*? Are you getting as much vitamin C to your tissues as you think you are? "Some nutrients are more stable than C, C is fragile," Johnston said. "I think the nutrient composition tables overestimate vitamin C intakes by what we consider to be significant margins."

And what about the *mega doses* some people shoot for, such as 40–50 times the RDA for C? "Vitamin C requires a transporter and you can saturate that pretty quickly," Johnston explained. "When you start taking over 200–500 mg you are really decreasing the amount you can absorb. I don't see a lot of benefit in consuming those high doses if you want to maximize tissue storage. You really need to take small amounts over the course of a day." For example, you might take 200 mg two or three times per day—if you think you need that dose.

The bottom line is just, "keep eating those fresh fruits and veggies."

During the 1941 siege of Leningrad in World War II, an epidemic of scurvy swept through Russian civilians, who'd been given only bread rations. Pine needles boiled in water (pine needle tea) helped stave it off, as pine needles are rich in vitamin C.[41]

The RDA for vitamin C is 90 mg per day for male adults and 75 mg for females, but supplements as well as fruits and veggies typically provide the body with far more than that amount. For children aged four and older, the

RDA rises incrementally from 25 mg to about 75 mg per day. Apples provide about 10 mg each, oranges about 68 mg, and a cup of lemon sections more than 100 mg, according to NutritionData.

I've taken to eating lemons raw or adding raw sections to smoothies, because they are very high in vitamin C and low in fructose (see Chapter 3 for a note on fructose) compared to a typical sweet apple.

A medium-sized apple contains almost 11 grams of fructose (and 8.4 mg of vitamin C), compared with a medium lemon (less than 1.5 grams of fructose and about 31 mg of vitamin C).

If you munched a clump of raw broccoli in a salad (however torturous that may sound to some), you'd derive about 66 mg of C, according to NutritionData.

Minerals

Essential minerals are inorganic substances from the earth that must be provided by the diet. They include calcium, phosphorus (phosphates), magnesium, sulfur, sodium chloride (salt), and potassium, as well as the "trace" minerals of which fewer milligrams are required per day. These include iron, zinc, copper, manganese, iodine, selenium, fluoride, molybdenum, and chromium.

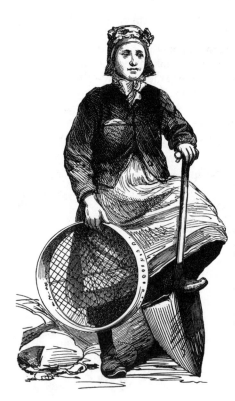

You can get minerals from your MVM supplement, as well as from both food and beverages. For example, drinking water from streams or aquifers (e.g., a commercial mineral water) could provide some of the minerals needed by your body.

The adequacy of the minerals you derive from food is directly related to the mineral richness of the soil the food was grown in. This is why we included a chapter in this book on the filial loyalty you should display toward all your local farms. Some processed foods are also fortified with minerals, such as bread fortified with iron or orange juice with calcium.

A whole-foods diet dominated by local vegetables and fruits that are in season or frozen at their peak of freshness, as well as healthy meats and cheeses, should provide many of the minerals you require in adequate amounts.

Minerals, like vitamins, play numerous roles in the body that belie the quantities consumed. Many minerals are constituents of life-giving molecules, like the iron in hemoglobin (red blood cells), which transports oxygen throughout the body; the phosphorus that is a part of adenosine triphosphate (ATP), which is the form of energy that our cells use; and the iodine that the thyroid gland uses to make thyroid hormone.

Chapter 4

Macrominerals

These are the major minerals that are required in the body in quantities of about 100 milligrams or more per day: calcium, phosphorus (phosphates), magnesium, sulfur, sodium chloride (salt), and potassium.

Calcium

About four percent of the body's weight is made up of minerals, with three quarters of that amount in calcium and phosphorus.[42] The vast majority of calcium resides in the bones and teeth, but calcium also plays a critical role in the extracellular fluid, among other places. Along with other biochemicals, calcium affects the permeability of cell membranes during the exchange of substances like oxygen, nutrients, and metabolic waste products.

Calcium's function is so important in the extracellular fluid that if you don't have enough calcium in your bodily fluids, the body will free up calcium from your bones, or "demineralize" them. This is why it is important to get enough calcium in your diet.

Vitamin D and calcium work together

Once the body senses a calcium deficit, it releases parathyroid hormone, which signals the kidneys to produce more of the active form of vitamin D. The active form of vitamin D, *calcitriol*, stimulates the absorption of calcium from any food in the small intestine, as well as the demineralization of bone if the latter source is inadequate. You can see how vitamin D and calcium work together.

Adults and adolescents should get about 1,000 to 1,300 mg per day of calcium (the RDA for pregnant and lactating moms over 18 years of age is 1,000 mg). Good sources of calcium are dairy (milk, cheese, and yogurt), as well as green vegetables like spinach and Swiss chard.

However, vegetables such as spinach, while containing a lot of calcium, also contain large amounts of oxalic acid, which can bind with and prevent the absorption of calcium. (See the upcoming sidebar "Going Against the Grains: Plants Contain Antinutrients.") Cooking breaks down the oxalates, which generally do not prevent the absorption of calcium from other foods you are eating at the same time, like cheese or yogurt.

Magnesium

Magnesium is required by the chemical reactions that make ATP, our primary energy currency, in the mitochondria of cells, according to the Linus Pauling Institute (*http://lpi.oregonstate.edu/infocenter/minerals/magnesium/*). The adult human body includes about 25 grams of magnesium, mostly in bones.

The synthesis of glutathione, a natural antioxidant in the body, requires magnesium. Magnesium also plays a structural role in bone, cell membranes, and chromosomes, according to LPI. And it goes on and on. Obviously, you have to get enough magnesium in your diet.

The magnesium RDA for males (i.e., the minimum amount you should get, give, or take) is 420 mg per day, and for females it's 320 mg per day. According to NutritionData, here are some examples of common magnesium sources:

- 2 cups coffee: 14.2 mg
- 2 squares baking chocolate: 190 mg
- 8 ounces grass-fed ground beef: 38 mg
- 8 ounces whole milk: 24.4 mg
- 1 cup spinach: 23.7 mg
- 1 cup Swiss chard: 150 mg
- 5–6 ounce filet of haddock: 75 mg
- 2 ounces cheddar: 15.6
- 2 Florida oranges: 28.2 mg

Cacao, a good source of which is high-cacao chocolate, is a rich source of magnesium. The surprising sources to me were chard and haddock, providing about half of all you would need in a day. Oranges are also a surprisingly good small source.

This exercise is also a good indication that you can derive your nutrition from commonly eaten whole foods, which obviously contain far more vitamins, minerals, and phytochemicals than just magnesium.

Phosphorus

Phosphorus is another major nutrient for your bones; about 85 percent of this mineral in the body is found there. A phosphates-and fatty acid–containing structure called *phospholipids* is a principal component of all body cell membranes. Last but not least, the primary energy currency of the body, a molecule called adenosine triphosphate (ATP), also contains this mineral, as do DNA and RNA, which are long chains of phosphate-containing molecules.[43]

Phosphorus has the same interaction with vitamin D as calcium when the body detects blood levels falling beneath a certain level. Parathyroid hormone sends the message to increase the generation of the active form of vitamin D in the kidneys, which in turn increases the amount of phosphates (and calcium) absorbed from the intestines.

People generally get enough phosphorus in their diets, which unfortunately includes the burden of food additives that contain phosphates. The RDA for phosphorus is about 700 mg per day for adults and 1,250 mg for children between 9 and 18 years old. Good natural sources (nonfood additives) of phosphorus are milk, yogurt, cheese, eggs, meat, and fish.[44] A vegan, however, eschewing both meat and dairy products, may have trouble getting enough phosphorus in her diet.

Potassium

People should generally keep their potassium to sodium (or salt) intake ratio at about 4 to 1. In other words, you should get about four times as many milligrams of potassium as salt. Researchers have pointed out that we're ultimately designed to have a high potassium-to-sodium ratio in our diet, and recent studies have underlined this point.

"Americans who eat a diet high in sodium and low in potassium have a 50 percent increased risk of death from any cause, and about twice the risk of death from heart attacks," according to a study published in July 2011 in the *Archives of Internal Medicine*.[45]

Here's a good list of useful potassium food sources with great potassium-to-sodium ratios:

- Medium-sized kiwi: 237:2
- 5–6 ounces salmon: 967:86
- One large stalk cooked broccoli: 820:115
- 4 ounces grass-fed ground bison: 353:76
- Medium-sized lemon: 80:1
- One cup raw spinach: 167:24
- California avocado: 689 mg:11
- One cup raspberries: 186:1
- One cup cherry tomatoes: 147:3
- One cup blueberries: 114:1
- One medium-sized banana: 422 mg:1

In other words, a small piece of wild salmon gives you about 1,000 mg (or 1 gram) of potassium, and confers a potassium-to-sodium ratio of more than 10:1.

So what does potassium do? The concentration of potassium inside a cell is about 10 times the concentration outside, and for sodium the ratio is reversed (other sources have different estimates for this concentration).[46] This creates a conveyor belt or "ion pump" across cellular membranes, a gradient that enables the basic machinery throughout the body: nerve cell signals, muscle contractions, the heart's cardiac output, as well as the transport of glucose fuel, for example, from outside to inside the cell.

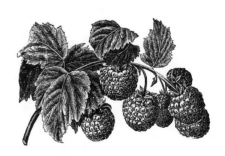

An endurance athlete can run dangerously low on potassium, and this is partly what causes any muscle spasms and cramps.

Adults require about 4,700 mg per day of potassium (children less than 14 years old need 3,000–4,500 mg per day). It is relatively easy to derive your necessary potassium from a whole foods diet, as the above list shows.

Sodium chloride (salt)

Along with potassium, salt makes up the *sodium-potassium pump* that is a basic part of cellular mechanisms (e.g., nerve transmission and muscle contraction).

You should consume less salt than potassium, at a ratio of about 4 to 1 in potassium's favor (see "Potassium").

Although conventional wisdom blames excess salt for high blood pressure and other problems, and most people on the Standard American Diet (SAD; note the pejorative expression) consume a lot of salt in their processed foods, it is still an essential mineral in physiology.

People have become sick and even died during long endurance contests by excessively diluting the salt content of their bodies with chronic excessive hydration (a condition known as *hyponatremia*). Even some of the best endurance athletes, marathoners, and long-distance triathletes have arrived at the finish line so depleted that they have to immediately receive an intravenous saline or sodium-chloride solution.

Along with potassium, salt is one of the important electrolytes of the body.

That said, it is easy to derive enough salt from whole nutritious foods (pastured eggs, high-quality cheeses, large salads, an electrolyte drink during a triathlon) without ever dusting your food with table salt.

Sulfur

The amino acids cysteine and methionine (two of the building blocks of proteins) contain most of the sulfur that the body uses. Therefore, if you're getting enough protein in your diet, you should be getting enough of the mineral sulfur.

Trace Minerals

Trace minerals are the minerals that we have to consume in our diet, drinking water, and/or a supplement in relatively small amounts. That's not to say they are unimportant, though; see the upcoming sidebar on zinc and *antinutrients*, for example, or consider that iron represents the "heme" part of hemoglobin, our red blood cells that carry oxygen, and that selenium is a major antioxidant in the body.

Like the macrominerals, the microminerals include common elements that you will recognize from the periodic table (if you ever paid attention in Chemistry class). We're just going to list the microminerals here, with helpful links for more details. The recommended levels for them range from around 10 milligrams to levels in the micrograms (1/1000 of a milligram, as in 55 mcg per day of selenium).

Copper

The RDA for this mineral is 890 to 900 mcg per day (*www.nlm.nih.gov/ medlineplus/ency/article/002419.htm*).

Iodine

The RDA for this mineral is 150 mcg per day for adults (*http://ods.od.nih. gov/factsheets/Iodine/*).

Iron

The RDA for this mineral is 8 mg per day for males and 18 mg/day for adult females (*http://ods.od.nih.gov/factsheets/iron/*).

Manganese

The AI level for this mineral is 2.3 mg/day for adult males, and 1.8 mg for females (*http://lpi.oregonstate.edu/infocenter/minerals/manganese/*).

Molybdenum

The RDA for this mineral is 45 mcg per day for adults (*http://lpi.oregon-state.edu/infocenter/minerals/molybdenum/*).

Selenium

The RDA for selenium is 55 mcg for adults, 60 mcg for pregnant women, and 70 mcg for lactating moms (*http://ods.od.nih.gov/factsheets/selenium/*).

Zinc

The RDA for zinc is 11 mg for adult males and 8 mg/day for females (*http://ods.od.nih.gov/factsheets/Zinc-QuickFacts*).

Okay, now you can take a deep breath. We're finished with the vitamins/ minerals, for the most part (but *you* shouldn't be). Following is a description of various web tools that you can use to manage your micronutrients.

GOING AGAINST THE GRAINS: PLANTS CONTAIN "ANTINUTRIENTS"

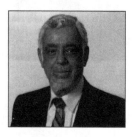

Despite their mute passivity, plants don't really want to be eaten. They don't have claws or teeth (at least most of them don't) and they can't run away as predators pursue them. In compensation, however, wheat, oats, rice, soy beans, various nuts, and many veggies like spinach are laden with chemicals scientists have labeled *antinutrients*. These phytochemicals are meant to help the plants play tough defense—i.e., to make them unpalatable to herbivores (like us).

Antinutrients are "compounds that prevent nutrients (e.g., minerals and proteins) from either being absorbed or utilized," according to Dr. Venket Rao, a professor with the Department of Nutritional Sciences at the University of Toronto who did some of the original research on these food chemicals several decades ago.

A cautionary event that placed antinutrients on the nutritional map was an "epidemic of dwarfism" in the 1960s in Egypt, Iran, and Turkey. It was caused by a poisonous combination of too much unleavened bread, like pita, and a lack of meats to provide the lost zinc.

Phytates, or phytic acid, in the bread bind with zinc in our digestive tracts and prevent the mineral's absorption. They also bind with iron and calcium. The unleavened bread (the leavening process breaks up the phytates) "caused massive zinc deficiencies," according to Rao. "Zinc is essential for growth."

Zinc supplements cured the epidemic, but the outbreak showed how insidious phytates and other antinutrients could be when consumed in a diet that lacks micronutrients from varied sources.

Soybeans contain antinutrients called *lectins*, which prevent carbohydrate utilization; *saponins*, a natural soapy substance that the plant uses as part of its own immunity against invading organisms; as well as a class of toxin called *protease inhibitors*.

Saponins can wipe out red blood cells if they come in contact with the blood system, rupturing the cell membranes in a very bad event called *hemolysis*.

Protease enzymes like trypsin are essential enzymes for the digestion of protein; therefore, consuming protease inhibitors in excessive amounts will deplete the amount of protein you can metabolize.

I asked Professor Rao about oxalic acid, which both raw spinach and dark chocolate contain (both of which I happened to have munched that day). "Oxalic acid binds to calcium, iron, and magnesium," he said. "Are you a coffee drinker?" (Oh, oh). Caffeic acid from too much joe will cause you to pee out excessive amounts of calcium.

On balance, the phytochemicals, which is a broad term that includes the specified antinutrients, are very good for us (see the "Antioxidants: Cultivate Your Inner Nerf" sidebar). Instead of consuming bushels of raw spinach and barrels of joe, keep your diet varied, mixed, and sensible. For example, I also asked Rao about someone who drinks soy milk every day because he doesn't get along with cow's milk (i.e., he is lactose intolerant). "Drinking one glass of soy milk on a daily basis does not pose any problem. The levels of the phytochemicals will not be too high."

"Many phytochemicals, vitamins, and minerals have deficient levels of intake, optimal levels, and doses that may not be good for you," Rao added.

Soaked, fermented, and sprouted foods involve preparations that will help remove most of the antinutrients. In fact, it's worth it to do a little research by Googling "sprouted and fermented foods." For example, here is an informative post from the excellent Whole Health Source blog: *http://wholehealthsource. blogspot.com/2009/01/how-to-eat-grains.html*.

Getting Micronutrient Information Online: Web Tools

The Web is organic and abounds with new tools for analyzing diet, exercise, and other aspects of health. We're going to discuss a couple of easy reference-oriented tools, meaning there's little busy-work involved in jumping in and finding out what you need. You might want to keep up with the new apps, which have their own approaches and philosophies. Here's a link tagged with "food" from Quantified Self: *http://quantifiedself.com/guide/tag/food*.

NutritionData

This indispensable tool is a user-friendly wrapper over the spartan but data-rich USDA National Nutrient Database (discussed momentarily, and in Chapter 2). Just search on any food, and you get a wealth of information on its protein, fat, and carbohydrate content (the macronutrients), along with very detailed information on micronutrients (vitamins and minerals). Figure 4-3 shows a browser window after a search on sweet potatoes.

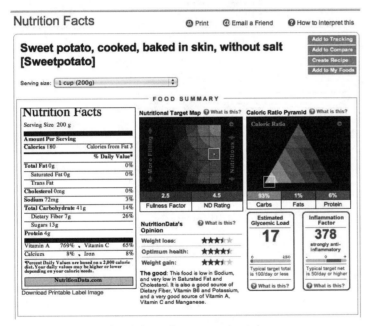

Figure 4-3. *Nutrition data information on sweet potatoes*

Just scroll down to the Vitamins or Minerals segments of this page and click on the More Details widget, and you'll likely discover many gems that you never knew before. For example, did you know that a large sweet potato contains about 1,922 micrograms of RAE for vitamin A? If you've already read the section on vitamin A, you know what an RAE is!

You can also reveal gaping holes in the nutrition department, as shown in Figure 4-4. This browser window shows the Vitamins frame of a NutritionData page after a search on Reese's Pieces. Not much there, but there are almost 15 grams of simple sugar in a 1-ounce portion of the candy.

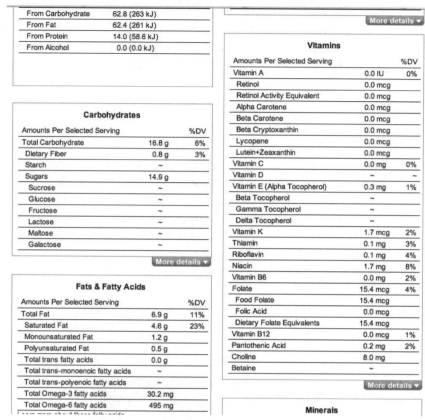

Figure 4-4. *Not many vitamins in an ounce of candy, but, no surprise, plenty of sugar*

See Chapter 2 for more details on NutritionData.

FitDay on Vending-Machine Fare

Although presented as a weight-loss and dieting site, FitDay (*www.fitday.com*) is a very useful tool for entering your foods for the day and finding out the associated micronutrient content, or lack thereof.

As a way of demonstrating how you can derive a vitamin and mineral profile for junk food—sorry, *treats*—from a vending machine and a fast-food joint, let's enter these foods into FitDay and see what results the software displays.

Imagine you start off the day with a 12-ounce take-out coffee for breakfast; then later on you raid the vending machine for peanut butter crackers, some potato chips, and a package of Reese's Pieces, which you mercifully leave only partially consumed. All this is washed down with a can of Red Bull. Finally, you top off the late afternoon by visiting the local fast food emporium and leaving with a Double Whopper and fries, with a vanilla shake in tow.

Figure 4-5 shows this fearsome lineup, as entered in FitDay.

Considering that only the bottom three items even remotely resemble an edible meal, one of the many data points that leaps off the page and begs for your attention is the calorie total: more than 3,000. The problem is that this chow-down represents a person's consumption for only part of the day.

Food Name	Amount	Unit	Cals	Fat (g)	Carbs (g)
		Total	**3,070**	**171.4**	**294.4**
Coffee, regular	2	coffee cup (6 fl oz)	4	0.1	0.1
Crackers, wheat, sandwich, with peanut butter filling	3	oz	422	22.7	45.8
Snacks, potato chips, plain, made with partially hydrogenate...	2	oz	304	19.6	30.0
Reese's Pieces	0.5	package (1.95 oz)	137	6.8	16.5
Red Bull Energy Drink	1	can	112	0.2	27.2
BURGER KING, French Fries	1	large serving	530	27.8	64.1
BURGER KING, DOUBLE WHOPPER, with cheese	1	item	1,061	68.1	53.9
BURGER KING, Vanilla Shake	1	small 12 fl oz	501	26.0	56.7
		Total	**3,070**	**171.4**	**294.4**

Figure 4-5. A FitDay.com breakdown of typical fast-food fare

A mere 3 ounces of wheat crackers with peanut butter filling packs a pretty good wallop at 422 calories, considering that this snack is just a prelude for the heavy hitters that come afterward.

The table shows a lot of fat here, but it's the type of fat that counts, as explained in Chapter 3. For example, the coconut milk that is part of a smoothie will tip the fat scale on FitDay, but this nutritious snack contains a portion of its fats in the form of lauric acid (which is a component of human breast milk).

More of the bad to middling news comes on the Nutrition tab, which you can click on at the bottom of the page. Figure 4-6 shows this revealing table, indicating that the substances you gobbled up and guzzled down bore little resemblance to the food our forebears sustained themselves on.

Calories	Nutrition	%-RDA/AI Graph	Cal. Balance	Custom Nutrition Goals

			RDA	% RDA				RDA	% RDA				RDA	% RDA
Vitamin A	0.0	mcg	900.0	0	Calcium	853.2	mg	1,200.0	71	Pant. Acid	8.4	mg	5.0	169
Vitamin A	0.0	IU	--	--	Cholesterol	279.9	mg	--	--	Phosphorus	1,485.2	mg	700.0	212
Vitamin B6	3.4	mg	1.7	201	Copper	1.5	mg	0.9	163	Potassium	3,216.9	mg	4,700.0	68
Vitamin B12	5.5	mcg	2.4	228	Iron	27.9	mg	8.0	349	Riboflav	3.5	mg	1.3	271
Vitamin C	19.6	mg	90.0	22	Magnesium	272.6	mg	420.0	65	Selenium	103.2	mcg	55.0	188
Vitamin D	0.0		10.0	0	Manganese	2.4	mg	2.3	103	Sodium	3,864.5	mg	1,300.0	297
Vitamin D	0.0		--	--	Niacin	46.7	mg	16.0	292	Thiamin	1.9	mg	1.2	160
Vitamin E	2.7	mg	15.0	18						Water	1,050.5	g	--	--
Vitamin E	4.1	IU	--	--						Zinc	19.4	mg	11.0	177

Description

This table lists your average daily intake for all nutrients. If a nutrient has an RDA (recommended dietary allowance) or AI (adequate intake) then the intake as a percentage of RDA/AI is displayed in the % RDA column.

More Info

- Set a Nutrient Goal
- Long-Term Nutrition Report

Figure 4-6. *Vitamins are no-shows in a FitDay profile*

The meal contains no vitamin A or D, and just enough C to perhaps prevent scurvy (but not for long). The table shows the RDA for each nutrient and the % RDA represented by the analyzed food. For example, the 201 adjacent to vitamin B6 indicates that the food contained about twice the recommended daily minimum amount of that nutrient. Deficits for a nutrient appear in red; it's all pretty simple to read and understand.

> *The good mineral profile here undoubtedly derives from the meat in the Double Whopper. This industrially mass-produced meat is far from a one-sided picture, however, as we saw in Chapter 3. For example, the meat probably came from a concentrated animal feeding operation (CAFO), and is not as healthy, to say the least, as meat from grazing animals that might be pastured near your town or city.*

This motley collection of packaged chow contained just a fragment of the necessary vitamin E, which, along with the dearth of vitamin C, leaves you with few antioxidants to clean up after the day's stresses (except for the selenium).

A diet like this will leave the body quivering and inflamed, given that the "fake" food contained almost zero phytochemicals with their associated antioxidants (see the "Antioxidants: Cultivate Your Inner Nerf" sidebar.) This means that some of the cellular damage, including of DNA, goes unchecked throughout the day.

The "meal" contained almost 1,200 calories' worth of carbs, many of which were represented by simple sugars like sucrose and fructose, jacking up the inflammatory effects of an excess sugar load.

Needs work: Potassium to sodium ratio

Another piece of data worth mentioning is the potassium to sodium ratio. Instead of the desirable ratio of about 4 to 1, this ratio was more like 0.84 to 1; in other words, the vending machine grazer is getting much more sodium than potassium, which has potentially dire effects down the road (see the "Potassium" section earlier in this chapter).

Of course, the point of this tongue-in-cheek exercise (no one really eats like this, right? Honest?) is to show FitDay's useful, revealing, and sometimes sobering metrics when it comes to micronutrients. Once you get over the tedium of entering foods, the tool is fun to play with, and it gives you a precise enough micronutrient picture of your current food intake. It doesn't deal with bioavailability (what quantities of these food nutrients actually make their way out of the gastrointestinal tract and to the body's target tissues), so you can only use tables like these for general guidance.

See Chapter 2 for more details on FitDay.

USDA National Nutrient Database

The search widget at *www.nal.usda.gov/fnic/foodcomp/search/* is the updated source of nutrition and food data that other tools, such as NutritionData (*www.nutritiondata.com*), use as an underlying data source. This database allows a simple search on terms like the name of a food or vitamin, as Figure 4-7 shows.

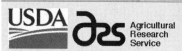

Search the USDA National Nutrient Database for Standard Reference

Enter up to 5 keywords which best describe the food item. To further limit the search, select a specific Food Group.

Certain codes can also be searched: NDB number (the USDA 5-digit Nutrient Databank identifier); the USDA commodity code; and the URMIS number for specific cuts of meat (enter the # symbol followed without a space by the URMIS code).

Keyword(s):   blueberries   Help
Select Food Group: All Food Groups
Submit

To view reports on foods by single nutrients, such as calcium or niacin, go to Nutrient Lists.

Use these links to access SR23 datasets or SR23 documentation.

Home   How to get information

Figure 4-7. *Up-to-date information on blueberries*

If you enter a certain food in the search space, the USDA nutrient database fires back a full page of data on that food's nutrient content, including carbs, fats, protein, vitamins, and minerals. The information is presented in a simple HTML table but has impressive detail, as Figure 4-8 shows.

The USDA site also has a large archive of PDF reports on single nutrients: *www.ars.usda.gov/Services/docs.htm?docid=20958*. In addition, the entire database is downloadable itself. See Chapter 2 for more details on the USDA National Nutrient Database.

Linus Pauling Institute Micronutrient Information Center

The LPI MIC (*http://lpi.oregonstate.edu/infocenter/*) has a wealth of useful information, including podcasts, comprehensive descriptions, and physiological background on individual micronutrients.

Nutrient	Units	Value per 100 grams	Number of Data Points	Std. Error
Proximates				
Water	g	84.21	12	0.672
Energy	kcal	57	0	0.000
Energy	kJ	240	0	0.000
Protein	g	0.74	12	0.019
Total lipid (fat)	g	0.33	12	0.018
Ash	g	0.24	12	0.005
Carbohydrate, by difference	g	14.49	0	0.000
Fiber, total dietary	g	2.4	4	0.124
Sugars, total	g	9.96	8	0.550
Sucrose	g	0.11	8	0.000
Glucose (dextrose)	g	4.88	8	0.275
Fructose	g	4.97	8	0.276
Lactose	g	0.00	8	0.000
Maltose	g	0.00	8	0.000
Galactose	g	0.00	8	0.000
Starch	g	0.03	4	0.027
Minerals				
Calcium, Ca	mg	6	12	0.785
Iron, Fe	mg	0.28	12	0.011
Magnesium, Mg	mg	6	12	0.197
Phosphorus, P	mg	12	12	0.508
Potassium, K	mg	77	6	5.450
Sodium, Na	mg	1	6	0.353
Zinc, Zn	mg	0.16	12	0.017
Copper, Cu	mg	0.057	12	0.014
Manganese, Mn	mg	0.336	8	0.028
Selenium, Se	mcg	0.1	2	0.000
Vitamins				
Vitamin C, total ascorbic acid	mg	9.7	4	0.890
Thiamin	mg	0.037	12	0.006
Riboflavin	mg	0.041	12	0.000
Niacin	mg	0.418	12	0.089

Figure 4-8. *Everything you wanted to know about chowing raw blueberries*

USDA Interactive Calculator

The USDA also has a handy calculator for estimating vitamin and mineral daily needs, based on your gender, height, and weight. Figure 4-9 shows the calculator's front page, found at *http://fnic.nal.usda.gov/interactiveDRI/*.

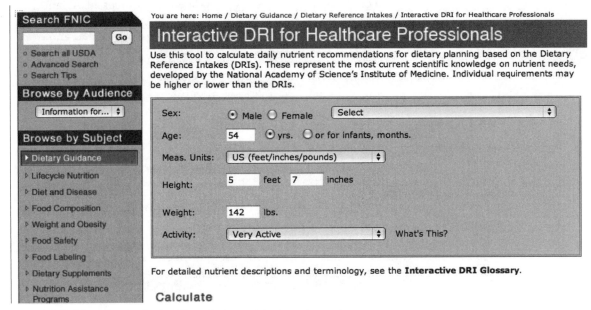

Figure 4-9. *Quick customized calculation of micronutrient requirements*

As an example of just drilling down to a few data points, I wanted to look at my own requirements for vitamins C and E, as well as for the mineral zinc. Figure 4-10 shows the result. This is a very good little calculator for checking the mineral content of an MVM supplement, for example.

National Institutes of Health, Office of Dietary Supplements Factsheets

Although still incomplete (they only cover, for the most part, vitamins), the NIH factsheets at *http://ods.od.nih.gov/factsheets/list-all/* contain all the necessary data on these micronutrients, including food sources, RDAs, and TULs.

You Entered:			
Male	Age: 54 yrs	Height: 5 ft. 7 in.	Weight: 142 lbs.
Very Active			
Results:			
Body Mass Index (BMI) is 22.3		Estimated Daily Caloric Needs: 3025 kcal/day	

• **About BMI**
Click on numbered footnote for more information.

Vitamins

Each reference value refers to *average daily nutrient intake*; day-to-day nutrient intakes may vary.

Vitamin	Recommended Intake per day	Tolerable UL Intake per day
Vitamin C	90 mg	2,000 mg
Vitamin E	15 mg	1,000 mg[1]

Click individual vitamin for fact sheet.
Click on numbered footnote for more information.

Minerals (Elements)

Each reference value refers to *average daily nutrient intake*; day-to-day nutrient intakes may vary.

Mineral	Recommended Intake per day	Tolerable UL Intake per day
Essential		
Zinc	11 mg	40 mg

Click individual mineral for fact sheet.
Click on numbered footnote for more information.

Figure 4-10. *Customized USDA calculator results*

SPORTS PERFORMANCE PROBABLY GETS A BOOST FROM VITAMIN D

Ever since the 1950s, when top German and Russian athletes were irradiated with ultraviolet light to boost their vitamin D levels, the European continent's scientific literature has shown that vitamin D biosynthesis and supplementation may provide a sports performance edge.

The active form of vitamin D is a secosteroid hormone that boosts athletic performance when the athlete is brought out of a D-deficient state, which probably applies to most athletes, according to Dr. John Cannell, the executive director of the Vitamin D Council. Cannell recently wrote a journal report based on the older European medical literature.

"Many of the papers came out of elite sports institutes run by Germans and Russians," according to Cannell, whose paper "Athletic Performance and Vitamin D" was published in 2009 in the journal *Medicine and Science In Sports and Exercise*. You can find it here: *www.ncbi.nlm.nih.gov/pubmed/19346976*.

"The higher the D level [they found in the athletes] the better their cardiovascular fitness."

The medical literature indicates that boosting vitamin D levels in athletes will improve speed, strength, balance, and timing; the athletes who can achieve optimal levels of 25-hydroxyvitamin D in their blood will have a better "choice reation time," according to Cannell.

Cannell told me in an email message that "lean body mass and strength are both increased with [better] D [levels in the body]," but that he did not know the exact physiological mechanism by which D exerted that effect.

"If you start with D-deficient athletes the effect is dramatic," Cannell said in a radio interview in August 2011. He views a 25-hydroxyvitamin D level of at least 50 ng/ml as optimal (higher than U.S. National Institutes of Health guidelines). "Most athletes are deficient" in vitamin D, Cannell speculates, since the typical tested person usually has a serum 25-hydroxyvitamin D level of far less than 50 ng/ml.

Most people require 5,000 IU per day of vitamin D3 to reach the 50-ng/ml level, according to Cannell. He "suspects that athletes need more than that" because of "metabolic clearance." A marathon runner or active cross-trainer is going to use up more vitamin D in her cells than a couch potato.

"Once you get over 50 ng/ml [in a person's test results] you start measuring some vitamin D (the inactive form that isn't typically tested for) in the blood, meaning the body has all the 25-hydroxyvitamin D it needs and is storing some for later use. It's also the level where pregnant women have [lots of] vitamin D in breast milk. It's often the level that lifeguards have, about 50 ng/ml."

Food Hacks: 5
Finding and Choosing Food

Before you get the wrong impression, this chapter will not be dominated by descriptions of power apps that go and find great healthy food for you. For this activity, we'll rely on the "wet app" that resides between our ears, and the accumulated wisdom that lives, metaphorically, somewhere in the vicinity of our solar plexus. The "gut feel," in other words.

> Sure, we'll mention a few food-choice apps later on, like Fooducate, GroceryIQ, and Restaurant Finder. You can find other food-shopping apps such as the ones that help with grocery lists at www.appbrain. com (see www.appbrain.com/search?q=food+shopping for a list of them), or www.apple.com/iphone/from-the-app-store/lifestyle.html for the iPhone.

The point is that a few rules of thumb, like "eat local, real food," or some of food author Michael Pollan's rules (summarized in the sidebar "Choice Food Rules from a Food Writer"), along with some well-known tips on managing a supermarket's tactics, will get you a longer way toward fitness than punching out choices on an app screen.

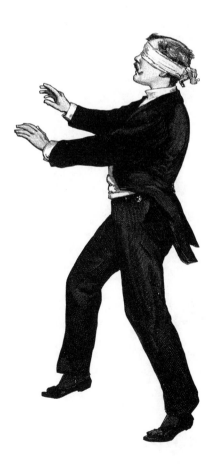

Ultimately, the best food app around would be the one that reads a label from your phone or recognizes a shape and simply spits out an accurate "Yes!" or "No!" But that one doesn't exist yet (Fooducate *does* represent a similar concept, though).

Eat Local: Leave the Big Boxes for the Extras

People apply a number of criteria when they seek food, including convenience, palatability ("It tastes good"), and cultural habit ("Mom always made me a PB&J for lunch, so that's what I'm going to make myself"). I'm going to add a fourth one: eating for fitness. This is a fitness book after all, and food is at least 50 percent of the game.

Our bodies have tens of trillions of cells, and millions of them turn over every day, even every second (your body makes millions of new red blood cells each day alone; the whole kit and caboodle of them turns over every four months!). In other words, you're constantly growing new parts of your body, specifically at the cellular level. Many of the ingredients for new cells, such as the fatty acids for cell membranes and the amino acids for new proteins (that go into everything, including the membranes), have to come from the foods you eat.

When done right, the eat-local strategy can take care of the first three criteria: convenience, taste, and habit.

There are also lots of environmental and energy-related reasons for eating local, and those certainly are legit. There are practical, even dystopian reasons too: what if the roads are washed out or destroyed by an extreme weather event, or there's a systemic collapse, and only locally produced or frozen food is available?

Eating local means for the most part *focusing on real food from farmer's markets, local farms, and even your own garden*. Then augment those purchases by getting other stuff (e.g., paper goods; big bags of rice; high-cacao chocolate bars; those avocados, kiwis, or lemons that aren't grown locally; or a glass container of OJ) at the big-box supermarket chains, if you choose to go to them at all.

Before you go ballistic and accuse me of hypocrisy (sure, I do patronize supermarkets once in a while—mea culpa), I do know people who get all their food from organic gardens, farms, and their own hunting.

This chapter also discusses:

- Navigating the shoals of the modern big-box supermarket

- Hacks for finding food when you are on the road

- Strategies for choosing food when you're on a really tight budget, which is the case for increasing numbers of us throughout the world

Eating local means for the most part focusing on real food from farmer's markets, local farms, and even your own garden.

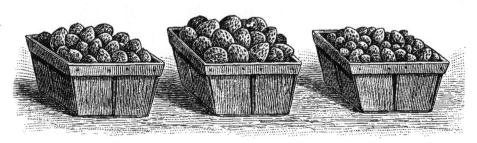

CHOICE FOOD RULES FROM A FOOD WRITER

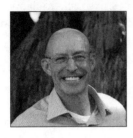

Photo credit: Alia Malley

"Every trip to the supermarket these days requires us to navigate what has become a truly treacherous food landscape," Michael Pollan writes in an October 2009 *New York Times* article called "Rules to Eat By" (*www.nytimes.com/2009/10/11/magazine/11food-rules-t.html?adxnnl=1&adxnnlx=1318334774-s68ZUNcP1I9Nbm0N-HDIQXA*).

"I mean, what are we to make of a wonder of food science like the new Splenda with fiber? ('The great sweet taste you want and a little boost of fiber.') Should we call this progress? Is it even food?

"How did humans manage to choose foods and stay healthy before there were nutrition experts and food pyramids or breakfast cereals promising to improve your child's focus or restaurant portions bigger than your head? We relied on culture, which is another way of saying: on the accumulated wisdom of the tribe. (Which is itself another

way of saying: on your mom and your friends.)"

Based on hundreds of entries from readers of the article, Pollan put together numerous favorite food rules, a few of which are reproduced below:

- "It's better to pay the grocer than the doctor."

- "Don't eat anything you aren't willing to kill yourself."

- "Avoid snack foods with the 'oh' sound in their names: Doritos, Fritos, Cheetos, Tostitos.

- "Eat foods in inverse proportion to how much its lobby spends to push it."

- "If you are not hungry enough to eat an apple, then you are not hungry."

- "Never eat something that is pretending to be something else: veggie burgers, margarine, artificial sweeteners.

- "Don't eat anything that took more energy to ship than grow."

Choosing Foods Locally

The main reasons for focusing on local farms and gardens are that:

- The food is probably more nutritious because it's not as old, it hasn't been transported thousands of miles (a variation of the latter point), and the soil richness of the small farm may be superior to that of big industrial farms that have depleted the minerals in their farmland through high crop yields over the generations (there are exceptions of course, and few farms are perfect—*wash all the food!*).

- For the same reason why you might consider getting a mortgage at the bank down the street, using the local car garage, or quaffing your morning joe at the Hippie Gal Café rather than the mall (sorry, Starbucks)—supporting local food producers makes for a stronger community.

A study of California's San Joaquin Valley from the 1940's compared corporate farms, small farms, and their effects on the surrounding communities. "Where family farms predominated, there were more local businesses, paved streets and sidewalks, schools, parks, churches, clubs and newspapers, better services, higher employment and more civic participation. Studies conducted since Goldschmidt's original work confirms that his findings remain true today" (see www.mindfully.org/Farm/Small-Farm-Benefits-Rosset.htm).

Almost every small to sizeable community has one or more local farms with a food stand. In recent years, many of these operations have grown in size and become year-round stores with expanded services, like pick-your-own, a dairy case (with all that raw milk, artisan cheese, and jerky based on regional game meat), and little farm versions of petting zoos.

A farm store I go to in Newburyport, Massachusetts has a bison that hangs around in a corral as the local mascot. Can Walmart do that?

Of course, in the winter months at northern latitudes, these operations have to ship in a lot of their produce, so the produce will often be no better than a supermarket's. However, in my experience, it's usually very clear which food is local and which is not, because the farm has an incentive to crow about its produce.

Local eggs that are pastured are also much more nutritious than a typical factory-bred egg, despite what its label says about "Omega 3 Eggs" and the like (and it's less disgusting to think about how the chicken that laid them lives). See the "Good Neighbor Sam's Eggs Are Healthier" sidebar and Chapter 3 on Omega 3 fats.

When your whole family goes to the farm, children in particular begin to finally learn where real food comes from, gradually recovering from the misconception of food as a shrink-wrapped "product" down the aisle from the DVDs, the motor oil, and the ammunition.

Farmer's Markets

Almost every small-town square and many cities now have farmer's markets on the weekends. New York City alone has 53 different markets throughout its boroughs.[1] Many of them, or their organizers, have websites and calendars.

To find these markets, just Google your location and "farmer's market," or check out the local paper. Fill up a bag or two with lettuce, carrots, potatoes, apples, eggs, honey, grass-fed beef and lamb, etc., on Saturday or Sunday, and that will keep you going at least through Tuesday.

The farmer's markets also tend to be park-like events in their own right—outdoors, kid-friendly places to hang out, with music playing, lots of dogs to pet, and even a few nearby Occupy Together folks to bat around some philosophical concepts with.

Community Supported Agriculture

Community Supported Agriculture (CSAs) programs allow consumers to buy a share of a farm's produce for a season. The farm relies on CSAs as a form of insurance (the consumer shares the risk that the crop could be limited that year), while the consumer has a steady supply of produce or meats and makes a small investment in sustainable local food production where she lives.

Almost every small-town square and many cities now have farmer's markets on the weekends.

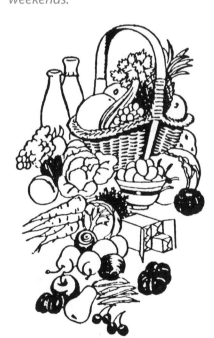

CSAs have become very popular; you'll see them advertised at many of your local farms and elsewhere.

These food arrangements come in all shapes and sizes. I had one during the winter that was meat-only, including a whole chicken once per month. CSAs usually offer full shares (for a family of four to six) and half shares (feeding about two). Sometimes they involve a stand of veggies to pick from (the usual case), or a crate of food that you pick up on a specified day once per week.

Some CSAs are a combination of small producers who band together to sell their wares. Many farms simply have their own CSAs, summer and winter ones, yet other CSAs grow no food but buy all their produce from a collection of farms.

Most of the time you get more produce than you can eat, so it becomes something you share with your friends (or you're impelled to glom all the produce together and make stews, which is good). A bit like the fitness gadgets discussed in Chapter 2, the CSAs have a "tail wags the dog" effect. Having a regular supply of fresh local produce that you've already paid for encourages you to eat more of it and therefore adopt a healthier diet, in terms of antioxidants and other phytochemicals (see Chapter 4). You know you've got food to finish at home, and thus shouldn't stop for that sub on the way back from work.

Local eggs that are pastured are also much more nutritious than a typical factory-bred egg.

Your Own Victory or Rooftop Garden

Victory Gardens are making a comeback, with the skyrocketing price of food these days. In the 1940s, the U.S. government was rationing foods like sugar, butter, and canned goods to aid in the World War II effort, so it urged the American people to plant their own gardens and provide as much of their own fruits and vegetables as possible. This led to an explosion of small, efficient food production in backyards and on city rooftops, as independent food production had a sense of purpose and history behind it.[2]

That all changed when we became Fast Food Nation, but a new direction seems to be in the air during our 21st-century version of hard times, where the "insta-food" might be cheap (and salty, and sugary), but the gas transportation and car ownership required to get there isn't. People are back to growing their own food, keeping their own chickens, and devising other solutions for cutting the costs of their daily calories. It's called survival. See "Code Crash: Choosing Food in Hard Times" up ahead.

Community Gardens

Another choice for people who don't have enough sunny property to plant their own gardens is the community garden. In this variation of growing food, a town or cooperative divides up some available land into small plots that you plant with vegetables or flowers. The cost of renting or acquiring a plot is usually very cheap. Depending on the community, you can get a 15-foot by 15-foot plot for around $20 total (and smaller plots for less). A friend of mine tells me that the only downside is that you might have neighbors that use nasty pesticides that you don't want near your vegetables, but that the overall effect is that you end up with more fresh food than you need, and the community-garden vibe is a pleasant and congenial one.

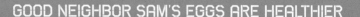

GOOD NEIGHBOR SAM'S EGGS ARE HEALTHIER

The next time you snicker at that frenetic gaggle of chickens your neighbor keeps in his front yard, consider their high efficiency as a food source. A "free ranging" chicken—one that scampers around pecking grass, seeds, and insects—lays much more nutritious eggs than a caged factory chicken.

Good neighbor Sam's eggs are virtually vitamin pills residing in a shell. According to the *Mother Earth News*, here's how pasture-raised eggs compare with "standard factory farm eggs": beta carotene—79 mcg vs. 20 mcg; vitamin A—792 IU vs. 487 IU; n-3 fatty acids—0.66 grams vs. 0.22 grams; and vitamin E—3.7 mg vs. 1 mg. The pastured eggs also tend to be much higher in vitamin D, according to the *Mother Earth News* tests. For more information, see *www.motherearthnews.com/eggs.aspx.*

Choosing Food in the Meat Space: Navigating the Modern Supermarket's Shoals

When you walk into a supermarket or a farm, both entities view you as a "food consumer" (they both need money, or perhaps some sort of barter or exchange in the case of the farm), but there the comparison ends. The farm hasn't hired a big-name consulting firm to polish its marketing tactics in order to lure the poor Mr. (or Mrs.) Moms dragging their two bawling kids inside to blow their hard-earned cash on more stuff they don't need.

Supermarkets have well-known strategies for manipulating the psychology of their customers. Most geeks, and food shoppers in general, resent any thought of being manipulated (they want complete control over their own behavior and purse strings); therefore, the purpose of this section is to recommend some alternatives to the supermarket's strategies, which, for the most part, are plastered all over the Internet anyway.

Mastering the Layout

Supermarkets have well-known techniques of positioning products at eye level on shelves, and even placing catchy cereal boxes and other junk foods at the eye levels of children. A retail-trade article I found on the Web even had a term for this form of using children as a bludgeon against their parents: the "pester effect."

Even though most people, by word-of-mouth or muckraking consumer news spots, know all about this strategy, it still works. I still see kids badgering their parents in the middle aisles to buy stuff for them: colored sprinkles or little boxes of sugar-flour admixtures that also contain plastic toys.

The solution, of course, is to *avoid the middle aisles of supermarkets*, which don't contain the essential foodstuffs anyway. You'll find most of the real food around the periphery of stores. Or, if you can, avoid bringing children to supermarkets. Bring them to a farm and go pick some apples. Physically exhaust them, in a good way, under the sun.

HOW TO READ FOOD LABELS

From a 20-pound bag of rice to a 100-gram can of sardines, just about everything you buy in a supermarket has a "Nutrition Facts" label and an "Ingredients" label. I'll give you a quick rundown on how to read these bits of packaging, as long as you realize that they don't contain a fraction of the useful information you could get on the same food from NutritionData or FitDay (see Chapter 2). Follow along with this brief discussion by taking a gander at Figure 5-1, a label from a can of vegetarian beans.

The purpose of Nutrition Facts is basically to show you the macronutrient ratio of the food (how much fat, carbs, and protein it contains). This small bowl of beans is mostly salty carbohydrate. The serving size is 140 calories with 27 grams of carbs, so we can find out its carb percentage using the following equation: $(27 \times 4) / 140 = 77$ percent. Carbs have about 4 calories per gram (protein has about 4 and fats have 9).

The rest of the macronutrients include only about 24 calories' worth of protein and a tiny amount of fat (a sign that this food is supposed to be *healthy*, along with the advertisement proclaiming "No Animal Products," but I'm not even going to enter that political minefield).

480 mg of salt is too high for such a small amount of food (with a calorie level of only about 1/15th of what a person would eat in a day), as is the 14 grams of sugar.

Now on to the Ingredients information located at the very bottom of the label. This shows the ingredients in descending order of weight. So, we have water and beans and tomato paste, then the not-so-good brown sugar, sugar, and salt. At least most grandmothers could explain many of the ingredients (mustard bran might leave a few of them scratching their heads). And modified corn starch—modified how? Turmeric is actually an extremely effective antioxidant spice chemical.

The bottom line is that you can use these labels as one minor criterion, and certainly not the only one, for choosing foods off the shelf.

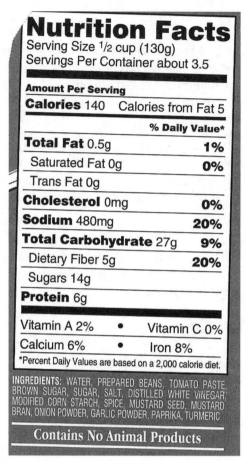

Figure 5-1. *Food labeling on a can o' beans*

It's the Positioning, Stupid

Believe it or not, companies have to pay supermarkets high fees to get prime spots on the shelves for their products. These are called "slotting fees." It gets more insipid. The front of the store is called the "chill" or "decompression zone." Items such as flower stands, greeting-card sections, and DVD and gift-card racks are designed to slow the customers down, so they'll start making impulse purchases.[3]

The primary reason for supermarket bakeries is to fill the air with a bready aroma so that you'll get hungry and buy more stuff (the store usually has enough bread on display from its favorite retail partners).

The dairy—milk, eggs, butter, etc.—is kept in the back, which is designed to force the people heading for their purposeful milk-and-egg purchase to make their way through the middle aisles, or past the gift-card and magazine racks, and the temptations therein.

You can defeat the common subterfuges of the supermarket, which are mostly designed to separate a fool from his money, with common sense.

Chapter 5

The fresh produce section is set up in front in order to convey an impression of freshness and health, even though a lot of the displayed food on top is the old worthless (nutritionally) stuff that the store is trying to get rid of first.[4]

Is this starting to sound like "truthiness" on The Colbert Report? *Conveying an impression or feeling of truth has a higher priority than the truth itself. Doesn't it make more sense to aim for food purveyors that have less of an incentive to hide their true purposes (and where most of the resources are applied not to manipulation or subterfuge but to growing quality produce and meat)?*

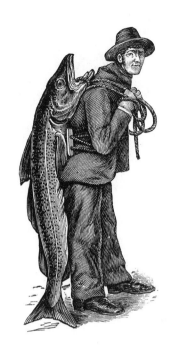

One trade article wrote about the use of "retail theater" to sell more fish from a supermarket fish counter. "You don't buy fish from a fish counter. You buy it from a refrigerated counter that is surrounded by trappings of the sea, images of trawlers and fishermen, and even the sound of waves and seagulls. You will leave the store with some fish, and your senses ringing from a trip to the seaside."[5]

Hmm. I buy most of my fish from a fish market in Newburyport, MA, where you see real piles of fish being processed just beyond the counter, with people wearing hats, boots, and gloves (they're not actors either!). A "fish-like" sound effect (fishiness?) isn't necessary because a real coastline exists about two miles away. Most people in America live on coastlines, and almost all of them have access to real fish markets.

You can defeat the common subterfuges of the supermarket, which are mostly designed to separate a fool from his money, with common sense.

It wouldn't be fair to pick on just supermarkets. Everyone is trying to make extra money off us eaters, including all those boutique "natural" health-food stores that cater to exotic diets and deep pockets.

Even a few smartphone tools lend assistance, if you need apps to stand between yourself and your impulses. Here are a few guidelines:

- *Stick to the periphery of a supermarket*, where most of the essential stuff is located, like produce, dairy, and meat. Just make one circumlocution, bang! And you're done. See the next tip.

- Try to *set and break records for the fastest time spent doing a supermarket errand*. Use a smartphone timer like Endomondo and try to break your last record. Make it a mission; "special ops shopping"—get in there and out of there as fast as you can. Endomondo will also accumulate your mileage as you dash purposefully around the store. I just used this technique, parking a nice walk away from the store (another fitness hack) and completing a purchase of fruit, nuts, coconut milk, and rice in less than 11 minutes (including waiting 3 minutes for checkout)—0.4 miles according to Endomondo on my Android phone.

- *Use local, specialized fish markets and local bakeries*, where the loaf was probably cooked that day (by somebody who lives in or near your town) and contains fewer if any additives or preservatives. If local bakeries used preservatives, why would they need "day-old" bread racks? (I used to love those for the day-old scones.)

- *Use a grocery list*, and stick to the list as you navigate the store. A smart-phone grocery-list app might be handy here (see "Choosing Food in the Digital Space with Apps").

- If you really want to program against your own impulses, *only leave enough money in your checking account for the amount you plan to spend on food*, before you even step into a supermarket. With online banking, this is very easy to do. Just transfer enough money into another savings or money-market account, leaving only the necessary sum in the ATM account, before you head off on your weekly shop. Don't bring any extra cash, and only pay with the ATM card. That way, you're punished for impulse buying by having to pay the bank an overdraft fee (now *that's* a negative incentive for spending extra money!).

Choosing Food in the Digital Space with Apps

As you can imagine, the app space abounds with food-finding and analyzing tools. One of them is Locavore, a simple app for finding nearby farms and CSAs. It grabs your location and displays the fruits and veggies that are still in season there. It further gives you an option for finding a farm or CSA that carries the specified produce, showing all the places on a Google Map (with location information like addresses and websites). You can find that app at *www.getlocavore.com*.

> *All apps are limited by the databases they load, which may fall quickly out of date—or were never comprehensive to begin with. Apps cannot magically pick farms out of thin air like they can magically pinpoint your location (using your cell phone's internal location software). I used Locavore in the parking lot of one of my local farms, and it did not locate or show the farm. It is free, however, so let's not nit-pick.*

GroceryIQ (*groceryiq.com/mobile.aspx*) is a pretty good free app for assembling and saving your own grocery lists. It's an app designed for a true grocery-list power user. The developers have thought about everything you'd want to do with a list, like email it and sync the list on your phone with your computer. They also have a nice barcode scanner for scanning in items, which are automatically categorized by aisle type (e.g., the deli counter) and added to the list.

For me, making any kind of list beyond the use of a pencil and paper, however, is too laborious and typing-intensive.

I just keep the "list" in my head and go on a fast-paced, "special ops" shop.

The Restaurant Finder (*www.therestaurantfinder.com*) is a spartan, handy app for finding restaurants based on your current location, which makes it useful while you're on the road. It gives you the option of searching for just seafood, Italian, or vegetarian restaurants, for example, in case you want to skip the flood of fast-food results. The app provides fairly accurate results and a Google Map for locating the restaurant.

Fooducate (*www.fooducate.com/barcode-samples.html*) is a barcode-scanning app that makes it pretty easy to get a snapshot with your smartphone of food quality in a grocery store. After a scan, it shows you a screen like the one shown in Figure 5-2, which gives the food a grade and points out some warning flags (like five+ teaspoons of sugar!).

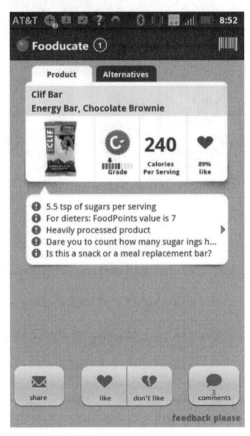

Figure 5-2. *A barcode scan result with Fooducate*

Fooducate will recommend alternatives along the bottom of the screen, as shown in Figure 5-3. This is a handy app for initial food screening from a nutritional standpoint. Most geeks, however, might want to get into more precise data such as protein, fat, carb, and micronutrient content.

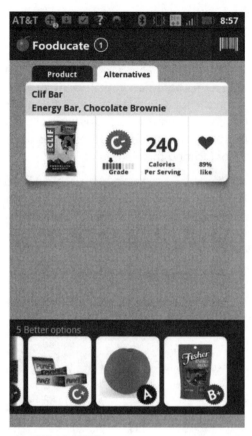

Figure 5-3. *Oranges get an "A" over Clif Bars*

As you can imagine, there are hundreds of these apps, mostly in free versions, for finding food, locating restaurants, making lists, and scanning barcodes. You can search for them at www.appbrain.com (for Android phones) and www.apple.com/iphone/from-the-app-store/lifestyle.html (for the iPhone).

Hacks for Finding Good Food on the Road

It can be tough finding fitness-oriented foods when you are on the road. When you don't want to settle for a lowest-common-denominator experience in airports (you know, your flight's cancelled, so you give up and aim for the martinis and a giant meatball sub), you can consider these hacks instead.

Search Google for "Whole Foods" wherever you are, if you have access to a computer or smartphone. One time I was in Seattle, WA, looking for food the day before a mountain climb (I was responsible for stuff like nuts, fruit, cheese, and chocolate bars). After getting general directions to a market from the hotel, I promptly failed to find anything food-wise but coffee shops and restaurants. Seattle can be hard to negotiate by foot, because it has a freeway running straight through the city.

> *Ironically, here I was seeking food to survive on a mountain, and I was falling flat on my face inside of civilization.*

I wandered around in the vicinity of my hotel and the Space Needle in a near panic, until I finally ran into a Whole Foods Market on Westlake Avenue. I could have saved myself some grief and time beforehand by doing a simple search on the laptop before I left my hotel.

Bring a nut-and-seed bag when you're in the plane, bus, or rented car. Fill up a large Ziploc bag and keep it in your backpack or duffel. Nuts and seeds are filling, nutritious, lightweight, don't require refrigeration, and won't go bad for an entire trip (dried fruit, by the way, is no better than candy). Choose raw nuts such as almonds, walnuts, and macadamias over the roasted and salted variety, as this is a processing method that compromises the nutrition of the nuts and seeds (the latter including sunflower and pumpkin). Apples and carrots are also more durable and transportable than other fresh foods.

Use travel time for fasting, particularly on planes. It's a "when in doubt, don't eat" moment (see Chapter 6). Just drink water and tea; you'll feel much better.

Search for the increasingly popular food trucks, in whatever neighborhood you find yourself in. These are little mobile food emporiums on wheels. A site called Roaming Hunger (*www.roaminghunger.com*) has food-truck maps for many major cities in the U.S.

Do a little homework on the Internet before you leave, and store the bookmarks for all the good food markets and restaurants around the places where you will be staying.

In the airport itself, *just subsist on fruit, tea, and water*, if you're not fasting. Food stalls in airports do sell fruit, albeit at a premium price.

Code Crash: Choosing Food in Hard Times

The Internet is chock full of sites, some of them very good, for finding and storing food for lean times, as demonstrated by the search results at *www.google.com/search?client=safari&rls=en&q=tips+for+finding+food+in+hard+times&ie=UTF-8&oe=UTF-8*.

Many of these sites have an apocalyptic tilt, which is so commonly embraced these days that, for the sake of originality, I won't make any references to societal collapse.

> *I do agree, however, with the old chestnut that we should hope for the best, prepare for the worst.*

It's becoming sadly more common to see the affliction of the richest countries in the world with regional food shortages. In the US, the state of affairs where one in four children are living in poverty and often going hungry is nothing short of shameful. At the same time, we're also bedeviled by a "quantity not quality" food consumption pattern.

What are good strategies if you simply don't have the resources to reliably acquire enough food? What are the good choices?

Barter with farms, or offer to work for food. When I was a student, and thus a waiter, dishwasher, and host in restaurants, I absorbed easily more than half my calories scarfing down the restaurant's food (it wasn't all that bad either—mostly meat, veggies, and salads). Go to your local farm and tell them you'll work once a week for a big box of fresh food.

Get the most bang for your buck. Buy healthy stuff in bulk that's filling. Examples are bags of brown, Basmati, or other kinds of rice; a sack of local apples and potatoes; whole fowl like chicken or turkey, where you can make broth out of the stripped bird; as well as big blocks of quality cheddar cheese (read: it's not a weird orange color and doesn't have salt as a separate ingredient). These foods are expensive but energy-dense and last a long time. Cram a big pot with stew materials and it will last several days. The supersized bags of crunchy snack foods are just a dead end; they might be cheap, but they're not nutritious or filling.

Go crazy with coupons. Enough said; there's so much already on the Web these days about coupon tips.

Eat only twice per day with apples or nuts for necessary snacks. It's healthier to eat only within narrow windows; say, 7:00 AM to 7:30 PM only (see Chapter 6). Ultimately, eating twice per day most of the time will be cheaper than trying to pay for three big meals per day. Of course, this advice is only for adults. Children should eat as much as they need to grow, fuel their active days, and fill their bellies.

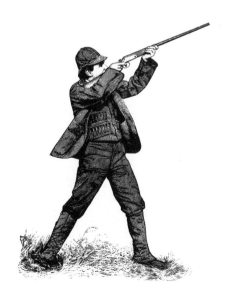

This is an obvious one: *hunt and forage for food*, beyond your own garden if necessary. A hunter who takes down a large game animal often has meat for the winter. Go fishing or gather blue mussels on the coastline (but check with the local health authority about any contamination or red tides first); see *www.motherearthnews.com/Nature-Community/1980-11-01/Mussels-How-To-Forge-Or-Farm-Them.aspx*. Find edible plants (handfuls of fiddleheads only go so far, however).

It's hard work, but we're evolved for this type of foraging behavior. That said, keep in mind *the basic math of not expending energy in calories that exceeds the amount of calories you forage.*

WHAT IF YOU LIVE IN A FOOD DESERT?

Food deserts are places where it's hard to get to a grocery store or supermarket to buy any fresh fruits, vegetables, seafood, and other healthy edibles. The desert could be a city where the grocery stores or supermarkets have closed down in large swaths of neighborhoods, or the countryside, where food markets are few and far between and people may not have access to public transportation or a car.

The Centers for Disease Control in the U.S. has a page on food deserts with links: *www.cdc.gov/features/fooddeserts/*. The USDA also makes available something called a Food Environment Atlas, a map depicting food availability throughout the U.S.: *http://maps.ers.usda.gov/FoodAtlas/*.

Chances are, however, if you live in a food desert, you already know it—no one has to produce a map to show that it's hard to find good food. What to do about it?

What do people do when they're stuck in a real desert? Survival experts know how to find water *in* the desert, from plants or rainwater that's been captured by pockets or depressions in rock, for example (they also know how to determine if the water is safe to drink). You can also figure out to how find food in your desert: farm-food distribution programs such as farmer's markets or food trucks may take place sporadically nearby; people may be growing food in community gardens; local churches and food banks may be distributing *healthy* foods (a new trend at best); and some of the "cheap eats" restaurants may have some healthy food on their menus (beyond the ribs, cheeseburgers, and fries).

When I was a student in New York City I often ate breakfast or dinner in a Spanish-style diner in my neighborhood. For a couple of bucks I could buy a complete dinner of chicken and rice, or eggs, bacon, and homefries, and the coffee was espresso served in small mugs. Of course, that was around 1980.

Step outside the shell of your favorite ethnic foods and try the food of other cultures. For example, there might be an Asian food market nearby with some healthy veggies and fruit.

People also try to *hike out of real deserts* if they're stuck there. So grab your backpack and bicycle, and ride to the food. You could come home with some meat, potatoes, and eggs, no sweat. I do this once in a while with my own backpack; I mountain bike to a farm and come home with some food.

It's worth it—you don't want to live out of the convenience store attached to the gas station and be stuck with a meal of orange cheese, beef jerky, and potato chips.

Consider the swallow-your-pride school of urban foraging—*freeganism*. "Dumpster diving" now has a cult following, and is far more productive and potentially nutritious than another fad called "planking" (I never knew what those folks were doing stretched out on their suburban banisters). An entire library of "urban and suburban survival" books exists, as hinted at by the few Amazon.com titles shown in Figure 5-4.

Customers Who Bought This Item Also Bought

Dumpster Diving: The Advanced Course: How to Turn... by John Hoffman
★★★☆☆ (9)
$15.60

The Scavengers' Manifesto by Anneli Rufus
★★★☆☆ (6)
$5.98

The Urban Homestead (Expanded & Revised Edition):... by Kelly Coyne
★★★★½ (54)
$12.21

Living Well on Practically Nothing: Revised a... by Edward H. Romney
★★★☆☆ (29)
$17.46

Possum Living: How to Live Well Without a Job and... by Dolly Freed
★★★½☆ (40)
$10.36

Editorial Reviews

Amazon.com Review

"Dumpster diving" is an unfortunate term for a noble pursuit: reclaiming and reusing perfectly good things that are being thrown away by wasteful or lazy people. It is also a political act highly frowned upon in materialistic societies because it removes one from obligate consumerism. And John Hoffman has written the ultimate guide for perfecting the art. A college graduate with a good job, Hoffman doesn't have to Dumpster dive: he loves to, and lives better--and more freely--because of it. In nations like America, there is an incredible amount of great stuff--often in great shape--thrown out every day. And Hoffman tells you how to claim it as your own.

At this point, I have a confession to make: I am a sometime Dumpster diver myself. Almost all of the furniture in our house has been found abandoned on the streets in our upper-middle-class neighborhood or nearby college campuses: sofas, tables, bookcases, lamps... you name it--even some of our several household computers! Personally, I wouldn't do some of what Hoffman advocates (such as diving for food), but as in the tradition of all Loompanics Press books, this is a no-holds-barred, tell-all book that assumes its readers can make decisions appropriate to their own lives.

Product Description

In step-by-step, illustrated detail, John Hoffman shows you how to use dumpster diving for food, clothing, appliances, furniture, books and other treasures. Discover how to dress for dumpster diving success, work your neighborhood dumpsters, dive a restaurant, use a "bag blade" and "dive stick", handle run-ins with the authorities, convert your trash to cash, and much more! While you are learning all these professional secrets, you will be entertained by outrageous anecdotes from a life-long master diver. --*This text refers to an alternate **Paperback** edition.*

Figure 5-4. *Dumpster diving and other freeganism urban scavenger titles*

Food Timing:
When to Eat, When to Fast

§

Fasting is a scary thought to some people. Food is deemed important for all kinds of reasons other than raw hunger. What's that line I keep seeing painted on restaurant walls and on websites: food is love? Fasting means *no* food, for hours on end (although at least half of the hours are spent asleep).

In the 2002 remake of the movie *Swept Away*, Madonna's character talks about the virtues of fasting, and that line is supposed to make you *hate* fasting, because she's promoting it, and her character is a snarling, narcissistic plutocrat. But fasting *is* virtuous, from a symbolic, religious, and ethical standpoint, and there's even good scientific evidence that a modified form of this practice, called *intermittent fasting*, is quite healthy.

> *People fast for lots of reasons: in solidarity with groups that are suffering persecution, for instance, such as the thousands of displaced people in the Darfur region of Africa (see http://fastdarfur.org). As for religion, in Judaism, for example, the Yom Kippur fast lasts 25 hours. During the Muslim Ramadan tradition, the fast takes place from dawn to dusk each day.*

Here comes that human-evolution angle again—we seem to be naturally evolved for fasting. Humans and mammals in general respond metabolically very well to it (see the sidebars covering the science behind fasting). This adaptation may have evolved from our ancestors' activity patterns. They had to constantly physically seek food, and must have periodically dealt with extreme swings in food availability (see the discussion in the sidebar "An Interview with a Scientist on Fasting and Metabolism" and this 2004 Journal of Applied Physiology article: *http://jap.physiology.org/content/96/1/3.full*).

It has become increasingly evident that we're actually *designed* to periodically fast.

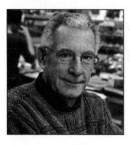

In October 2011, I interviewed Dr. Thomas Seyfried, a biology professor at Boston College whose research program has the goal "to manage complex diseases through principles of metabolic control theory." His contact page is at *www.bc.edu/schools/cas/biology/facadmin/seyfried.html*.

How did you first become interested in implementing research on intermittent fasting, caloric restriction with adequate nutrition (CRAN), metabolism—in the context of genetics and the environment?

We have researched for many years the therapeutic benefits of calorie restriction and calorie-restricted ketogenic diets for managing several neurological diseases like epilepsy, autism, lipid storage diseases, and cancer. Inflammation underlies the progression of many diseases. Both calorie restriction and fasting target inflammation.

Are we humans designed for intermittent fasting—in other words, does it turn on pathways that promote health? Does it express genes in a positive way? Many have speculated that our evolutionary ancestors (such as from the Upper Paleolithic) may have experienced extreme swings of food availability, thus intermittent fasting or the equivalent became built into our genes.

Humans evolved as a scavenger species. Scavengers generally experience a "feast-famine" existence. I agree that our physiology evolved to function during extreme swings of food availability. Humans are genetically programmed to survive for long periods (months) with little or no food. This information is elaborated further in Herbert Shelton's book *Fasting for Renewal of Life*.[1]

A number of studies have shown consistently interesting and positive results from fasting and lab animals. Is it safe or sensible to extrapolate the results from the smaller mammals to humans?

We (and others) have shown that calorie restriction in rodents is not the same as calorie restriction in humans. The basal metabolic rate of rodents is about seven times that of humans. Consequently, the health benefits seen in rodents from a 40% calorie restriction are realized in humans from a seven-day water-only therapeutic fast.

What are the types of metabolic changes that take place during an intermittent fast (i.e., insulin levels go down, glucagon goes up)? Can we assume that there is a lot of variability in how humans and mammals respond to it?

The physiological changes associated with fasting are conserved across mammalian species. Insulin goes down because blood glucose goes down. Glucagon goes up in order to mobilize fats and to produce glucose (gluconeogenesis) from stored proteins. Fats are metabolized to ketone bodies, which replace glucose as a major fuel for the brain. Ketone body metabolism reduces inflammation and enhances metabolic efficiency of most cells.

Are there any interesting long-term metabolic adaptations that take place after many weeks or months of fasting?

Yes, energy efficiency increases. This means that the energy stored in the chemical bonds of consumed foods is maximally oxidized for ATP synthesis in all body cells. Energy efficiency increases up to a point, however. Prolonged fasting can lead to the pathological effects of starvation.

Is there a rule of thumb for when an intermittent fast becomes starvation (i.e., a number of hours), and therefore not healthy (it's causing micronutrient deficiencies and too much harvesting of muscle for energy)?

It is important to distinguish the differences between fasting and starvation. Water-only fasting for a week or two is therapeutic, as the body enhances metabolic efficiency. Starvation is pathological and occurs after about 40 days of no food for most normal-weight people. Starvation damages the body in metabolizing needed muscle tissue for energy. Obese people, however, can survive without the pathological effects of starvation for many months. George Cahill and Oliver Owen show this in their many studies of obese patients.

AN INTERVIEW WITH A SCIENTIST ON FASTING AND METABOLISM (continued)

Can I ask if you fast? (I'm an intermittent faster, about 15 hours a few times per week.)

I usually fast for 24 hours at least once a week and up to 18 hours several times a week, but I have not engaged in prolonged fasting for several days or a week. I would definitely conduct a more prolonged fast if I were diagnosed with diabetes or cancer. Our extensive research shows how fasting deprives the glucose needed to drive cancer cell growth. Fasting will also enhance insulin sensitivity and reduce the symptoms of diabetes. It is not necessary to use toxic drugs to manage these diseases.

I would be remiss if I didn't ask: do you have a favorite fitness gadget (a pedometer; HR monitor, etc.), and if so, which one?

No, I do not use fitness gadgets. However, we do use blood glucose–ketone meters to monitor our blood glucose and ketone body levels following short fasts. Blood glucose levels in the 55–65 mg/dl range and ketone levels in the 2–3 mmol range are indicative of high metabolic efficiency and health.

Intermittent Fasting

Intermittent fasting is a hot topic, particularly among weightlifters and resistance trainers.

An intermittent fast is a short-term fast (usually lasting a part of a day) that you include in your lifestyle throughout the week. It's a part of the whole matrix viewed as your fitness routine, taking place alongside the various modes of exercise and rest periods that are dispersed throughout a training regimen.

Intermittent fasts are good for your metabolic health, increasing the burning of fats for energy, improving insulin sensitivity, lowering inflammation, and increasing growth hormone levels (while fasting). Its proponents even advocate undertaking an occasional training session while fasted.

Intermittent fasts represent a shift of traditional thinking among athletes and coaches. For decades, athletes have experimented with various *overfeeding* strategies for fueling exercise (such as carbo loading, uncommonly high protein intakes, and even heroic images of Rocky Balboa guzzling down a dozen eggs).

From the "don't try this at home" file: as Chapter 4 (on micronutrients) points out, excess consumption of raw egg whites can cause a severe vitamin B7 (biotin) deficiency, because of avidin, a protein in egg whites that binds with biotin and prevents its absorption.

There are no hard and fast rules on how to implement an intermittent fast, and later in this chapter we provide a few tips on getting started.

WHAT HAPPENS IN YOUR BODY DURING FASTING

Your metabolism undergoes a number of positive changes during an intermittent fast, including the increased burning of your fat stores for energy:

1. *Insulin levels go down*. Insulin is the messenger hormone that the pancreatic beta cells secrete in response to a rise in blood glucose. Insulin acts as the key, permitting the entry of glucose and amino acids into cells. If the muscle cells or fat cells, for instance, sense too much insulin in the blood all the time, they become resistant to it (because too much glucose or sugar is toxic to the cell). Fasting and exercise help the body retain its sensitivity to your own insulin. Insulin also inhibits lipolysis and promotes fat storage, rather than the metabolizing of fats for energy.

2. *Glucagon levels go up* during fasting. The pancreas secretes both glucagon (when glucose levels are low) and insulin (when blood glucose is high). A hormone, glucagon carries the message to release fats, or free fatty acids (FFAs), into the bloodstream so that the body's cells can start utilizing FFAs for energy, since the blood glucose levels have dropped. The fancy term for the burning of fats is *lipolysis*.

3. *Glucagon also tells the liver to break up or "depolymerize" its stored starch* (called glycogen) so the body can use the stored glucose for energy. The liver-glycogen stores are easily replenished after fasting, by eating carbs, because the liver only stores about 70 grams or 280 calories' worth of glucose. The muscles store up to another 200 or 300 grams or 800–1,200 calories' worth of glycogen (which is actually long polymers made of glucose molecules bonded together). Some estimates put the body's total storage of glycogen at up to 2,000 calories; see the sidebar "Where Did You Get All That Energy?" in Chapter 10. The latter amount varies based on how big and muscular a person is, and other factors. On the other hand, prompting your body to burn fats more efficiently is a great thing; we store about 100,000 calories' or more worth of fat.

To roughly determine how many stored calories you have in the form of adipose tissue or stored fat, figure out your body composition first. Say you're a male, weigh 165 pounds, and have 15 percent body fat. Your body has about 165 x 0.15 x 16 ounces of stored fat: 396 ounces or 24.75 pounds. There are about 28 grams in an ounce and about 9 calories per gram of fat, so the total stored calories

would be 396 x 28 x 9, which equals 99,792 calories. Compare this to only about 1,200 calories of stored glycogen, give or take, and roughly 12 pounds' worth of muscle protein that you could harvest for energy. At any one time, our bodies are using all three sources of tissue for food, but there's a limit on how much protein harvesting you can do. If your body uses about one third or more of your muscle mass, (i.e., muscle wasting), you will die. Still, the body has a remarkable ability to generate energy from stored tissue, which perhaps tells us something about how we evolved.

4. About 10 to 15 percent of energy during fasting derives from catabolizing or using protein as an energy source, the fancy term for that being *gluconeogenesis*. The body has a mechanism for catabolizing protein into amino acids and, via a certain chemical pathway, making glucose or sugar from the amino acids. It's normal to use some of your muscle protein, for example, for energy, and the body has internal feedback systems to protect your hard-earned muscle from being excessively harvested. It's just that we've evolved to have a variety of internal methods to generate cell fuel when we're not gobbling up carbs all the time (a food source that's only been in virtually limitless supply for about the last 50 years or so). After about a week of fasting (as an intermittent faster, you'd never fast for a week anyway), the body cuts way back on gluconeogenesis.

Let's say your body generates 12 percent of the energy it needs during a fast by converting amino acids to glucose (gluconeogenesis). This is a reasonable speculation, but we know that the vast majority of intermittent-fast energy will be provided by free fatty acids and stored glycogen. You might expend 1,000 to 1,500 calories during a typical intermittent fast. This equates to perhaps 120 to 180 calories or 30–45 grams of protein, which is not significant. A whey protein shake plus other protein sources during the post-intermittent-fast meal will take care of that, and then some.

WHAT HAPPENS IN YOUR BODY DURING FASTING (continued)

5. *Human growth hormone (GH) levels go up* during fasting, as they do during exercise and during deep sleep. GH also has a lipolytic effect; it binds to fat cells and imparts the instruction to "release fats for burning and don't store as much fat." GH has an important anabolic effect on building muscle and cartilage. GH stimulates the liver and other tissues to secret a "minion" hormone, IGF-1, which in turn sends the protein or muscle-synthesis message.[2]

6. *Ketone body levels go up.* Ketone bodies, or ketones, are the biochemicals that result from the burning up or oxidation of fats (free fatty acids) for energy. As your use of FFAs goes up, your ketones go up. The body,

particularly the brain, can use ketones as energy in the absence of glucose; rising ketone levels are the direct result of burning more fat for energy. Dr. Tom Seyfried has done interesting research on the inability of many cancerous tumors to use ketones for energy, for example (see the previous sidebar, "An Interview with a Scientist on Fasting and Metabolism").

This is just a selection of changes the fasting body undergoes, and I derived some of them from a 1982 physiological analysis of a religious fellow who underwent a long-term fast.[3]

For the most part, during intermittent fasting, you only fast during one chunk of the day (such as when you're sleeping plus a few hours), and you can even start out initiating an intermittent fast during just one or two days of the week.

Variations: 19/5 and "Eat Stop Eat"

Some people respond well to sticking with a specific intermittent fasting protocol that is part of a bigger fitness routine, usually with an experienced trainer/athlete behind it and with the help of books or a website. Some examples of these are:

1. The "Fast Five," or 19/5, a setup that involves fasting for 19 hours every day, then eating whenever hungry for 5 hours: *www.fast-5.com*.

2. Leangains (*www.leangains.com*), a 16/8 setup with additional protocols for training and eating.

3. Alternate day fasts (ADFs) that involve fasting for a full 24 hours and eating an unrestricted (within reason…) amount of calories the following day. One variation of ADF is "Eat Stop Eat," which was invented by Brad Polin, a sports trainer who wrote a book of the same name.

Interestingly, the fasting benefits tend to accrue with ADF even if the total amount of calories consumed is no different than what people used to eat before they went the ADF route (e.g., no fasting, three meals a day). See the sidebar "What the Studies Say About Fasting."

Most fitness geeks have plenty of leeway for determining the type of fasting that works best for them.

WHAT THE STUDIES SAY ABOUT FASTING

A number of studies have focused on the positive effects of intermittent fasting and caloric restriction (CR), sometimes referred to as caloric restriction with adequate nutrition (CRAN). The latter practice involves substantially restricting the usual calories taken in by about 15 to 40 percent in order to take advantage of the longevity and health benefits that a number of lab tests have indicated (at least with animals like rats, mice, and monkeys). CR is one of the few proven longevity extenders. But most people cannot stomach (pun intended) CRAN, because it begins to look and feel like chronic starvation, and you certainly could not make any athletic gains like new muscle on it. The good news is that *studies have found similar metabolic benefits with intermittent fasting*:

- A 2007 study in the *American Journal of Clinical Nutrition* found that alternate day fasting (ADF)—that is, a day of feast and a day of fasting—lowered risk factors for cardiovascular disease, diabetes, and cancer, and helped some subjects lose weight. The review found more compelling animal evidence and speculated that human trials exploring these issues hadn't lasted long enough (in some cases, only a few weeks). The authors speculated that three mechanisms may be at work with fasting: 1) the cells become more stress resistant; 2) the mitochondria in the cells produce fewer free radicals, the metabolic "storm" that creates oxidative stress and DNA damage; and 3) CR may induce a built-in program that slows down metabolism in the presence of scarcity. "Indirect evidence suggests that the two regimens [including CRAN] may share mechanisms."[4]

- A 2005 study in the *Journal of Nutritional Biochemistry* found that intermittent fasting also increased lifespan in lab animals, even when caloric intake had not been reduced overall. Various diseases (in animals) such as cancer, diabetes, and kidney disease were delayed or prevented by CR and intermittent fasting. The suggested mechanisms (in humans as well) were decreased insulin resistance (lower glucose and insulin concentrations in the blood), reduced oxidative stress, increased cellular stress resistance, as well as enhanced immune function. Intermittent fasting imposes a mild stress on brain cells, which respond by "enhancing their ability to resist more severe stress." The "cellular and molecular effects of IF [intermittent fasting] and CR on the cardiovascular system and the brain are similar to those of regular physical exercise, suggesting shared mechanisms."[5]

- A January 2011 article in the *Journal of Applied Physiology* found that cycling in the fasted state four times per week was more efficient than cycling with high-carb fueling. The study examined 20 young men, half of whom received about 1,000 calories of carbs before and during the 60- to 90-minute cycling bout, while the other half fasted during the session. Fasting had a number of effects that did not take place with the carb-fueled athletes: greater amounts of intramuscle fats were utilized for fuel, exercise intensity increased more in the fasted cyclists, metabolic enzyme activity was "upregulated" among the fasters, and fasted training "prevented the exercise induced drop in blood glucose" (surprisingly enough…).[6]

The Basics of Intermittent Fasting: Getting Started

You probably want to give intermittent fasting a try. At the very least, it provides a default choice in the face of any confusion about whether what you are eating is counterproductive or not: "When in doubt, don't eat." Here's how to get started:

1. Map out a day where you can go at least about 14 hours without solid food (water, tea, and black coffee are okay). This usually involves the period after you've finished dinner and then throughout the night. But you can use whatever setup is easiest to implement, given your life schedule. The actual time blocks depend on your personal work and sleep routine, of course.

2. The fast cannot usually involve any calories (unless you're doing a partial fast); this would disrupt the fasting metabolism (in which your blood-sugar or glucose levels are maintained without the input of food—see the sidebar "What Happens in Your Body During Fasting"). Tea or coffee without cream or sugar is generally okay, but a purist might insist on no caffeine, which exerts a powerful effect on the central nervous system (thus, you could argue, changing the hormonal milieu for the fast). Most of us have to work or have responsibilities during most fasts, so a little coffee or green tea during the intermittent fast is a reasonable compromise and poses no harm.

3. Upon awakening, in the usual fasted evening scenario, you skip breakfast and, if so inclined, start the day only with a cup of joe or tea. As we mentioned, a lump of sugar and big splash of cream in the coffee will tend to send the food signal to the body, in part by raising insulin levels, so that's generally considered a "cheat," or you might consider this a partial or moderate fast.

The USDA Nutrient Database does indicate that tea and even black coffee are not 100 percent calorie-free (two calories per eight ounces, in fact). An intermittent fasting purist may insist on only water or reliably calorie-free drinks during the fast, but we might be splitting hairs a bit too finely here. You'll still be getting some of the metabolic benefits of fasting by restricting calories a lot.

---

4. The science also supports *a fasted workout*. Therefore, the next step would be to hit the gym hungry for your favorite high-intensity weight regimen. To many beginner and veteran athletes, this might seem counterintuitive, even scary, but it actually feels good and the athlete tends to adapt to lifting weights on just sleep, water, and coffee (in my case). *What is the science?* For one, a 2010 study in the *Journal of Physiology* took three groups of young men and fed them a high-fat, high-calorie diet for more than a month. They divided them into three groups: one group fasted and trained (four times a week cycling); another group trained on carbohydrate fuels, like a high-carb breakfast followed by energy drinks during exercise; and the third (control) group did nothing. The control group gained about seven pounds in six weeks, predictably. The carb-fed group gained about three pounds, but the athletes training in the fasted state didn't gain any weight, even when they were pigging out around the training and fasting. Among the fasters, several biomarkers improved at a higher rate than in the carb group, including insulin sensitivity and the muscle adaptations for quickly turning over the increased fatty acids in the diet.[7] For more intermittent fasting–related study results, see the sidebar "What the Studies Say About Fasting."

---

5. You can also do endurance training in the fasted state (this was actually the training protocol for two of the fasting studies we cite in this chapter). This appears on the face of it, and from my experience as a former endurance athlete when I usually stuffed food like gels or bananas in my pocket, to be much harder to do when fasting than short-term high-intensity weight training. After 80 minutes of, say, hard riding, you could *bonk*, and there are good physiological reasons for that, such as because all the glycogen—your internal storage depot of starch in the muscles and liver—has been depleted by the fasting and exercise itself. It does depend on the intensity level of the exercise, and how well you have previously adapted to fasting. You could also save this kind of training for the nonfasting days, unless you're very adapted to it.

6. Or, you don't have to train; you'll still enjoy some of the benefits of intermittent fasting.

INTERVIEW WITH THE "WARRIOR DIET" AUTHOR

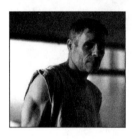

Ori Hofmekler is an author, a former member of the Israeli Army, an acclaimed artist, and a well-known nutrition and muscle-building researcher. His most recent book (2011) is *Unlock Your Muscle Gene: Trigger the Biological Mechanisms That Transform Your Body and Extend Your Life* (for more information, see *www.warriordiet.com* or *www.defensenutrition.com*). He answered a few questions for us on the research he has done on fasting and metabolism.

What was your inspiration for creating the warrior diet and writing the book?

What drove me to write the *Warrior Diet* book is a combination of factors—my personal experience, the historical evidence, and the science that provides evidence for its nutritional strategies.

I've been enjoying the benefits of this diet regimen for many years. Nonetheless, what inspired me the most

was the realization that the same dietary principles were followed by some of the healthiest and most culturally advanced early warrior societies, including the Greeks, Spartans, Macedonians, and Romans.

In addition, growing scientific evidence points to the outstanding benefits of this diet for human health and longevity. Based on evolutionary biology, we now know that the human body evolved to thrive on specific foods and a certain feeding cycle. The premise of the warrior diet is to revive these primal dietary features and provide guidance on how to apply them in your diet.

What is the rationale for the 20/4 structure of fasting-eating? Are we humans evolved for this "famine/feast" cycle?

Accumulating evidence indicates that we are evolved for intermittent fasting, based on a feeding cycle of one meal per day. And the proof is in our bodies. If you take a close look at how the human autonomic nervous system operates, you'll realize that it's inherently designed to accommodate this feeding cycle—hence, fasting (or undereating) during the day, and feeding at night. Let me explain.

INTERVIEW WITH THE "WARRIOR DIET" AUTHOR (continued)

The autonomic nervous system is divided into two parts: the sympathetic nervous system (SNS), which regulates your activities during the day, and the parasympathetic nervous system (PSNS), which regulates your activities during the night. These two parts of the autonomic nervous system have opposite effects on your body. During the day, the SNS promotes alertness, fat burning, and action, whereas during the night, the PSNS promotes relaxation, energy conservation, and sleepiness.

Note that the SNS is promoted by lack of food and inhibited by large meals. The PSNS, on the other hand, is promoted by large meals and inhibited by lack of food.

This means that the human body is not programmed for large meals during the day. Large meals inhibit your SNS. And every time you eat a large meal during the day, your body shifts into a nightly mode—conserving energy rather than spending energy, and getting fatigued rather than keeping alert. This is why you feel sleepy and sluggish after a big lunch.

Meal timing is a crucial factor that cannot be overlooked. All the evidence shows that biologically we evolved for nocturnal feeding. We digest and utilize nutrients better at night, when relaxed, under the domination of the PSNS. Daytime meals such as the typical breakfast and lunch are counterproductive, as they suppress cognitive functions, inhibit fat burning, and disrupt normal metabolic functions. Daytime overfeeding seems to be a major contributing factor behind the current epidemic of obesity, diabetes, and related diseases. But there is more to it…

A frequent intake of large meals during the day suppresses critical metabolic pathways responsible for detox, repair, and rejuvenation. The human body evolved to benefit from fasting in a similar way that it evolved to benefit from exercising. Periodic fasting puts the body in a survival mode, which is crucial for maintaining prime health. Animal and human studies have shown that fasting resets the metabolic system to improve insulin sensitivity, increase energy-utilization efficiency, restore hormonal balance, destroy cancerous cells, repair tissues, counteract disease, and block the aging process.

The lack of food triggers a cellular recycling mechanism, which digests and recycles broken proteins and damaged cells to be used as building blocks for cellular and tissue repair. Technically, fasting activates growth factors that signal stem cells to commit and regenerate new cells in the brain, muscle, bone, and connective tissues.

It has been suggested that early human adaptation to this famine-feast cycle was an evolutionary advantage that improved our species' gene pool through natural selection (survival of the fittest), and kept us alive and thriving on this planet.

The purpose behind the warrior diet's 20/4 structure of fasting/feeding is sheer simplicity. This structure helps illustrate and clarify the ratio between fasting (or undereating) and feeding.

You get a window of four hours for your main meal, which is about the optimal time needed to fully nourish your body. The other 20 hours include 6 hours required for complete digestion. This leaves you with about 12 hours of net fasting, where your body shifts into a survival mode—hence, you enjoy 12 hours of detox, repair, and rejuvenation every day. And the accumulating effect of this rejuvenation process will be manifested in your state of health, physical shape, and biological age.

The 20/4 structure is just a suggested model. In real life there is no need to calculate hours—the premise of this feeding cycle is simple: have one main meal per day at night.

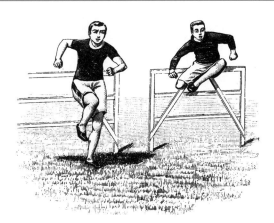

Eating in Blocks or Windows

When you're taking part in regular intermittent fasts (essentially, every day), you have narrowed your window for eating. You might only eat in an 8-hour window during the day (fasting for 16 hours). There are good reasons why some of the prescriptive intermittent fasting regimes are based on this narrowing of the eating window. You take advantage of all the benefits of fasting (e.g., better blood-sugar control, more fat burning, higher glucagon and growth hormone), and you can eat based on hunger level whenever you want during the window.

Chances are, this eating in a narrower window means you only eat two meals a day, but they can be big meals that include supplements (like a whey protein shake) if you're actually trying to put on muscle. Other people will simply eat fewer calories without breakfast and lose extra pounds. After fasting and exercising, you should break the fast within about an hour and eat. Eat quality protein, like branched-chain amino acids (BCAAs), now that you've started the muscle-building process by fasting and lifting weights. There is also evidence that fasting preferentially catabolizes (uses for energy) the BCAAs the body harvests from muscles,[8] so it makes sense to restore them with quality whey protein (which contains BCAAs) or meat afterward.

The rest of your meal, which is likely to contain some carbohydrate (veggies, fruits, rice, potatoes, bread, etc.), will quickly replenish the liver glycogen, since the body preferentially refills that glucose-storage depot once it's been depleted.

Don't Be a Hungry Vampire

Eating in blocks and windows after a fast also prevents other kinds of bad habits, like the unnecessary night eating (because you ate during the day), or constant snack-eating, which we're not designed for. Middle-of-the-night eating is notorious for generating unneeded body fat; if you stop eating at 7:30 PM and initiate even a minimal fast of 12 hours each night (eating again at 7:30 AM), watch for the probable difference it will make in cutting unnecessary fat and in how you feel.

Fasting might not be a good idea if you're taking medication and/or struggling with a chronic medical issue, so make sure to *consult a physician in these circumstances* before you try intermittent fasting. Because of the difficulty of making wise choices while being saturated with unhealthy pop-culture images of celebrities whose bodies have been augmented by Photoshop, fasting may also not be a good idea for young men and women who might seek weight loss as a goal, as opposed to metabolic improvements.

ONE ATHLETE'S EXPERIENCE WITH FASTING

I asked Bob Watson, a teacher, athlete, and cross-country coach, to provide some details on his own experience with intermittent fasting. He mainly combines intermittent fasting with resistance training and, when he's coaching, running.

I've been doing the Martin Berkhan/Leangains-style 16-hour daily fast for a while now. I toyed with 24-hour fasts once or twice/week a couple times this summer, but honestly it feels too long—not that I get overly hungry, but when I break the fast the food would sit heavily in my stomach and the joy of eating was diminished. Also, I think the 16-hour daily regimen works well for me because of my personality (I like routines) and my regular work schedule.

Others might find longer fasts once or twice a week easier to do. Most days it's no problem to make the 16 hours, but if I'm famished and haven't hit 16 hours yet, I eat. When I travel I play around with different fasting protocols so I don't have to eat airport food.

I usually don't get too hungry, and when I do, it's very manageable. I used to get hungry and get headaches, my stomach would growl, etc. Now, if I'm hungry, I can eat right away or I can wait an hour or more with little to no discomfort. There is one aspect of the fasting that I keep a mental eye on, and I think this is very much linked to my detail-oriented/concrete thinking personality: I worry a bit that I obsess about timing my meals and feel pressured to always be on top of fasting/eating times. I would like to start adopting a looser stance like you talk about—doing it a few times a week. I will keep playing around until I find something natural, but for now the 16-hour fasts fit nicely into my schedule.

My usual schedule is:

Wake up 6:30. In the morning, I drink 2 pints of water upon waking. Then I make a half mug of strong black coffee that I sip on the way to work and into my first period class. I drink another pint or more of water around 9–9:30.

I usually eat lunch between 11 and 12. This is usually a pretty big meal, as I'm ready to eat at this point. Leftover pot roast, 6-egg omelets, things like that. If it's a workout day, I'll add a starch—usually a large sweet potato. I also have a shake with lunch on workout days. I make a "fat bomb" smoothie à la Richard Nikkoley from *freetheanimal.com*: coconut milk, water, frozen berries, protein powder, cocoa powder (100%), and one or two raw egg yolks (from my chickens in the backyard). I usually drink half of this at lunch and the other half after dinner as dessert. Water with all meals and throughout the day—I try to keep my intake up. I probably drink about 4 or 5 pints during the day.

Apps for Fasters

You can use any digital timer to show you how long you've fasted (or you could just look at your watch). For example, you can use the Endomondo app with an unspecified fitness category of "other," as shown in Figure 6-1 (we talked about this app for measuring sports fitness training in Chapter 2).

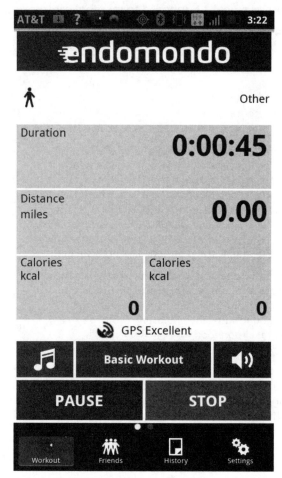

Figure 6-1. *Time your fast with Endomondo*

An iPhone App named IF Timer is also available, but I haven't used it yet (Apple user, alas, with Android smartphone). Check it out at *http://itunes. apple.com/us/app/if-timer/id414565808?mt=8&ign-mpt=uo%3D4*.

The Fitbit gives you a pretty good picture of how many calories you've burned during the fast (we also discuss this device—a pedometer with a website—in Chapter 2). I'm not too sure how useful that is, as "calories in, calories out" is probably a crude measure of what's happening physiologically during a fast (and your weight will be affected by how well you're hydrating during the fast, among other things).

At any rate, while I'm not privy to the algorithm the Fitbit software uses, the calorie calculation probably goes something like this: your basal metabolic rate (say, 70 calories per hour for me) x number of hours of fast + extra calories expended by activity (say 300 calories, during a 4.5-mile walk on the beach).

Your basal metabolic rate (BMR) represents how many calories you expend to maintain internal physical systems in the absence of additional activity—say, if you laid on the couch all day.

So, given the latter equation and a 16-hour fast, the fast would have expended or "cost" about (16 x 70 + 300), or roughly 1,420 calories. This gives you an idea of how much you should be eating during the chow-down window, to replenish your body and even add lean mass (in that case, you probably should eat *more* than the fast expended).

The Other World:
A.K.A. Outside

7

We geeks just don't get outside enough. After a while, "outside" begins to be defined as the carpeted hallway outside the main office where the restrooms are, or the food court emporium downstairs.

I once worked in a software house in a beautiful, historic seacoast community. People worked hard there and seemed to like the company and their jobs. The trouble was, no one went outside. People were so fond of their cushy positions, it was as if they were afraid to leave the environs after 9 AM rolled around. Even at lunch break, most of them would stay in their cubicles or repair to the cafeteria for the meatloaf and mashed potatoes.

What do you expect from a company that still held "casual Friday," during which management wore jeans (they probably called them "dungarees")?

Of course, it wasn't exactly the company's fault that no one was going outside (even though they were a little chintzy about vacation time). Everyone had simply forgotten their roots, or had been dissuaded by antisun dogma.

Outside the company were beautiful hilly walks that you could take in the sun. I took them every lunch break, and they made me forget about the somewhat dun-looking brick offices. A whole new world existed out there, including a coffee shop I'd hit up for a to-goer on the way back. The shop was partly managed by a former Sherpa for Mt. Everest expeditions, believe it or not (he was now working at about 50 feet above sea level). He would chat with me about climbing Everest, I would look at his maps, and from there I would dream. I never would have discovered his shop if I never went outside.

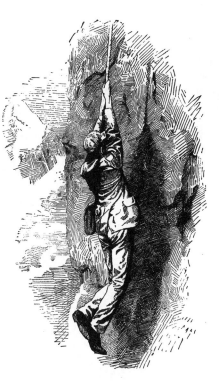

The Sun Is Our Friend

To keep a theme going from Chapter 1, we have built-in software code that expects us to be companionable with the sun. We were not designed to sit in a dark room all day and night, typing code. This has become the norm in some software outfits, but once you discover the negative fitness implications of being a shut-in, you might look askance at this sunless office existence.

Simply being in the sun, or at least outside, first thing in the morning, then at least sporadically throughout the day for an indoor worker and for a long time during the weekend, is healthy.

The problem is, we've been inculcated with advice and dogma that the sun is our enemy. It causes skin cancer; therefore, we should always cover ourselves with clothes and sunblock. A very good doctor in every other way once told me to apply sunblock whenever I was out in the sun for more than 10 minutes, even in New England during the winter.

The sun is healthy for a number of reasons:

- It helps you make vitamin D (a lot of it, if you're a young lifeguard in a bathing suit or a youngster running around in the sun—sun *burns* are bad though, so watch the dosage).

- Vitamin D and/or increased sun exposure may actually prevent many cancers, possibly beyond the vitamin-D effect. According to Dr. john Briffa, "Higher levels of this nutrient and/or increased sunlight exposure are associated with a reduced risk of several cancers."[1]

- Sun exposure first thing in the morning stimulates a part of the hypothalamus in the brain called the *supra-chiasmatic nucleus* (SCN) to send signals to the rest of the body, helping control body temperature and the release of hormones such as cortisol and melatonin (which has a delayed release, until evening). These actions control your internal clock (when you feel wakeful and sleepy—see Chapter 9).[2]

- Sunlight has a mood-elevating effect for most people.

- Heck, we might find out, down the line, that a little sun exposure positively effects gene expression.

And it goes on and on.

Our ancestors spent a lot of time outdoors in and out of the sun, and it's even surmised that as we migrated to northern latitudes from Africa, the evolution to lighter skin was designed to admit more sunlight and vitamin D.

GO OUTSIDE FOR *FRILUFTSLIV*: ASK THE SCANDINAVIANS

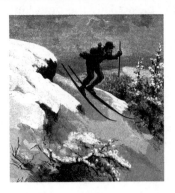

Why *should* I go outside, when I have work to do? Well, ask the Norwegians and Swedish people, with their centuries-old *friluftsliv* (roughly pronounced, "free-loofs-leave") tradition. As a writer who has just come upon this concept, I realize that I have strongly embraced this tradition (without conceiving of it concretely as "tradition"), even though I never knew that a cultural philosophy had been framed around it. The term translates loosely as "free air life" or "free open air."

It is a philosophy of basically making a spiritual connection with nature by walking and skiing in the wilderness a lot (please hold the sarcasm about communing with nature; there really is something to this philosophy fitness-wise). "Nature" could just be the local park or coastline—whatever you have available. You don't have to jump on a plane bound for an expensive holiday in the Alps or Himalaya to enjoy it. The idea is to take long walks (or ski trips) whenever you have the free time, with people you enjoy or just on your own, and that this activity is intrinsically beneficial for your body and soul, and makes you spiritually stronger by helping you appreciate your environment and understand your ecological niche.

Since way before the iPad, *friluftsliv* has been thought of as an escape valve for modern industrial lifestyles that jam us inside all the time and somewhat warp our views of our place on the earth. There is a philosophical connection between *friluftsliv* and the concept of "Deep Ecology," an invention of the Norwegian mountaineer and philosopher Arne Naess (see *www.deepecology.org/movement.htm*).

Both the Swedish and Norwegians have cultivated their outdoor traditions by implementing laws allowing the free use of uncultivated land and wilderness for hiking and skiing, no matter who owns it. Too often, as one essay about *friluftsliv* points out, we have commercialized the wilderness as an "arena" for testing ourselves and our gear.[3]

Not to mention the fact that long walks outside are healthy and a good remedy for stress. *Friluftsliv*, hmm, it's hard to say, but count me in.

A recent study in the British Journal of Nutrition *examined the vitamin-D levels of two traditional cultures that live near the equator and spend a lot of time outside—the Maasai and Hadzabe hunter-gatherers of Tanzania in East Africa. The mean vitamin-D level (25(OH) D) in the blood of about 60 study participants, men and women, was 115 nmol, or about 46 ng/ml, all obtained naturally by exposure to sunlight. The people typically avoided the sun at its strongest, during midday. "Populations with traditional lifestyles having lifelong, year-round exposure to tropical sunlight might provide us with information on optimal vitamin D status from an evolutionary perspective," according to the study.[4]*

So, now we've established that being outside is healthy (see the sidebar on the Scandinavian philosophy of *friluftsliv*).

Exercising Outside

Obviously, *exercising* outside is healthy, too—particularly the right kind of exercise. Simply being outside during parts of the day, such as first thing in the morning as the sun rises, enhances your overall outlook and fitness in its own right. Now we're going to add some descriptions of outdoor fitness techniques and tools, beginning with good old walking.

Walking

Back when I was putting in mega miles as a runner and biker, I used to have a somewhat snotty attitude toward walking. I used to see lots of people taking their habitual morning walks, and snicker. My attitude could be summed up as "Hey, we're bipedal by nature, so how can *that* be a 'workout'? You gotta kick it up a notch to get really strong!"

Little did I realize that I was the one who was wrong, or know that this was the whole point, and elegance, of walking in the first place. We're perfectly designed for walking, we can go many miles without tiring or breaking down, and the motion itself has a variety of beneficial effects. It's healthy, simply because walking *isn't* sitting.

You don't have to put in mega miles to reap the benefits of walking. As mentioned in Chapter 2 on tools, we seem to be designed for a steady oscillation of movement throughout the day (not sitting all day). Thus, little walks spread throughout the day, particularly as mental breaks, have a perfect place in our fitness strategy while working. Not to mention the fact that they get us outside, under the sun (or maybe if you're in Seattle, at least the view is good), and off the mechanistic treadmill.

> *It's possible that walking helps burn fats, the chief source of fuel for striding, from peripheral fat depots of the body, where you want to reduce it. Jogging, on the other hand, may burn fat predominantly within the muscles' fat storage sites, where you don't mind having fat.*

Walking raises the heart rate, but not to the extent where you kick your metabolism up to a level where you stop burning fats predominantly (we'll discuss walking and weight loss when we cover our Endomondo fitness walk). The cardiovascular benefits particularly accrue when you're carrying a little weight like a backpack and the walk itself is hilly (see "Hiking and Climbing" just ahead in this chapter).

You can combine walking with many other fitness techniques, such as pull-ups, push-ups, jumping, and sprints. We'll discuss all of these combo fitness techniques throughout this chapter.

Recovery plan

Walking is the perfect recovery plan for resting from a sprint or especially a resistance-training or weight workout. You're getting the rest that's required following those types of training sessions (if you're doing them correctly), yet ideally, you're outside, getting *some* movement, as well as enjoying Mother Nature.

Walking is also good preparation for any big efforts that you have planned (e.g., climbing your first 14,000-foot mountain, or doing your first triathlon), yet it doesn't leave you overtrained, unrested, or with muscles that lack their stored glycogen. It is essentially a form of rest that still qualifies as exercise, if you catch my drift.

Sports nutrition–wise, the big muscles are likely to retain their glycogen stores, since during a slow walk you are mostly going to burn fats from fat storage sites (so don't bring stuff to eat on a walk, or your body will leave the fats alone and burn the carbs you're eating for energy!).

Simply being outside during parts of the day, such as first thing in the morning as the sun rises, enhances your overall outlook and fitness in its own right.

Family stroll

Walking is the "training" you can do with other companions, whether it be an 80-year-old grandparent, a child, or a dog. What is that saying? "Want to lose weight—get a dog." There are hundreds of benefits to walking. Like swimming, you can even do it injured (unless the injury is to your legs).

Walking is great for people whose jobs require long or frequent cell phone calls. Just do it while walking; you've killed two birds with one stone, and converted a health-negative behavior (yakking on cell phones) to a net positive. As long as you keep the cell phone a safe distance from your head, that is! Do most phone calls while walking— the calories will add up.

Walking tools

Other than your walking stick, of course, a phone with the Endomondo app loaded onto it and a camera are perfect tools for tracking and capturing your walk. Go to *www.endomondo.com* if you haven't acquired the free app yet.

When you launch the app on your phone, you'll see the screen shown in Figure 7-1. This is the screen that tracks your walk. Notice that the type of activity with the little hiker icon has been set to Fitness walking (just tap that area of the screen to show different types of exercise routines). Start the timer and off you go.

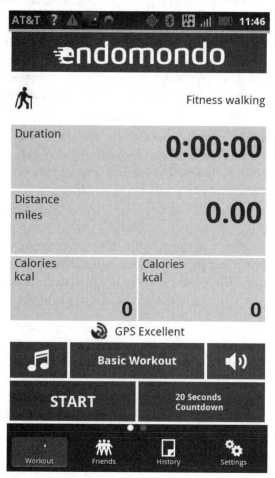

Figure 7-1. *Set Endomondo for a walk*

The app will grab all the statistics and mapping data for your walk (and we'll show you how to load that data into Google Earth later, in the "Hiking and Climbing" section). Figure 7-2 shows the statistics for the short walk I took to start off the morning. It wasn't very long—1.45 miles and about 28 minutes—but notice that the calories or kcals burned were estimated at 130. I'll include a bit more information on that in a moment. The buttons at the bottom allow you to upload the session to Endomondo's website, where you have a personal page, or to Facebook.

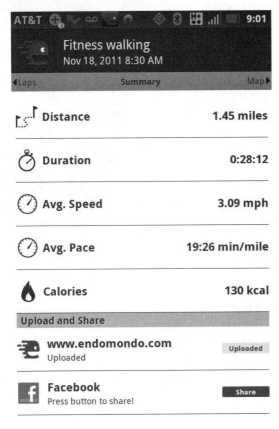

All details at www.endomondo.com

Figure 7-2. *All the Endomondo stats for your walk*

You can scroll to another screen for a map of your walk, but you can view an even better one on the website itself. Figure 7-3 shows the map for my flat walk and the profile graph, which displays the miles-per-hour and elevation data for every step (no pun intended) of the way. Endomondo will store all your walks, runs, cycles, hikes, etc.

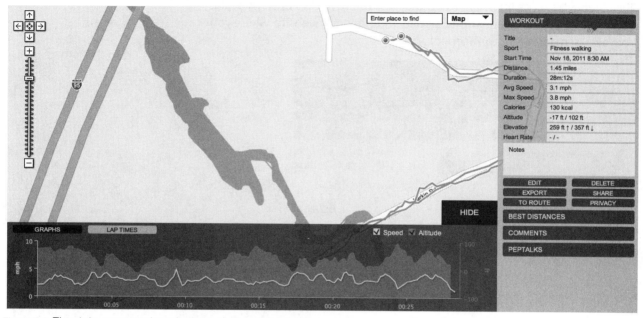

Figure 7-3. *The stats, maps, and graphs for an Endomondo stroll*

The calorie count is, of course, an estimate, which probably includes your basal metabolic rate (BMR). See the sidebar on BMR for more information. For example, my BMR is roughly 70 calories per hour, meaning I'd burn off about 1,680 calories while prone in bed all day. So, during a 28-minute walk, I burned about 130 kcal according to Endomondo, or about 100 kcal extra on top of my BMR.

WHAT'S YOUR BASAL METABOLIC RATE?

The BMR represents how many calories humans expend to maintain their vital organs and functions. This is the amount of fuel in calories that is required to run your brain (which represents about 20 percent of your energy), your heart, lungs, liver, kidneys, skeletal muscle, and on and on. It does not represent the calories you expend running or lifting weights, or even digesting food (food-related thermogenesis).

It is usually expressed as calories or kcal per day, as in 1,680 kcal per day or 70 kcal per hour. The BMR is roughly the amount of calories you would burn in a day if all you were doing was lying on a couch.

An easy calculation to figure out your BMR per hour is kilograms (kg) of weight (1 kilogram = 2.2 pounds) times 1 if you're a man, or times 0.9 if you're a woman. So a 70-kg, or 154-pound, man has a BMR of 70 kcal/hour, or 1,680/day; and a 60-kg, or 132-pound, female has a BMR of 60 kcal/hour or 1,440/day. There are other, more complicated, BMR formulas (see *http://en.wikipedia.org/wiki/Basal_metabolic_rate#BMR_estimation_formulas*), but they pretty much reach a similar conclusion.

The body-composition (BC) scales that many athletes and health-conscious people use, such as the Tanita BC scales, use a slightly different formula that attempts to take into account the different levels of lean body mass each person has.

Lean body mass is the weight of your body, not including its fat tissue. Strip all the fat off your body, even the adipose tissue you need to survive, and that's your lean body mass.

A pound of muscle burns more calories per day (about 6 to 10) than a pound of fat (about 2), so more muscular people have above average, but not *that* much higher, basal metabolic rates. For example, if you gain five pounds of muscle (which is hard to do, depending on where you are starting from), your BMR goes up by about 30–50 kcal per day (a couple of big bites of a corn muffin). Despite former claims that adding muscle will cause your BMR to soar to the tune of 50+ calories per pound per day, this is not true. Muscle building has many other substantial health benefits, however, including better strength, balance, injury prevention, positive gene expression, and insulin sensitivity.

Little things add up

If you're trying to drop a few extra pounds (and who isn't these days, among us geeks?), and you take two of these pleasant, easy walks per day (no big deal), you will expend an extra 7 x 200, or 1,400 kcal for one week (if you don't quaff a pint of India Pale Ale during the walk, or chow down a corn muffin). This would add up to 8,400 calories in six weeks, or about 2.4 pounds (8,400 / 3,500).

There are about 3,500 calories in a pound.

As mentioned previously, the section on hiking shows how to load captured Global Positioning System (GPS) data into Google Earth to view an even cooler and more memorable panorama of your route (except we'll show something more exciting, as in a wilderness mountain hike).

Sprinting

We are all natural-born sprinters. How many times did you sprint as a child—after a friend, a dog, a baseball, a Frisbee, a dream, a phantom? Forgot, didn't you? It had to have been thousands of times. Study after study has shown how effective and efficient sprinting is for fitness. We won't bore you with all the technical details behind sprinting, except to mention a few eye-opening studies, then we'll move straight to some cool sprinting techniques and protocols.

One of the most impressive aspects of sprinting, or *interval* training, is that studies show it tends to slow the aging process in terms of the cardiovascular system and the specific leg muscles involved with sprinting, such as the Type II "fast twitch" fibers in your quadriceps or thigh muscles. Your skeletal muscles include Type I slow-twitch muscle fibers, which are less powerful but take longer to fatigue, and the faster-fatiguing "fast-twitch" fibers—Type IIa (slightly longer to fatigue) and Type IIx.

One of the most impressive aspects of sprinting or interval training is that studies show it tends to slow the aging process in terms of the cardiovascular system and the specific leg muscles involved with sprinting.

> *Interval training means short, often all-out sprints followed by short rests, and then additional sprint repetitions. Intervals are a common training technique in a number of sports, including cycling, Nordic skiing, swimming, and even weightlifting.*

One 2006 study did a detailed analysis via muscle biopsies of the legs of sprinters of varying ages. They studied men aged 18 years all the way up to 84. The results were surprising; the 84-year-olds (yeah, people that age and older are still sprinting!) had fiber-power values that greatly exceeded those of untrained 70-year-old men. Even more impressive was that the octogenarians had the equivalent sprint power of untrained 40-year-old men, less than half their age.[5] So get granddad out there!

The study also emphasized the fitness gains and antiaging aspects of explosive-type exercise techniques: "Although our findings are not directly applicable to untrained people, they tend to favor the view that, to minimize the effect of aging on the neuromuscular system, optimal overall physical training might require actions that impose explosive-type overload on muscle."[6]

Sprint efficiencies

Sprinting produces high fitness levels in a more time-efficient manner compared with long endurance workouts. Study after study indicates this benefit, including the original research behind the now-famous Tabata Protocol (see the "Tabata sprints" section).

A 2006 study in the *Journal of Physiology* studied the fitness difference between athletes who had undergone short-term interval training and others who did long-distance cycling. They split up 16 men to perform six training sessions over 14 days. The "sprinters" did four to six all-out 30-second sprints on a bike with 4 minutes rest between them. The long-distance cyclists did 90-minute to 2-hour cycles each workout, at a moderate pace.

The study scientifically analyzed the athletes after the study period to measure their progress in improving cardiovascular strength. Even though the total difference in cycling time was 2.5 hours for the sprinters (over six workouts) versus 10.5 hours for the longer-distance cyclists, the training benefits were about the same.

"Given the large difference in training volume, these data demonstrate that SIT [sprint-interval training] is a time-efficient strategy to induce rapid adaptations in skeletal muscle and exercise performance that are comparable to endurance training in young active men."[7]

The long and the short of it

"So what?" you might reply. "I like riding my bike for long distances—I don't want to go home after getting my butt kicked for 28 minutes." So be it—I often have the same attitude. Long-distance endurance training, what some have dubbed "chronic cardio," does have it downsides, however, in terms of eating up lean body mass (a.k.a. your muscles) and generating more wear-and-tear injuries to the feet, knees, and hips, as well as a greater production of oxidative stress—the "reactive oxygen species" that you're eating all those antioxidants in your meals to deal with.

On the other hand, one of the upsides of "long slow distance" is its relaxing, contemplative quality—its positive influence on reducing stress. Sprinting, by contrast, sometimes feels like another form of stress.

It is "good stress", though—see Chapter 11 and its segment on hormesis.

As a practical matter, not everyone can jump right into sprinting, particularly someone who has weight issues or is bouncing back from injury or illness and has just begun an exercise program.

This past weekend, I took advantage of a mild winter in New England to put in about 30 miles on my mountain bike, under the sun. It felt wonderful (I did throw in some cycling sprints in high gear on the first day), and provided a welcome relief to higher-intensity skiing in some of the subArctic temperatures we had experienced of late.

The consensus advice is, at least once a week, substitute a sprint workout for one or more of those long hauls, and you'll be fitter and better off.

Sprint protocols

Sprinting offers all kinds of combinations or ways of structuring the workout. Thankfully, everyone knows how to do it (just run, and imagine you're being chased by a grizzly bear!). It all depends how fit you are when you start

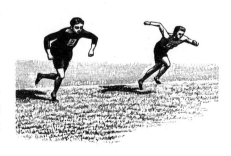

Sprinting offers all kinds of combinations or ways of structuring the workout.

sprinting. I'm an advocate of going to a track or a soccer field where the distances are known and/or marked off. A beach is also a great place to sprint, because it offers the extra resistance of sand and the opportunity to do the runs barefoot, along with the sublime seascape itself.

We're talking about running sprints here, but the same protocols can be applied to intervals in other sports.

Sprinting a soccer field

A regulation soccer field is about 100 yards from goal line to goal line (some are 110). Here's a routine I use sometimes.

I have a soccer field about two miles from my house (given the popularity of the sport, just about everyone does these days). As a warm-up, I pull on a pair of sneakers, hop on a mountain bike, and ride around effortlessly for 10 or 20 minutes, ending at the field. A warm-up is necessary—it doesn't have to be too extensive—because you're going to be using your "highest gear" for sprinting, and you don't want to tear anything.

I get to the soccer field, park the bike, and do a little more stretching and warm-up as I jog over to the goal line. Since it's grass, I often do these sprints barefoot. In the beginning of the season, when I'm not up to sprint shape, I dash no more than 50 yards, to the center of the field. Even a few 25-yarders to get in the proper state of mind and to prime the big leg muscles for an all-out effort will do the trick.

Maximum effort, not steady state

Another common technique for sprint warm-ups on a field or basketball court is "shuttle runs." Sprint 5 yards, turn around and jog back; sprint 10 yards, turn around and jog back, sprint 15 yards, and so on.

I sprint to the 50-yard line four or five times, with each sprint a little stronger than the one before. Depending on how you feel, you can just walk back to the goal line after each dash. The idea is not to keep the heart rate high *all* the time, but to produce a maximum effort that lasts just a few seconds.

The mental game

All forms of exercise are "mental" in nature, and involve a lot of emotional engagement and visualization. Sprinting is no different. I imagine I'm fleeing from a predator, or trying to save a loved one (yikes, that train is coming and they need to be dragged off the tracks in time!). When you hit the final 10 yards, you really open up; imagine an Olympic sprinter who starts in a crouch, but by the final yards she's in a straight-up stance, taking short powerful strides and pumping her arms.

Time to go all out

Sprinting involves a lot of upper body engagement to propel the body forward.

If a few 50-yard sprints feel good, it's time for an all-out 100. Do one complete soccer-field sprint all out, leaving nothing left. Time yourself, and use that metric for future runs. As you get stronger, all your sprints will be 75 to 100 yards, barring a few warm-ups.

I try to keep 15 seconds or less as a benchmark, for example.

How do you know you've gone all out for 100 yards? This is kind of a personal, almost primordial feeling, a mixture of fatigue and fear. Most of the time, you simply can't go any faster. Once you get used to sprinting 100 yards, the final 25 yards will feel liberating, but *you can't wait* to hit the finish line. Your body should feel like it is undergoing an intensive, good stress. Once there, you commonly can't talk at all as you catch your breath. Your heart rate probably hit its maximum level, roughly 220 minus your age, then went back down, rapidly if you're in good condition. Sometimes after the final rep of an interval you feel ever so slightly nauseous. This passes very quickly. I don't advocate sprinting until you barf!

To get yourself psyched, watch Usain Bolt of Jamaica run a sub-20-second 200 meters: www.squidoo.com/Usain-Bolt-The-Track-And-Field-Athlete-Biography.

You can walk back slowly to the goal line, with runner's high and all, calmly savoring the maximum effort. You're the healthier for it.

Specific sprinting protocols

There are all kinds of protocols you can use for structuring your sprints, including ones of your own invention (see the "Make it up" section).

We just mentioned a study that used *four to six repetitions of 30-second all-out sprints*, with four minutes of rest between them. This is a good protocol for the beginning of your sprint program. The rest period seems like a long time, but that's the point. Being rested for each repetition allows you to reach the proper level of intensity for each interval.

As we'll get into in our discussion of resistance training in the next chapter, the purpose of the sprint is to stimulate or stress the big, fast-fatiguing Type IIa or IIx muscle fibers. These muscles are not trained by slow to moderate jogging; that kind of locomotion will be taken care of by the less powerful, slower-to-fatigue Type I fibers of the leg.

Type II fibers include a few subclassifications—IIa and IIx.

If you don't blast through your fast-twitch muscles, you won't stimulate the adaptations and metabolic changes that you want.

Another protocol involves *10 one-minute intervals at 60 percent of your maximum capacity, with a minute rest between each one*. This routine came from Clarence Bass's website (www.cbass.com); he's a totally ripped septuagenarian who has written many books on bodybuilding and health, and knows of what he speaks.

The latter routine could be used as a moderate introduction to hard sprints like the Tabata Protocol.

Tabata sprints

The now-famous (among interval and CrossFit geeks) Tabata protocol is a remarkably simple (but hard!) method for increasing your cardiovascular strength and health. It is becoming very popular in several sports, as it's become quite common for runners, cyclists, Nordic skiers, and CrossFit aficionados to adopt this technique.

The Tabata Protocol is named after one of its inventors, a professor and researcher in Japan named Izumi Tabata. His studies determined that this interval protocol allows you to have your cake and eat it too: the routine strengthens both aerobic fitness and sprint strength. It derived from work he originally did with speed skaters.

The intervals involve *eight repetitions of 20-second all-out efforts, with 10-second rests*. In other words, a total of four minutes, not including warm-up and cool down. The key is the shortness of rest, which is minimal while you're doing these sprints, if you do them correctly (meaning, you don't exceed the rest interval). Izumi himself, in an interview, pointed out that this four-minute maxed-out routine is "more than enough to make even a fit person exhausted . . painful." In fact, for this reason, he doubted that Tabata would ever be popular beyond hard-core competitive athletes.[8]

The protocol has nevertheless become wildly popular, even among resistance trainers, probably because of its proven effectiveness, its short-term duration, and the challenge it presents. I think people simply love running as fast as they can, as if this behavior triggers a kind of Paleo pathway with which we are instinctively familiar.

For example, I introduced Tabata sprints to a cross-country team about a year ago. We jogged over to a dirt path in the woods. Knowing that a typical soccer field length would be good for Tabata sprints, I jogged along, roughly measuring that distance (counting a yard for every one of my strides), then marked the end with a stick I pulled out of the woods. This was a decidedly low-tech introduction to Tabata sprints, taking place in a woodsy, less sanitized environment than a track.

Then we broke up into two separate groups, one the slightly speedier and more fit and the other slightly less so. I did the sprints with them, then looked at my watch to count off the 10-second rest. They turned out to love the workout, and it became their favorite training session throughout the week. The cross-country coach, a friend of mine, noted that the team made rapid strides in overall strength and fitness once they started using Tabata. It was noticeable after just two sessions.

One of the runners told me later that she kept doing them throughout the summer once a week on her driveway.

Could it be that one of the reasons this routine is popular is the catchy name itself, with its funky internal rhythms that seem to suggest "keep to the beat"?

Make it up

You don't have to jump right into Tabata sprints. You can just make up your own routine, and it will make a difference. It's the all-out effort that matters. Here's what I did the other weekend. I didn't have the flexibility to go to a track or the beach alone, as I was looking after my son at home.

I used Endomondo to measure a 100-to 120-yard length along the flat driveway that runs in front of my house. This is easy to do: just set Endomondo for a Fitness walk, and begin walking until you reach .07 mile (roughly 123 yards; the app will increment the miles by hundredths of a mile). 100 yards is about .056 of a mile, so you can pace out .06 of a mile and place a marker a bit shy of that milestone. Now you have a 100- and a 120-yard course to sprint on.

You can also set the Endomondo app for a kilometer unit of measure in its settings segment.

I did six 120-yard sprints with a leisurely walk back to the starting line in between, accounting for a rest between reps of about 1:15. I was doing each rep in about 19 to 21 seconds, not quite all out, but maybe 80 to 90 percent. Then I did the final 100 all out, a little faster than I did the previous sprints. That was just what I felt like doing that morning, no more no less. In the old running days we used to say, "Do one less interval than you think you can do" (don't run to failure). In other words, when you finish an interval and your body is telling you that you have just one left, that's the time to go home.

I cannot point to a scientific study that underlies the latter strategy, but it's folk wisdom that works well.

Run/Cycle/Sprint Hybrids

Sprints can easily be incorporated into steady-state training sessions. This is typical of cycling when you head off at your usual "spin" or cross-country pace, then initiate sporadic all-out sprints along the way. Fartleks and body speeds are two ways of incorporating sprints into long runs.

Fartleks

Fartlek means "speed play" or "speed game" in Swedish. It is nothing more than fast runs or sprints between landmarks during a long run. The technique has been around since the running boom started in earnest decades ago, and was designed to add a speed workout to mileage.

The way I always did fartleks was to sprint between telephone poles. City or suburban runners can sprint a block sporadically; or you can use whatever milestone you want, such as running hard up every hill. You can also mix up the number of repetitions and the intensity of each. If you run a fartlek really hard, you may have to walk the next tenth of a mile or so.

Fartleks matter even on a short run, like two to three miles. Instead of just plodding along on a rather inefficient jog workout, you've done your routine run plus sprints.

Body speeds

Body speeds are a kind of technique drill for runners. They are good preparation for doing sprints if you're just getting back to running all out (because we do let that inborn skill go stale!).

You head out on a flat run or a track, and then for 50 or 100 yards or so run at about 75 percent of your maximum rate or sprint speed. While you're running, you visualize being graceful, balanced, and smooth in your stride. You try to improve awkward aspects of your running, like rocking back and forth and not using your arms enough.

In other words, you're *not* going fast enough to be thinking exclusively about how hard the effort is and only getting to the finish line. Your pace is slower, so you have the luxury of focusing on body and spirit as you glide along—it's "mindful sprinting."

The idea is that by practicing your fast-running technique, you will become a smoother runner, and the more graceful sprinting will become second nature during your all-out intervals. Body speeds are also fun to do because you are going fast (and fast is fun), but they don't hurt as much as all-out sprints. They seem to work.

Body-Weight Exercises

These are exercises that are designed to make you strong by pulling or pushing your own weight around. They can be performed inside or outdoors, but for most people it's more fun to do them outside. That way you can get some sun and fresh air while you're huffing and puffing, and you can combine these exercises with runs, hikes, and bikes.

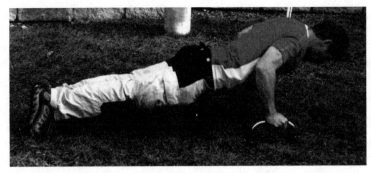

Figure 7-4. *Doing pushups outside with pushup bars*

Push-up training, particularly in the beginning, shares some features with sprinting. If you can't yet do a lot of push-ups at once (e.g., 30-50 without resting), work up to them in sets, with a decent rest between sets.

Push-ups

Most people know what a push-up is (as well as a pull-up), ever since Coach McConnell barked at them in gym class, "Down and do 10!" Figure 7-4 shows what a pushup looks like.

Figure 7-4 shows a person using push-up bars, which provide some variation when doing the exercise. For some people, the pushups are a little easier and the position more comfortable with the bars. For others, they are harder. The conventional push-up involves palms flat on the ground.

Push-up training, particularly in the beginning, shares some features with sprinting. If you can't yet do a lot of push-ups at once (e.g., 30–50 without resting), work up to them in sets, with a decent rest between sets.

Push-ups are a great warm-up exercise, as well as a strengthener for your arms, shoulders, chest, and back.

You can improve your push-up and overall strength by actually making them harder by adding more weight. I do push-ups with my young son lying on my back, which is kind of a nice way to get a workout in while you are horsing around with kids. You can also do push-ups with a weighted vest (a vest you put on that suddenly makes you 40 pounds heavier!). For the sake of "empathy training," all men should be required to walk around in these vests before their wives ever enter into a pregnancy.

All kidding aside, the vests are adjustable by four-pound increments.

The idea is that when you've done push-ups with a greater amount of weight resisting you, your muscles (and everything else that is involved with pushing your weight, such as the neural mechanics) will adapt to the harder weight and the "normal" push-ups will be easier.

Inverted Push-ups

Other ways to "resist" a typical push-up is by doing inverted ones, with your feet on a bench, step, chair, or couch. Or, even harder, place your feet on the small inflatable exercise balls they have in gyms and do inverted push-ups that way.

Combine push-ups with sprints/weights. After each sprint interval, drop down and do 10 push-ups. This is a CrossFit-type routine. Or include push-ups with weightlifting. I often finish my final set of bench presses by turning around and doing inverted push-ups on the same bench. Bench presses are covered in Chapter 8.

Pull-Ups/Chin-Ups

Most people can do at least one push-up with no practice, but pull-ups? This is a tough one. It's a challenge worth meeting, though, because once you reach the point where you can perform several pull-ups, you know you have reached an impressive level of conditioning, strength, and health.

Pull-ups are a challenging but fruitful exercise. This exercise strengthens the arms, chest, back, and even abdominal muscles. Chin-ups are very similar, but involve the grip with your palms facing you, or facing each other (as in the grips on certain pull-up bars in gyms).

Outdoors offers the ideal setting for doing pull-ups. I start off most mornings at home with some sun (if it's out) and a set of pull-ups on a small jungle gym in my yard. You can obviously do them on any conceivable bar or beam from which you can hang, including a tree branch.

Figure 7-5 shows a setup for outdoor chin-ups. The grip involves the palms facing toward me.

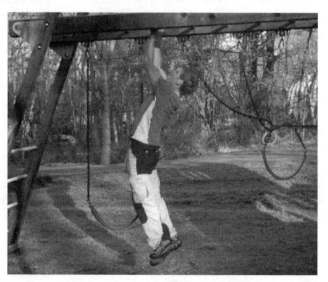

Figure 7-5. *Palms in, a chin-up outdoors, with one foot hooked behind the other*

How to do a pull-up

Warm up first by doing something with your arms and shoulders that is easier than a pull-up (which includes just about anything) such as a dip or pushup. Grip the bar above you and hang by the bar, palms facing away from you about shoulder-width apart. Cross one foot behind the other and try to keep your back straight, your body aligned and balanced. Pull yourself up so that your chin meets or exceeds the bar height. Then go all the way back down and do it again. Yeah, right!

You can experiment with different grip variations, wider or narrower on the bar.

Try to do as many as you can. Imagine not only your chest and arms providing the propulsion, but also bring in your upper back and abdomen with a recruitment of many muscle groups. The same concepts hold true for chin-ups, but this time the grip involves the palms facing in.

You can get stronger for pull-ups by implementing any exercise that strengthens the upper body, such as push-ups, bench presses, or military presses (see Chapter 8). Another way to increase the number of pull-ups you can do is to offer resistance in some manner, as in increasing the weight you are lifting, beyond your body weight. Use a weighted vest or belt and try to do as many pull-ups or chin-ups as you can.

Another recommendation comes from Stew Smith, a former Navy Seal, whose website includes a lot of valuable fitness information.[9] He suggests using the pyramid method: do one pull-up, rest, two pull-ups, rest, etc. until you can't do anymore. Then work your way back down (say you were able to do five): 1,2,3,4,5,4,3,2,1.

Trick or program yourself for more push-ups and pull-ups

Let's say you have a bad habit you want to break, or you simply want to draw attention to it. You can't keep your hand out of a bag of cookies or potato chips, or a refrigerator full of beer. You have a weakness for watching vapid TV broadcasts when you could be reading or getting more outdoor exercise. Every time you eat a cookie, you have to do 5 pull-ups, a kind of penance. Or 10 pull-ups; make it progressively more difficult. Every minute of imbecilic TV or web surfing is translated into another pull-up. Or better yet, simply turn off the TV and other screen devices unless you have something purposeful to do with them (like finish a book!).

Planks

Pull-ups strengthen your entire upper body, and so do *planks*. You've heard people mention the importance of strengthening your core (i.e., lower and upper back, abdomen, hip extensors, etc.). The plank is a good exercise for this.

The plank position is similar to a push-up position, but you are balanced on your forearms and toes. Keep your body aligned in a level position; don't let your back sag down. Use your abdominal muscles to keep your back and hips in a straightforward position. Try to hold the position for a minute, and do several repetitions.

Figure 7-6 shows what a plank looks like.

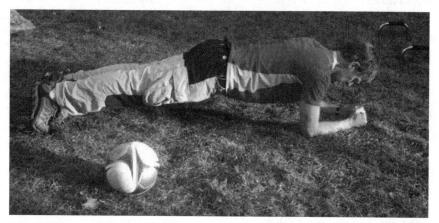

Figure 7-6. *A plank outdoors in the sun*

Obviously, you can do planks both inside and outside the gym. Another variation is to do inverted planks, similar to an inverted push-up, in which your feet are up off the ground on a bench or chair. I don't fancy this position, however, because it seems to turn into an upper-body workout. Another plank variation is the *kickback*; when you're in the plank position, pick up one of your feet about five inches and hold that position for a few seconds, as Figure 7-7 depicts.

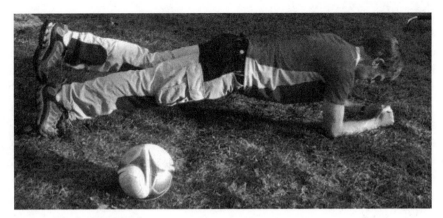

Figure 7-7. *A plank kickback*

Running Jumps

Jumping falls into the sprint category as an exercise we are designed for, but that quickly goes stale as we age. It's an explosive movement that will keep the powerful Type II, fast-fatiguing, fast-twitch muscles of the leg in tune. I like to do various jumping drills outside. Walking along a trail in the woods, I'll find a fallen tree and do sets of five standing jumps as high as I can onto the fallen trunk.

You can combine a short sprint with leaping. Go out to the beach and do a running jump as far as you can into the sand, similar to an Olympic long jump. We're often too static and programmed with our exercise routines. We go to the gym or "facility" and train robotically or let an instructor put us through our paces; we lose the creativity and playful nature of exercise.

Just make something up that requires different kinds of leaps under the sun. I have a stone wall that I jump on top of after a 30-yard or so run. It's almost 40 inches high, and I've found that the upper-leg weightlifting has helped augment my jumping ability.

Hiking and Climbing

Hiking is a perfect combination of cardiovascular and weight-bearing exercise, if you're carrying something on your back. Most hikes don't peg your heart rate at an incessantly high level (which isn't recommended for frequent exercise bouts, because it wears you out and depresses your immune system, among other things).

The exceptions are the occasional hard climbs such as Mt. Washington's Tuckerman Ravine in New Hampshire, Mt. Whitney in California, Mt. Rainier

Hiking is a perfect combination of cardiovascular and weight-bearing exercise, if you're carrying something on your back.

in Washington, or countless other climbs in the Rockies, Alps, Andes, Scottish Highlands, or other places. It's not like you're going to do these climbs every weekend, unless you're a mountain guide. Particularly concerning the Whitney Mountaineer's Route or Rainier, you will be baked afterward, and sore. Better to rest for a couple of weeks after these kinds of efforts.

Escape valve from the "thousand little stresses"

Hiking is generally a low-level effort ideal for strengthening the upper legs, recovering from harder efforts such as sprints or weights, as well as enjoying Mother Nature. It provides a break from "screen life" and the thousand little stresses of our modern lives.

I've moved to using trekking poles for hiking in recent years, and I find that they help me establish a rhythm, as well as taking the pressure off my knees and lower back during any steep descents.

Figure 7-8 shows me following my guide Braden Downey on Mt. Whitney's Mountaineer's Route in 2010. Quite a spiritual journey!

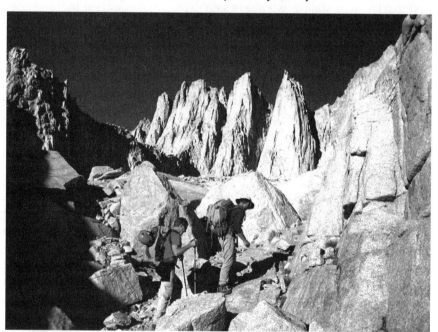

Figure 7-8. *Hiking is a great form of outdoor exercise and adventure*

Hiking as training is great for you, whether you are planning an upcoming climb or not. Pack a heavy backpack, anywhere from 20 to 40 pounds, and hit your favorite trail, or even some stadium steps. If the pack isn't heavy enough, put rocks or other heavy items inside it. When I'm training for a hard hike or climb and I can't get to Vermont's Green Mountains at the moment, I'll hike wearing a 40-pound vest.

> *Lugging around a weighted vest is not as fun as hiking a mountain, but it's better than nothing.*

Tools for hiking and trekking

There are numerous GPS-related tools and apps that augment a great hike (along with a good camera!). You can use Endomondo to track your hike and measure all kinds of aspects, such as your pace at different segments of the climb and the various elevation grades.

You can use Backpacker GPS Trails, another app for cell phones, to map out a hike with waypoints, as well as load preexisting treks into the software to guide your own trip.

Endomondo mashed up with Google Earth

We discussed Endomondo's mashup with Google Earth briefly in Chapter 2, but here I'm going to go into a little more depth on each application's features. These are great combinations of software tools, tailor-made for trekking geeks.

Figure 7-9 shows a late-autumn wilderness hike I took in Vermont's Green Mountains. This was actually the descent part of a hike into the woods from the top of a small mountain. The figure shows the screen Endomondo will display in your browser after you click the Workouts menu choice, then choose one of your climbs in the calendar view.

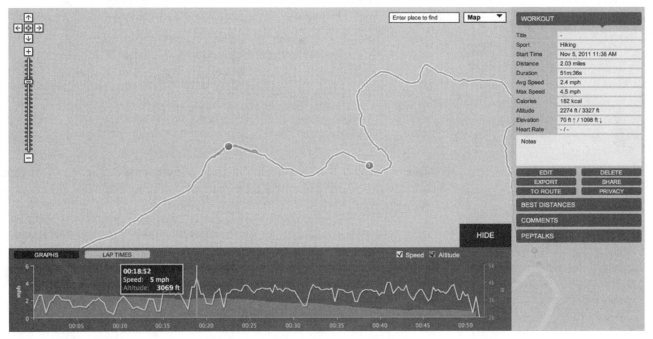

Figure 7-9. *The Endomondo graph shows speed and elevation*

As Figure 7-9 shows, you can trace the line on the graph at the bottom of the page with your cursor, and it will show the accumulated time at that point, the speed at which you were moving, and the elevation. The little blue circles are mile markers along your route.

The right-hand column shows all the juicy statistics for the hike. Click the Export button to store a GPX XML file, specifically a *.gpx* file, on your computer's hard drive.

> *GPX stands for GPS Exchange Format. It is a "light-weight XML data format for the interchange of GPS data (waypoints, routes, and tracks) between applications and Web services on the Internet" (www.topo-grafix.com/gpx.asp). See the "Inside the GPS Exchange Format File" sidebar for more GPX files).*

The free Google Earth application can then import this *.gpx* file.

It's a text (actually, XML) file with a name such as *no name.gpx.xml*. Open up this file in your favorite, XML-capable text editor and save it as *myhike.gpx*, or something like that, to make it friendlier for Google Earth (I use the BBEdit text editor on the Mac for this task).

The GPX file contains a bunch of track segments and track points in XML markup, which looks like the following code:

```
<trk>
    <src>http://www.endomondo.com/</src>
    <link href="http://www.endomondo.com/workouts/kEWNFeprngg">
      <text>endomondo</text>
    </link>
    <type>HIKING</type>
    <trkseg>
      <trkpt lat="44.147904" lon="-72.915766">
        <time>2011-11-05T15:38:39Z</time>
      </trkpt>
      <trkpt lat="44.147904" lon="-72.915766">
        <ele>1013.6</ele>
        <time>2011-11-05T15:38:44Z</time>
      </trkpt>
    </trkseg>
</trk>
```

This is the way the GPS device records a route: as a sequence of latitude and longitude points associated with a point in time, as well as an elevation figure.

INSIDE THE GPS EXCHANGE FORMAT FILE

The GPS Exchange format is "a light-weight XML data format for the interchange of GPS data (waypoints, routes, and tracks) between applications and Web services on the Internet."[10] You usually see a GPX file as a text file that is in the form of XML. If you don't know what XML is, it's just a structured method for describing the data contained by the text file with a markup language (similar to HTML and especially XHTML, which provide most of the underlying code for web pages).

Chances are, if you download a file from your GPS device, it will be in GPX format (with a suffix or extension that looks like *.gpx*). The file can be uploaded to other devices that want to read the route it contains. Garmin Connect, (*connect.garmin.com*) Endomondo (*www.endomondo.com*), and Backpacker GPS Trails Pro (*www.backpacker.com*) all allow the downloading of your recorded routes as a GPX file.

Viewing the file in a text editor, it's pretty obvious that it contains the information on a route or path over the earth. Here's an example from a GPX file from recorded ski runs on the Endomondo app: a "track" contains "track segments," which contain "track points":

```
<trk>
    <src>http://www.endomondo.com/</src>
    <link href="http://www.endomondo.com/workouts/
iSbBGiVz9CQ">
        <text>endomondo</text>
    </link>
```

```
<type>SKIING_DOWNHILL</type>
<trkseg>
    <trkpt lat="44.135844" lon="-72.895998">
        <time>2011-12-13T14:19:24Z</time>
    </trkpt>
    <trkpt lat="44.135844" lon="-72.895998">
        <ele>522.1</ele>
        <time>2011-12-13T14:19:32Z</time>
    </trkpt>
    ...
</trkseg>
</trk>
```

A track point (`<trkpt>`) is just what you would expect it to be: a point of latitude and longitude or geographical point on a map, a timestamp (the second when you happened to be cruising over that point), and your elevation at that time (feet above sea level). In XML parlance, the `trkpt` element has a `lat` and a `lon` attribute that represent its latitude and longitude. It contains nested `ele` and `time` elements, representing the elevation and captured time.

Put thousands of these points together in a GPX file, and you can draw a fine-grained line on a topographical map, which is what most applications do with them. You can also use your favorite computer language, such as Java or PHP, to read the XML off the file and do something else with it, such as save every track point you have ever recorded and display them on a map of the world.

For more details on GPX, see *www.topografix.com/gpx.asp*.

Launch Google Earth (there's a free version), then open up your *myhike.gpx* file from within Google Earth, using the File→Open command.

If you've resaved the file Endomondo exported in your text editor (with a .gpx extension), Google Earth shouldn't have any problem recognizing it.

Figure 7-10 shows a sky-high view of your hike in Google Earth. Just a few easements; not too many roads in there!

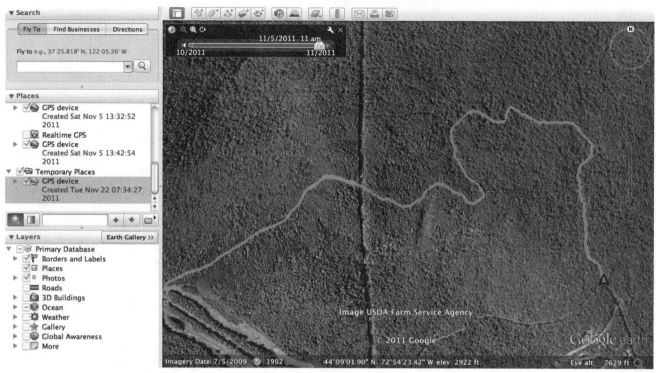

Figure 7-10. *A bird's-eye view of your hike in Google Earth*

If you ⌘-click the blue line tracing your path in Google Earth, you can choose the Show Elevation Profile feature. This opens up the graphic display along the bottom of the page, showing all kinds of useful elevation data that you can examine. Figure 7-11 shows this graphic display.

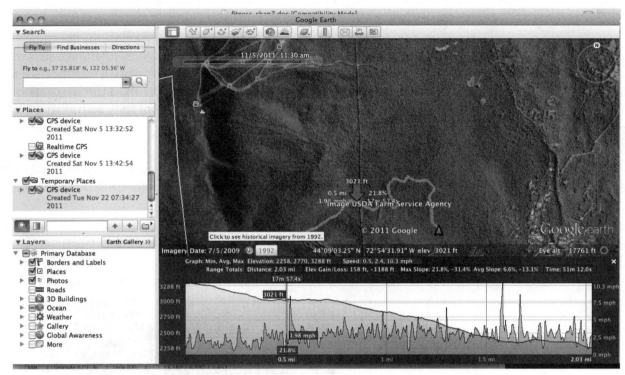

Figure 7-11. *The nifty elevation profile graphic in Google Earth*

This is a fun mashup with a practical purpose. Suppose you have forestry- or land-management responsibilities and you need to map out routes through complicated terrain, or you simply want a record of a route through the wilderness. This combination of applications will give you most of what you need. The elevation profile in Google Earth will indicate the elevation grade (e.g., 21.8%), the elevation measurement, and the miles per hour at which you were moving, at any point in the hike. Cool!

> *GPS is notoriously inaccurate, in terms of different devices giving different mile measurements (they sometimes differ by tenths of a mile). This drives runners crazy, for example. You should never really use GPS to measure off an important race route or provide a profile for a newly discovered peak. The elevation grades and miles per hour are estimates. For the vast majority of our purposes, though, the GPS data is good enough.*

So, between the Endomondo app on your smartphone, its export feature, and Google Earth, your ability to capture all kinds of hikes, bikes, runs, treks, or whatever with advanced visualization tools is unparalleled. You don't have to be climbing Mt. Everest either to use this stuff; it will embroider even one of those short urban walks you took during a break from work.

Backpacker GPS Trails

Another nifty software tool that you can use for hiking is the Backpacker GPS Trails app. Unlike Endomondo, this app is specifically designed to record a shareable, GPS-enabled trip with recorded waypoints. A waypoint is a milestone on a route; it can be annotated with icons and a text description. You can mark a waypoint on a route at any important spot, such as where a trail veers in another direction.

The Backpacker app also provides other ways of annotating a map, such as text comments and images. It even has an associated mapping application, for generating printed Topo maps (for a price, however). Figure 7-12 shows the screen on my Android phone.

Backpacker GPS Trails Pro (there's a Lite version too) has an associated website at *www.backpacker.com*, with a map and statistical data similar to that provided by Endomondo (the latter is more thorough at capturing the exercise aspects of the hike, and keeping a running count of all the data).

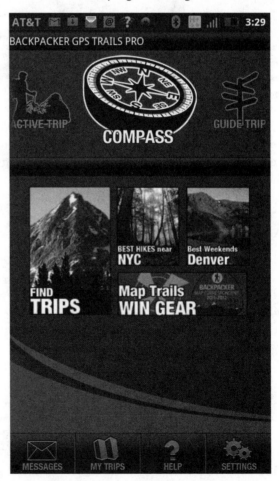

Figure 7-12. *Record a hike or make a Topo map with Backpacker GPS Trails Pro*

GPS Trails Pro is also designed to plug in preexisting hikes and waypoints, thus allowing the hiker to use his phone as a GPS navigator.

Figure 7-13 shows the page at *www.backpacker.com* after you've stopped recording your trek and (automatically) uploaded the waypoints to the Web. This was a little four-mile walk on the beach at Plum Island, Massachusetts.

A waypoint is marked as a set of geographical coordinates for a location, such as 42.781893, –70.804734.

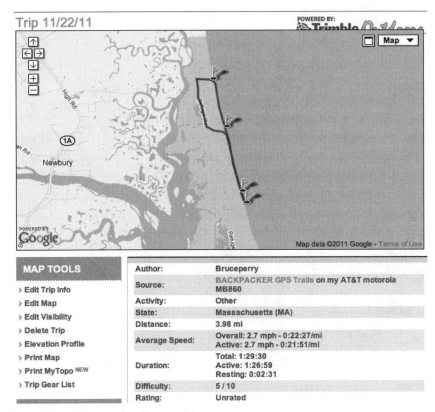

Figure 7-13. *An island walk with waypoints*

The little flags in the figure represent the waypoints that I set during the walk. You can annotate the waypoints to provide more information on the hike. The software allows fairly extensive editing of the map and waypoints online. Like Endomondo, it allows the download of a GPX file (with the extension *.gpx*) that you can plug into another GPS tracker, as well as a KML file that will open up directly in Google Earth.

A KML file is just another kind of XML file that Google Earth knows how to read, with an XML namespace of http://earth.google.com/kml/2.1.

Like Endomondo, Backpacker GPS Trails allows the download of a GPX file (with the extension .gpx) that you can plug into another GPS tracker, as well as a KML file that will open up directly in Google Earth.

Another feature I like, although it's commercial, gives you the option of generating a printed topographical map from the hike you recorded, as depicted in Figure 7-14.

Your Map Preview

Preview map thumbnail: click on the map image to download the full preview.

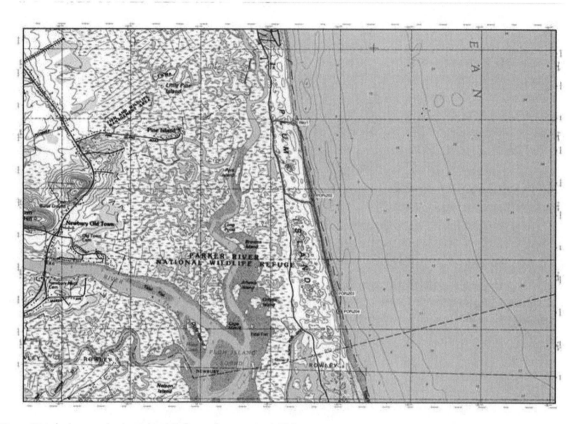

Figure 7-14. *An impressive topographical map from a coastal hike*

This relatively inexpensive app seems promising as an easy way to use your phone and GPS to record and share hikes.

Outdoor Cross-Training Routines

The woods, beaches, and even deserts provide unlimited opportunities for outdoor exercise of a structured (e.g., parcourse) and unstructured nature.

A parcourse or "fitness trail" is an outdoor trail that has various stations set up along the way to do stretching, balancing, and strength exercises. I've encountered a number of cool parcourses in Switzerland.

Using the theme of just "making things up" as you go along, I've trained with a cross-country team by using what one might call "wild runs" through the woods. This was our own version of MovNat (see the accompanying sidebar). We'd start off with scrambling and pull-ups on a sturdy, low-lying tree branch. This tests all-body strength, flexibility, and, for lack of a better term, tree-climbing ability. There's nothing like climbing trees for maintaining strength-oriented fitness, and it falls into that "what we're born for" category. Why have country kids over the ages been so good at climbing trees? How come they don't have to be taught or coached first?

WE'RE BECOMING "ZOO HUMANS": MOVNAT TO THE RESCUE

You may have noticed a recurring theme or paradigm in this book that goes something like this: we modern geeks, programmers, and office inhabitants are designed for a completely different set of behaviors and environment than those we find ourselves, here in 2012, confined to.

This is one of the simplest explanations for why we feel so lowly so often. If you took a lynx out of the Vermont woods and put it in a cage, well . . .This realization among many has launched what I would call an antimodernist movement, both recreational and philosophical, similar to the Sixties, but not necessarily laden with politics. You might also call it a "back to our nature" movement. *Friluftsliv*, discussed earlier in this chapter, also falls under this paradigm.

An athlete, sports trainer, and outdoors philosopher named Irwin LeCorre puts it very succinctly in his description of the popular "Movement Naturelle" or MovNat workshops that he has designed and taught throughout the world. Take note of this, from *http://movnat.com/about/the-zoo/*:

The "zoo" is a modern, global, and growing phenomenon generated by the powerful combination of social conventions, technological environment, and commercial pressures. Increasingly disconnected from the natural world and their true nature, zoo humans are suffering physically, mentally, and spiritually. Are you experiencing chronic pains, are you overweight, do you often feel depressed or do you suffer from frequent illnesses and general lack of vitality?

These symptoms indicate that you are experiencing the zoo human syndrome. Modern society conditions us to think that this is normal and unavoidable. We don't think so. Our true nature is to be strong, healthy, happy, and free. We have designed a complete program that empowers zoo humans to experience their true nature.

He describes MovNat as involving: "the combined training of walking, running, jumping, balancing, moving on all fours, climbing, lifting, carrying, throwing, catching, swimming and defending."

Here are some more tidbits from MovNat's web descriptions of its approach to fitness (*http://movnat.com/about/the-pillars/*):

* "In nature, any animal unable to move is condemned. As civilization leads us to increasing physical apathy, it is crucial to underline that constant physical idleness leads inevitably to loss of physical function and innumerable health problems."

* "MovNat is primarily based on rediscovering and optimizing instinctual movement patterns. It is in the first place about re-wiring the entire system of the human body back to its original mode and function."

The MovNat group offers a number of workshops and fitness retreats: see *http://movnat.com/train-with-us/*.

"We evolved from apes" would be the clichéd, somewhat cheeky response. The point is, we are designed to move naturally over the landscape that surrounds us. It's just that we go stale sitting inside and in our vehicles all day.

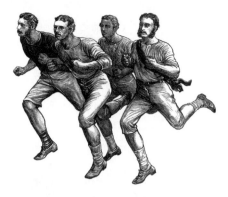

Then we would head off for a trail run, always interspersed with fartleks and *pick-ups* (dynamically picking up the pace then slowing down). We would stop, go off into the woods, and do balance drills on fallen trees, but extemporaneously. This kind of training is vastly superior to conventional static cross-country training (e.g., do jumping jacks then run till you drop, then do it again).

The runners would always look forward to these wooded romps because they were fun. By the way, they were very strenuous, too.

Beach Fit Workout

If you're lucky enough to live near or visit an open-ocean coastal area, you'll find out that the seascape provides all the gym you need. Just take off along the sand: running, sprinting, walking (Endomondo tracking is optional). A beach is usually covered with driftwood of varying sizes and weights. This derives from storms that rip trees and manmade structures off the coastline and carry them out to sea.

> *Unfortunately, the beaches are also covered with an astonishing amount of trash. Ocean pollution is a huge problem in the world. Take part in as many beach clean-ups as you possibly can, organized and on your own. Consider bringing trash bags when you take a walk on the beach.*

Use a log or piece of driftwood for jumping drills. Find a piece of wood shaped like a spear and hurl it like a javelin (watching for any beachcombers, of course). My occasional "beach fit" mornings are usually quite remote and during the winter; few other people are around, except maybe my son. Find a heavy piece of wood (those salt-laden and waterlogged pieces of debris can get pretty heavy). Starting in a crouch, pick up the log and push it end over end several times. See Figures 7-15, 7-16, and 7-17.

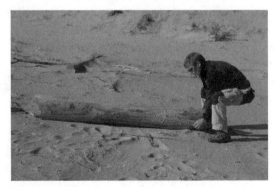

Figure 7-15. *Log flipping on the beach*

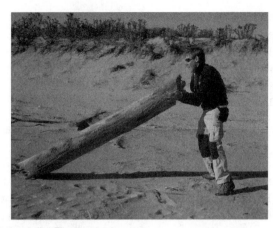

Figure 7-16. *Hoist that bale! Flip that log!*

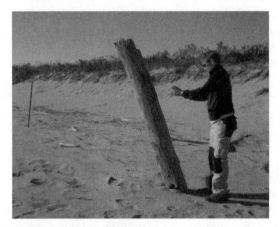

Figure 7-17. *Complete the drill—rest—do it again*

Heavy carrying is great exercise, because it uses so many of the big muscle groups, upper and lower body. Instead of just walking a mile on the beach, walk a mile carrying a heavy piece of driftwood on your shoulder. Team carries are popular, in which a group of people hoist a log onto their shoulders and carry it along the beach. This activity fosters camaraderie and teamwork. One slipup or lazy attitude, and the whole team suffers from the misstep.

Another sequential teamwork drill on the beach involves taking turns carrying a common load across the sand. The cross-country team I worked with, under an excellent coach and athlete, Bob Watson, lined up and took turns carrying a piece of driftwood as fast as they could a specified distance on the beach.

If you're lucky enough to live near or visit an open-ocean coastal area, you'll find out that the seascape provides all the gym you need.

The person carrying the heavy item (like a chunk of driftwood) returns, passes it to the next person in line, then goes to the back of the line to await another turn. This represents another fun teamwork-oriented exercise that involves components of high-intensity resistance exercise and appropriate rests between each carry or rep, not to mention a lot of razzing from the temporarily idle teammates.

Again, the young teammates usually love it, for obvious reasons. It's a "go with the flow" type of routine, with an element of playfulness. These types of workouts are by no means less effective than traditional, structured training ("Today we're doing eight 200-meter dashes, six of which must be under 30 seconds"). The playful workouts in pretty, outdoor settings are a good accompaniment to something more difficult to tolerate mentally, such as Tabata sprints.

Obviously, this chapter by no means covers every type of exercise you can do outside. We generally left out team sports, as well as specific sections on the various forms of long-distance running, cycling, and skiing (see Jack Fultz's run-training methods at the end of this chapter). Space limitations do not allow for this kind of coverage, but all of these specialized outdoor sports can use the techniques described herein to augment their own specific skill requirements and regimens.

Alpine Skiing/Snowboarding

Alpine, or downhill, skiing and snowboarding are fantastic forms of outdoor winter exercise. They are conducive to adoption by all ages; it's common to see kids of 5 and sprightly codgers of 70 or older kicking up their heels on the slopes. My ski area has an "80-year-old club" with special parking spaces for them (and yes, the club has a few members).

I've taken up downhill skiing more in earnest over the last five years, and it's been a reminder that there is so much variety and nuance to this sport—there's even a form (called Alpine touring) that involves hiking up a mountain carrying your skis, then hitching into the skis and shooshing down.

This is commonly called "backcountry" skiing or snowboarding, because a groomed resort is not required (but, especially in the Alps and the western US, avalanche training is required). Variations on free-heel skiing include Randonee, Alpine touring (AT skiing, as the lingo goes), and telemark skiing.

Alpine skiing and snowboarding have a number of special benefits:

- They foster leg strength, overall body balance, and improved *proprioception*, or awareness of your body or physicality in space (and your ability to make fast, coordination-oriented adjustments).

- Downhill skiing is a great form of aerobic and anaerobic training; for beginner to expert-level skiing, a hard top-of-the-mountain to the bottom run is like a long sprint.

- Skiing allows you to adapt to the cold temperatures; be outside during the winter (which drives many of us inside), often in the sun; and burn tons of extra calories as your metabolism ramps up to keep your body temperature stable (my pre-ski breakfasts always include one or two extra eggs, or I lose too much weight or lean mass). Cold-weather sports in general increase thermogenesis, or the burning of extra calories to maintain the homeostasis of your temperature at about 98.6.

- It's a fantastic, "mindful" activity (like Nordic or cross-country skiing) that allows you to join people of all ages in doing something healthy, or to be alone in a wilderness environment and escape urban-type lethargy and stress. Yes, it's *friluftsliv*!

- It's not a slow, endurance-focused type of activity with consequent higher oxidative-stress levels and risk of overtraining. Alpine skiing is more like sprinting.

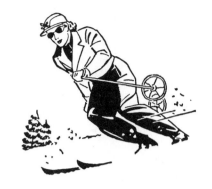

Downhill skiing is a great form of aerobic and anaerobic training.

Yes, you can use your tools to track Alpine skiing, with very interesting results.

Alpine Replay

Alpine Replay is an app for both Android and the iPhone that is specially designed to track your ski or snowboard runs, and much more. Similar to the other tracking gear we've discussed, you basically load it up on your phone, switch it on, and put it away as you begin compiling your runs, turns, jumps, and aggregate total vertical feet. Later, you log into the site at *www.alpinereplay.com* to view an impressive collection of statistics, including the total time of active skiing, sustained speeds, fastest speed, aggregated vertical feet skied, number of runs, where you rank in these categories, etc.

Figure 7-18 shows the Alpine Replay screen on my Android phone, in recording mode.

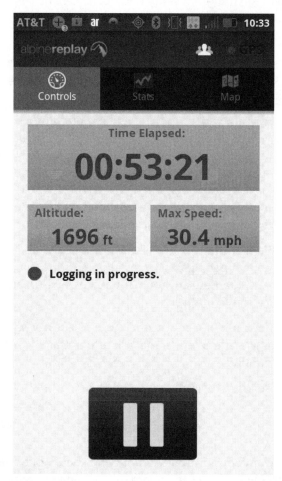

Figure 7-18. *Begin recording your ski runs with Alpine Replay on a smartphone*

Along with the skiing, the fun begins when you view your stats afterward at *www.alpinereplay.com*. Figure 7-19 shows the charts on a bunch of downhill ski runs, including fastest run, fastest sustained speed, where you rank among all users (including just within the resort where you skied), the routes you took on a Google Map, and more.

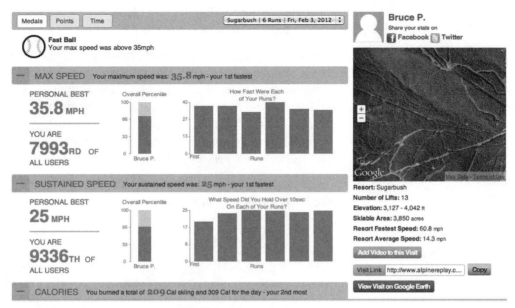

Figure 7-19. *Alpine Replay provides the stats, maps, and ranking for each ski run*

More charts caress your eyeballs after you depart the slopes. Figure 7-20 shows the total distance skied, the vertical drop, the maximum speed, the estimated calories burned, and other data. Through the app's settings, you can even have the runs automatically posted to Twitter or Facebook.

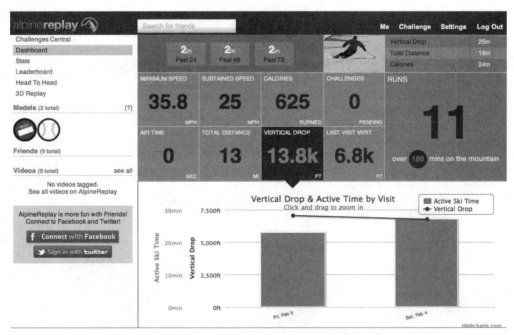

Figure 7-20. *You can automatically post skiing statistics to Twitter and Facebook*

The app sports a few differentiating details compared with other tools, according to the Alpine Replay website:

> *We measure speed, airtime, vertical, calories, distance and more, on any mountain in the world. Compare and compete with anyone, including yourself, with the click of a single button on your iPhone or Android. You will see a basic set of stats right on your phone or log into the AlpineReplay.com [site] to see even more detailed stats, compare and compete between friends, push your stats to Facebook and Twitter, or virtually compete against your friends in 3D.*

It even boasts of a "patent pending jump detection technology" that's designed to measure your jumps and how much "big air" time you attained.

> *I'll have to measure that one with my son, Scott, as my own "big air" time is limited these days. I'm a fairly conservative "stay grounded" skier. Alas, Alpine Replay told me I got 0.04 seconds of air on my last couple of days—hey, but I did hit 36 mph.*

More ski tracking

I have also used Endomondo and Google Earth to track my Alpine ski runs. We already described this combination in detail in the "Hiking and Climbing" section. In this section, we'll quickly show you what kind of data and imagery these apps can generate for skiing. Figure 7-21 shows Endomondo's Workouts screen based on a brief, hard alpine ski I initiated in Vermont.

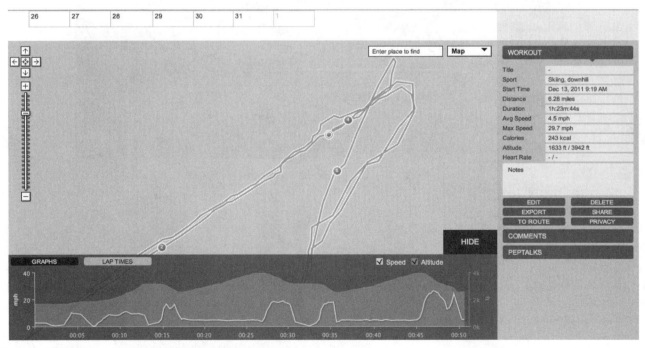

Figure 7-21. *Each ski run is graphed, with speed and elevation*

The browser view shows a profile of all your runs. You can trace, with your cursor, the yellow line representing each one of your ski runs, finding out the speed and elevation. This aspect was actually a bit risky for me, because of the natural inclination to beat the last run's speed rate. Normally a conservative, under-control skier and still getting the kinks out of my technique, I hit around 30+mph on one of those curvilinear runs. I've since hit about 42 mph on Alpine Replay, but the various phones can be error-prone when reporting maximum speed. You can, in other words, gather a lot of interesting trivia on your ski runs.

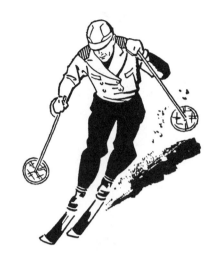

> *An Olympic Nordic skier can routinely hit 50 mph, and a downhill racer 70+ mph!*

Again, all you have to do to track ski runs is launch the Endomondo app on your smartphone, set it for downhill skiing, and tuck it in a pocket. Once in a while you'll hear the sultry voice tell you that you've completed another lap. Finally, in the Workouts section of the Endomondo website, export the ski runs as a GPX file (with a *.gpx* suffix). Then open that file up in Google Earth, for some more interesting stats and imagery.

It doesn't matter what kind of name you give the file in your text editor—*skiruns2.gpx* would be fine. The data tends to be richer in Google Earth, as Figure 7-22 shows. It even has me going 36.8 mph as a top speed (not sure how Endomondo and Google Earth are drawing different conclusions about speed, using the same data; they apparently use different algorithms).

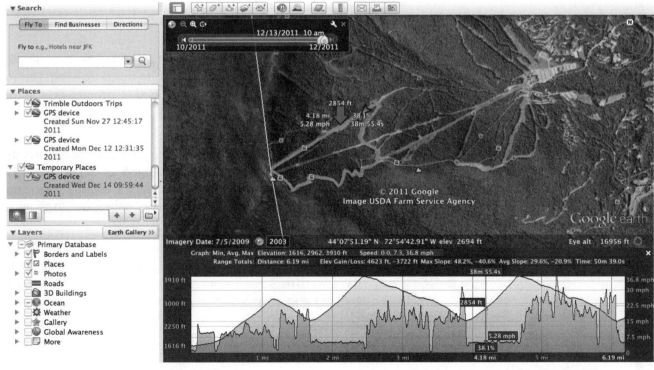

Figure 7-22. *Analyze your ski runs in Google Earth*

The GPX file, which is XML markup, includes track points and time-stamps every few seconds. Using the latitude and longitude points (which the tool also captures as XML elements), as well as the time-stamps, the software tries to capture the speed at which you moved from one geographical point to another, just as a GPS watch for running would do to estimate your pace. People who use GPS for precise measurements have tended to complain about the variances in data produced by different devices.

Google Earth gives you a nice illustration and overview of your ski runs, in terms of the blue line on the mountain. Google Earth will compute your total vertical for the ski runs, or the total number of feet you skied down, as the elevation loss figure—here, about 3,722 feet. A good day of skiing might earn you 15,000 feet or more of vertical.

Another interesting data point is Max Slope, which represents how steep the ski runs can get. Here it was an elevation grade of 48 percent—that's pretty steep. These tools are excellent for analyzing all your downhill ski days, and spending the day on impressive mountainous terrain such as Big Sky, Montana, Whistler Blackcomb, British Columbia, or Zermatt, Switzerland would generate very interesting visuals.

The total vertical for a ski day is similar to the volume for weightlifters— the total amount of pounds or kilograms they lifted during one session.

Airport Fitness Hacks

We include an airport fitness section in this chapter because an airport is kind of outside of our accustomed realm. If you do much traveling, you've probably spent a lot of time waiting in or stranded at airports. Let's see a show of hands for people who've been trapped at an airport and felt like crap!

You can generally get around the forced sedentary behavior of airports by crafting your own exercise routine, or perhaps using an airport gym. By using the Airport Gyms website (*www.airportgyms.com*), you can try to find a gym or health club at the airport where you will be hanging out. In general, good luck with that!

Testing this app, I got three hits for Boston, but two involved 10-minute taxi rides, so they're not really located at the airport; they're in hotels that allow you to buy a day pass to use their weight machines, which is worth it only if you have a very long wait at an airport and want to cough up the taxi and gym-pass fare.

Not very practical. You're usually waiting to board, or if your flight gets bumped, you're hustling, trying to get on another one.

You can generally get around the forced sedentary behavior of airports by crafting your own exercise routine, or perhaps using an airport gym.

As for the gym that was within walking distance, a comment included with the search result pointed out that one of the hotels was no longer allowing day passes, so you do have to check with these facilities beforehand, such as by email.

Denver also produced three hits on airport gyms, but all of them required taxi rides. A note stated: "Denver's airport is located such that it can take some time to get on and off the 'compound.'"

San Francisco had a number of possibilities, yet all involved taxi or BART subway rides. These aren't really airport gyms!

I only found gyms located at airports in big hubs like Chicago, so I assume for most travelers who don't want to jump in a cab and actually leave the airport for a lengthy time (and expense), these airport gyms do not yet have a lot of practical value (the website will be a good resource, however, once airports start getting their acts together). Some of the more elite clubs at airports might have small workout rooms, which their members can use when they aren't elsewhere in the club drinking scotch and getting massages.

Create Your Own Airport Exercise

Notice a recurring theme in this chapter?

You can create your own routine at the airport, which is always a good idea since we know that endless sitting is very bad in the long run. Plus, all that lousy food, stress, jet lag, and lethargy feels crummy in general, right? First, just constantly walk, ideally outside, and try to take your carry-on stuff in a backpack. This makes it easier to convert your airport waits into weighted hikes, which are a good form of exercise.

Always take the stairs instead of the escalators, *always*, and walk instead of lounging on the conveyor belts or moving sidewalks.

Constantly drink water and refrain from stuffing your gullet with all that crappy airport food, like mass-produced pizza, old cellophane-wrapped sandwiches, vending-machine junk, and er, um, wine and margaritas. Just bring some nuts or grab a piece of fruit once in a while. Fasting is perfect for airports.

Beware of the Terminal Zombies

Along with walking, use the hard seats for inverted pushups, meaning push-ups with your feet off the ground. Do some Hindu pushups on the rug. They don't last long enough to break a sweat, unless you're waiting in an airport in Jakarta, Indonesia (even then, they might be blasting the AC), and just a few sets of these pushups are great exercise.

You can probably also find a place to do pull-ups, and who cares what the other passengers think! You'll probably inspire them. Do some deep knee bends or "air squats" with your backpack on, and if you're outside in the cool weather on tarmac, try some jumping jacks (but with your backpack *off* for those). The trip will be far pleasanter and healthier if you avoid becoming just another "terminal zombie."

JACK FULTZ: THE 1976 BOSTON MARATHON WINNER'S COACHING TIPS

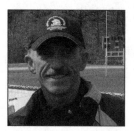

We interviewed Jack Fultz, who won the Boston Marathon in 1976 in triple-digit heat, then ran a personal best 2:11:17 in 1978. He provides personal coaching services and teaches at Tufts University.

Can you provide a little background on your Boston Marathon coaching experience—e.g., how many runners, how long you've been doing it? Do you still run in Boston or any marathons?

I train individuals for Boston and other marathons. The Dana-Farber Marathon Challenge team for which I develop online training programs and oversee runners' training-related issues is comprised of more than 500 runners each year now—though we've grown to this size over our 23 years, starting in 1990 with 19 runners.

I was diagnosed with osteoarthritis in my hip in 2000. I had it resurfaced in the summer of 2010. Despite some infection complications, I'm healthy once again and I work out every day—but I run only very sparingly. Biking is my primary aerobic activity now, though I swim/ERG/elliptical somewhat regularly as well.

How long is the training program (say, in weeks)?

I created 18-week training calendars for the beginner, intermediate, and advanced marathoners on our DFMC team. That's pretty much what I do for individual clients as well.

What's the basic routine (I assume it's molded to the particular runner)? How many miles per week? What kind of runs (long, slow vs. shorter-tempo runs)? How many rest days per week?

My beginner and advanced programs include only four running days each week. Two of the non-running days include some form of running simulation workout—elliptical machine, especially the Cybex Arc Trainer, which I believe to be the single best running simulation machine on the market when set and used appropriately, stationary biking, and/or deep water running.

A lot of variety over various terrains and different speeds of training, gradually building over the 18 weeks in terms of quality and quantity. My advanced program only includes three runs at 20 or more miles but also a few runs at 18 miles, so there are plenty of long runs—and I encourage my runners to run a portion of their long runs at marathon race pace if they're feeling good and strong.

Do you add any interval or track work?

I encourage all my runners, beginners as well, to include some form of speed training. That can be as simple as including 100-meter long "strides" of quicker paced running near the end of most of their training runs. But I also encourage them to have include at least one run/week where they include some running that is quicker than their regular steady pace, whether that is just some light fartlek running or structured track workouts. Even beginners will benefit from the variety and slightly greater challenge that "speed" training provides. For a 12-minute miler to run 11 or 10-minute pace for 200–800 meters constitutes "speed" training, even though it isn't all that fast. It is to them.

Do you have the runners do any races during the training period (e.g., 5k or 10k)? Any cross-training (biking, weightlifting)?

Training races are always a good idea to include, especially for the novice racer. The novelty of registering for a race, pinning on a number, starting en masse with a starting gun/horn, and "speeding" over the course against the clock can be intimidating. Running a few races before the big marathon eliminates the novelty factor of racing and the runner will [be] less nervous or intimidated on marathon day. The race also provides a greater training effect than most workouts possibly can.

Do you use any of the new technology gizmos and GPS tools for endurance athletes, like Nike+?

I use a Garmin Edge with HR for much of my biking. I'm staring to consider using HR for some of my individual clients but the larger team is left to their own devices. Many use GPS and some of those use HR—but very few use HR as an exclusive training guide. But it can be very useful if one is well versed on how to use it.

JACK FULTZ: THE 1976 BOSTON MARATHON WINNER'S COACHING TIPS
(continued)

Is there a dietary component to your training program?

I use the standard "see food diet"—I see food and I eat it. I believe that eating behavior is often just as important as "what" one eats—eating more, smaller meals and healthy snacks throughout the day and when eating a complete meal, to eat slowly and not overeat at any given time. By eating slowly, savoring the flavors of the food, we assist our digestive system by swallowing our food in near-liquid form and we're much more likely to stop eating when our hunger has been satiated rather than when we're uncomfortably full.

If you were competing in Boston in 2011, what would you do differently compared with your regimen in 1976?

I'd include a lot more of the alternative training I mentioned above. At the height of my racing career I'd average 125 miles/week for 10–12 weeks in preparation for a marathon. That's a lot of pounding and I'm sure most national and world-class marathoners suffer through a lot of overtraining injuries and lesser overtraining symptoms of fatigue and body ache that could be eliminated by replacing some/many of the body-pounding road miles with time on a Cybex Arc Trainer or doing deep water running. That's where we go now when injured—but they could serve a runner much more as a preventative tool. I'm an absolute believer in this and I believe I could train a healthy runner for a marathon just as effectively, and maybe more so, by having them do the majority of their training via these safer modalities. They'd require less recovery time between hard workouts, thus being able to do more intensity training and significantly reduce the likelihood of losing training time due to injury.

Hello, Gym!
Finding Your Way Around the Fitness Facility

8

Your friend, the guy or gal who you can tell you *anything*, wanders into your cubicle, clearly with something on his mind. "Dude, get in shape," is all he says, then unceremoniously walks away. You figure he's right; the encounter had a "right on the money" vibe to it. What's the first thing you do?

You join a local gym, the one that everyone's joining lately, or that one on the way to work that you got a couple of guest passes to but never bothered to visit. "Gym" is also considered an antiquated term for it; the numerous fitness franchises are running out of brand names for their fitness facilities, and they all have a different angle, and machines, and gizmos.

Now What?

So you've joined up and shown up. Now what? You see crowds of people milling around and on machines. It's like that scene in the film *Gattaca* with Ethan Hawke trying to pretend he's Jude Law on the treadmill, except there are ellipticals, cycle spinners, StairMasters, and more. You haven't even ventured into the football-field-sized mecca of stationary weight machines and barbells. It's kind of scary, jarring, but you want to do more than sit down at the juice bar, order a 12-ounce "Seattle's Best," and ogle the people sauntering by in their Lycra.

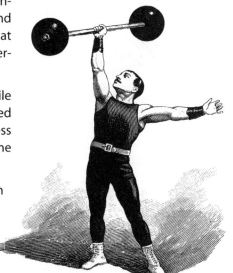

You can get one of the in-house trainers to show you around, but while that's a good idea for the first time, you don't necessarily want to get sucked into their way of doing things, and it costs a lot more. Besides, these fitness facilities aren't really *that* different from each other, and a fully equipped one commonly has everything you need to get strong and fit.

This chapter describes the kinds of exercises and routines you can focus on in a typical modern gym. There are dozens of them, in reality, so we're only going to get you started with about 15 of them, including photos, then point you in the direction of good websites that contain many exercise descriptions and demonstration videos.

We're also going to introduce a few smartphone apps that make a good accompaniment to working out in a gym, or home, or hotel room—but only if you have the patience and time to make screen choices and enter data, during or after a workout.

These include *Men's Health Workouts*, Fitocracy's mobile app, and a workout tracker at *www.bodybuilder.com* (there are dozens of fitness apps, however, so we recommend if you're an app aficionado that you do some exploring on your own). We'll also briefly discuss the CrossFit philosophy and facilities that are cropping up all over the place.

Before you hit the gym, it's of paramount importance to get some instruction on the proper technique for lifting weights. The excellent site *Bodybuilder. com*, for example, has a comprehensive collection of demonstration videos on just about any exercise with weights you can think of.

Before we get into all that, though, let's get some lightweight philosophy and terminology out of the way.

Lifting Is a Good Focus

By now you might be wondering why the chapter focuses on the "lifting weights" angle. A gym offers all kinds of routines, including all those cardio machines, not to mention Yoga, Pilates, Zumba, and countless variations on those movement scenarios. Since we realistically cannot cover everything you can possibly do in a gym or fitness place, we're not going to try. We're also going to venture out on a limb and recommend resistance exercise or strength routines as the main activity to focus on in the gym.

You can, of course, use any piece of equipment, machine, or class you want upon entrance to a facility (such as for a warm-up), but in terms of health and fitness, a solid resistance-exercise routine will get you the most bang for your buck, for the following reasons, among others:

Adding lean mass or muscle counteracts one of the principal effects of aging, which is the loss of lean mass or muscle.

- Adding lean mass or muscle counteracts one of the principal effects of aging, which is the loss of lean mass or muscle. If we age in a Western society without doing anything to resist the typical influences of the lifestyle, our body composition changes: we lose muscle as we gain fat. It can begin happening fairly early in life, such as the late 30s or 40s. This development is, by definition, unhealthy. We need fat to survive. A normal distribution of adipose tissue is an amazingly efficient form of energy storage and regulation. However, lots of extra fat is evidence that the calories you consume exceed your total energy expenditure (TEE, or the amount of calories you burn off each day) and that your metabolism has begun to go south on you. Extra fat is bad for your internal organs; a robust distribution of extra muscle is healthy for your internal organs. The medical community has even invented a fancy, disease-sounding name for this condition of losing muscle: *sarcopenia*. It's considered such a threat to the health of an aging population that—you guessed it—the pharmaceutical industry is going all out to invent a pill to combat sarcopenia. You don't need a pill. Just lift weights.

- Resistance training is another fertile area for geeks gathering and analyzing data, on routines, weight lifted, reps, total volume, and progress—and that might be the most stimulating aspect of lifting weights, at least in the beginning.

- For the younger among us, resistance training helps you to realize your athletic goals, whether it's sprinting on a track or bicycle, a team sport, or using your upper body to hit or throw a tennis ball, baseball, or lacrosse ball. Resistance training, when done correctly, will increase your strength, by an impressive magnitude—possibly 100 percent, depending on the baseline you start from. Yes, you can double your strength.

- Resistance training helps *avoid injuries* by strengthening muscle fiber, connective tissue (such as ligaments and tendons), and bone mass (yes, a person who lifts weights has greater bone density than someone who doesn't). Ever gotten a serious injury, one that happened while you were doing something relatively innocuous such as bending over to lift something or stepping on stairs the wrong way; one that took you out of school, work, *life* for weeks or months? Ever considered an easy-to-adopt routine that makes sure this never happens in the first place, or ever has to happen again? (Losing excess weight is also an injury-preventive measure.)

- The practical effects of being stronger cannot be overemphasized or quantified—think of all the "heavy work" you have to do in ordinary life, from lifting items around the house (including people and children) to performing physical tasks around the yard or at work. Ever since I got back into weights with greater seriousness a few years ago, I've noticed a huge difference in this area.

- Resistance training counts as *anaerobic* and *aerobic* cardiovascular training. In other words, resistance training will give you significantly better oxygen capacity for walking up hills and stairs, carrying loads, and just getting around in life. Anaerobic training means utilizing energy in the absence of a continuous replenishment of oxygen, as in sprinting. Aerobic exercise involves utilizing a more or less continuous supply of oxygen as you breathe and run, bike, or swim, for instance. Weightlifting helps both areas. Ever noticed how much you're huffing and puffing after high-intensity resistance training? (We'll explain that term in more detail shortly.) It follows that *if a muscle has more capacity for pulling a given weight, you will use less oxygen doing so.* In addition, your cardiovascular mechanics—the heart, lungs, capillaries, and veins, along with the brain, liver, even the endocrine system (all of the glands that secrete the all-important hormones that rule what goes on in your body, such as growth hormone, testosterone, and the adrenal hormones like

Resistance training will give you significantly better oxygen capacity for walking up hills and stairs, carrying loads, and just getting around life.

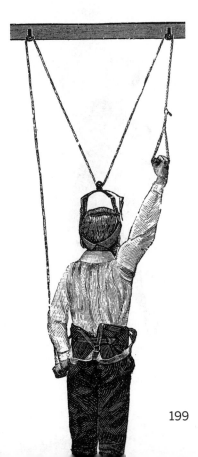

epinephrine and cortisol)—all of these systems must upregulate to support this new muscle fiber you are adding.

- New muscle fiber increases your basal metabolic rate (BMR—see Chapter 9), or the amount of calories you burn at rest or during normal activities, but not by the degree that people typically assume it does. If you add 10 pounds of muscle to your body, for example, your calorie burn increases by about 60 to 100 calories per day (about 6 to 10 calories per pound of muscle per day). The benefits of new muscle and weight training are greater strength, injury prevention, balance, and metabolic health, *not necessarily* more calories burned per day.

- Cardiovascular work is usually initiated at the expense of resistance training. Unless you're running or biking at a high intensity (such as doing Tabata sprints), the value of these exercises for most people is minimal. Excess cardio, for example, actually burns up or catabolizes your lean mass (so it can contribute to weakening during the aging process). "Despite increased testosterone, hypertrophy does not typically take place with aerobic endurance training. In fact, oxidative stress may actually promote a decrease in muscle fiber size in order to optimize oxygen transport into the cell. Without the proper exercise stimulus, the cellular mechanisms that mediate muscle fiber growth are not activated to the extent that hypertrophy [muscle growth] occurs."[1] This means that too much running or biking could make some of your muscles smaller.

Negative Weightlifting Biases: Get Over Them

If you're reluctant to try weightlifting because it seems like foreign territory for you—a clique or cult you do not want to join—I urge you to rethink your decision and try to expel the negative stereotypes. Try to ban these biases and images from your head—that weightlifting is just for adolescents (including adolescent-acting adults) who are trying to look like the Incredible Hulk or young Arnold, or people who are incarcerated and trying to make their tattoos look bigger by increasing the surface area of the underlying muscle.

Weightlifting is for everybody, including octogenarians and nonagenarians—people between the ages of 90 and 99. Most gyms could probably give you some great stories about elderly people who have gotten stronger and healthier (physical strength does equate to health) since starting a resistance-training program.

> *I didn't know I was a quinquagenarian (between the ages of 50 and 59; if you want to see all those fun names for ages, go to http:// en.wikipedia.org/wiki/Ageing#Dividing_the_lifespan).*

Weightlifting, including high-intensity training, is also absolutely *very good for women*. They often turn out to be better at it than a lot of men are.

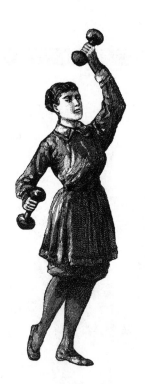

The benefits of new muscle and weight training are greater strength, injury prevention, balance, and metabolic health, not necessarily more calories burned per day.

WHEN WEIGHTLIFTING IS *WORK*: TWO NFL FOOTBALL PLAYERS' PERSPECTIVES ON TRAINING

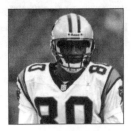

Jim Turner was a wide receiver, returned kicks, and played special teams with the Carolina Panthers about 10 years ago, and Chris Crocker, a safety with the Cincinnati Bengals, is a 10-year veteran. He's played for three other teams: Cleveland, Atlanta, and Miami. Both of them, obviously, know their way around a gym and strength building. Turner ("J.T.") is 6′ 4″ and played at about 210 pounds; Crocker is listed on his Bengals web bio page at 5′ 11″, 197 pounds. I interviewed them at separate times during the winter of 2012, near the close of the National Football League (NFL) season.

What was your greatest thrill as an NFL player?

J.T.: I got to meet Jerry Rice on the field before we played the 49ers my rookie year. Even when you're in the NFL you still looked up to these guys when you were young.

What kinds of off-season strength routines did you do?

J.T.: We spent the off-season working out—back in the old days they actually *had* an off-season; [but for us] even the workouts that were not mandatory had a high attendance. The type of strength routines you did depended on your strength coach; I had three different coaches with three different strategies.

For upper-body day (typically Monday) the routines involved triceps work, pushups, pull-ups, deadlifts, machine pull-downs with the Smith machines; and "curls for girls"—guys like to look good in their uniform. For leg days, we [did] not do squats with the bar because of the back issue—we did more push squats, the leg press, one-legged squats, calf raises, a lot of hamstring and quad exercises because that's where a lot of injuries come from. You have to make sure those muscles are strengthened and balanced.

With pro sports and resistance training, we fundamentally [design workouts] that will help us do what we have to do during the game: sprints (e.g., short sprints like 40s; "two-mile runs would be distance training for an NFL player"), squats, deadlifts, a lot of people do deadlifts—because that's the stuff that makes you strong. That's the core stuff that works. I see people do esthetic stuff that really doesn't help them, when I go to the gym now.

Crocker: In most teams that I've been on it's mandatory that you lift twice a week, one upper body, one lower body. Some of the guys do their own thing and lift three to four times a week.

Its different everywhere—this is the fourth team I've played on and my 10th season. You go through different phases—the older you get, the fewer heavy weights you use—you try to focus on elasticity and flexibility; you're still trying to be explosive, but you're going about it in a different way. Things like TRX bands come into play [*www.trxtraining.com/*]. We're using a lot of the same things [amateur athletes] use. You do a lot of things that require muscle-memory—football-specific stuff.

Looking back, would you have done anything different training-wise (e.g., rest for athletes seems to have greater appreciation nowadays)?

J.T.: Yes, yes, yes, more rest, more sleep. I got into yoga later, but I would have implemented more flexibility into the program earlier. I would have warmed up better. I ran track in college and high school and one thing I learned from that sport was that you almost have to warm up to exhaustion. I would have integrated more warm-up into my NFL routine, practice-and game-wise.

Another thing is that the guys don't really like to work out. Everyone is self-motivated, but there's a reason why the NFL fines you for missing workouts. Just because they're professional athletes, don't think that they wake up in the morning and say "Wow, I can't wait to get to the gym." That's far from the case.

Tell your readers, everyone's in the same boat. Human beings don't like to [do those kinds of workouts]—it doesn't feel good for anybody; it's not supposed to feel good, but at the end of the day the results are there.

Crocker: I'm satisfied [with the approach his strength coaches used]. [When I asked him whether it was true that the resistance training isn't very fun, he answered:] I would say that it's not fun trying to maintain the strength—when you're younger you lift and gain strength *fast*. When you're older you have to work twice as hard [to maintain the same level of power]. You're already consumed with trying to play the sport, the last thing you want to worry about is maintaining [muscle-specific strength]. That's why later on I have focused on trying to be flexible and explosive. [With weightlifting] you can get into areas where you're too big for your position; you don't see quarterbacks bench pressing 500 pounds, like an offensive lineman.

Do you use any of those Super Slow techniques that are popular in some weightlifting circles?

Crocker: We don't do anything slow in football.

A Few Jock and Physiology Terms, as Promised

A term you're usually going to come across while analyzing your gym workouts is *total energy expenditure* (TEE). We have previously defined basal metabolic rate (BMR) as the energy expended keeping your brain and basic systems going—in practical terms, the amount of calories you would burn if you were motionless all day. It's basically a calculated figure to help determine your daily caloric needs—you don't really want to be motionless all day!

Your TEE is your BMR plus the calories you burn moving and exercising all day. If you want to be really specific, the TEE equals your BMR plus exercise-oriented thermogenesis (generating heat by moving about) plus the calories expended by *non-exercise activity thermogenesis (NEAT)*.

The latter term means "the energy expended for everything that is not sleeping, eating, or sports-like exercise."[2] For example, all that activity that I've mentioned that doesn't have anything to do with a formal workout: walking places, going up and down stairs, chasing the dog, answering the door, doing chores and taking the trash out. What the Fitbit tends to measure is NEAT.

TEE is the most practical measure of the amount of energy you're expending in a day, and it's a useful number to compare to your total caloric intake. Generally, you will gain weight if your caloric intake, as measured by a tool such as FitDay (*www.fitday.com*), exceeds your TEE. This isn't always a bad thing. If you want to put on a substantive amount of muscle, you will have to provide the raw materials in the form of food and calories. You will not only have to consume quality protein and plenty of fats to burn off, you will generally have to be in a calories-surplus state to add muscle weight to your body.

TEE Formula

A journal article from October 2006[3] (*Preventing Chronic Disease*; *www.ncbi.nlm.nih.gov/pmc/articles/PMC1784117/*) provides us with a couple of equations or formulas that give a close approximation of how many calories you are burning by just humming along throughout the day and perhaps hitting the gym afterward.

The largest portion of these calories is referred to as the *basal energy expenditure* (BEE), also known as the BMR. Remember, this is the amount of calories your body expends just keeping its own cells and systems going for about 24 hours. The formula is long, but not *that* complicated:

BEE = 293 − 3.8 × age (years) + 456.4 × height (meters) + 10.12 × weight (kg)

I plugged in my age, weight, and height and came up with about 1,500 calories. Of course, the various formulas and tools you use for estimating the BMR will not always spit out the same number. My Tanita body-composition scale specifies around 1,680 for my BMR, and a previous formula we discussed estimated 1,440. It's often a fairly rough estimation.

For women, the formula from the article looks like this:

BEE = 247 − 2.67 × age (years) + 401.5 × height (meters) + 8.6 × weight (kg)

What about a more realistic figure for the amount of calories you are going to burn off via all of your gym activities? You figure out the TEE by using this formula:

TEE = 864 − 9.72 × age (years) + PA × [(14.2 × weight (kg) + 503 × height (meters)]

What's PA? It represents a physical activity rating for the day (I've condensed that aspect of the formula for the sake of brevity; the scientific article describes a more lengthy way of scoring separate activities by their metabolic equivalent of task—MET—and thus reaching a PA level for them). Here are the numerical options for the PA part of this equation:

Men:

Sedentary: PA = 1.0

Low active: PA = 1.12

Active: PA = 1.27

Very active: PA = 1.54

Women:

Sedentary: PA = 1.0

Low active: PA = 1.14

Active: PA = 1.27

Very active: PA = 1.45

Assume that I downhill-skied all day in the cold, or did a lot of walking plus my hardest bout of high-intensity weight training. With my age (55), height (1.7 meters), and weight (65 kilograms) plugged in, here is what the formula looks like (some sets of parentheses added by me).

The formula itself: TEE = 864 − 9.72 × age (years) + PA × [(14.2 × weight (kg) + 503 × height (meters)]

With values: TEE = ((864 - (9.72 × 55)) + ((1.54 (PA)) × [(14.2 × 65 + 503 × 1.7)])) = 3,068 calories

That's a close enough approximation of how many calories I would burn during a high-activity day, but the number seems to inhabit the low end of the range. It would not be surprising if the various tools that people use to estimate their TEEs use this and similar formulas.

Top 40 HIT: High-Intensity Training

High-intensity training, or HIT, is generally the kind of weight training that uses high weights and low reps. As resistance training has many different formats and camps, and triggers much web forum debate, the HIT routines tend to have their strong advocates and committed detractors (the opposite of HIT would be using light weights, multiple sets, and high reps).

Setting aside the hyperanalysis among the lifting cognoscenti (just Google the term "high intensity training," and you'll see plenty of lengthy discussions and articles), I tend to apply HIT to weights, as well as sprinting for runners or cyclists—anything that is conducive to intensity.

Any short-term exercise that is anaerobic in nature and tends to hit the big muscle groups with an all-out effort is HIT, as far as I'm concerned. I suppose it's an issue of semantics; you can drill down to more specific applications of this term if you'd like. When performed correctly and falling far short of causing injury, the HIT routines are some of the most effective fitness regimens for any program.

MOUNTAINEERING GUIDE: WHEN YOUR JOB IS YOUR FITNESS ROUTINE

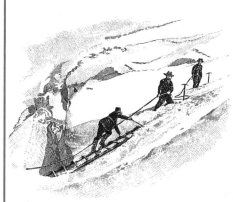

Only in recent history have humans created separate time segments in their lives for workouts and fitness. Right up until the modern era (when the running and outdoor-rec booms began in earnest, during the seventies), many people had ordinary lives that kept them in pretty good shape by default. Now you have to look for such lifestyles. I emailed Matt Hegeman of Alpine Ascents (Seattle, Washington), who was my lead guide on a 2011 Mt. Rainier climb, about whether he had a fitness regimen for keeping him ready in the big mountains. In a word, "No."

"My fitness regimen may not be very easy to put a finger on since I don't really have one," he said. "My fitness comes by doing. For example, in the summer for work I climb Rainier and on my days off I'll go rock climbing. No time for training. If I want to get in better shape for rock climbing, I go rock climbing 3–5 [times] per week. If I want to get in better shape for skiing, I go skiing 3–5 [times] per week. My lifestyle allows me to do this. I guess you could say that my lifestyle is my training regimen."

Hegeman recently participated in a guided climb of Aconcagua in Argentina, the highest mountain outside the Himalaya at 22,841 feet above sea level. He called it "Aconslogua" due to the merciless uphill but not often technical terrain of the climb. I can attest to the fact that the lifestyle will keep you in shape, simply based on our final Rainier day: about 3,400 feet up at midnight, followed by a 9,000-foot descent. On guiding days, a guide will burn thousands of calories, perhaps up to 7,000. And what did Hegeman and some of the other guides have planned for the following week (after maybe half a day's rest)? Another five-day guided tour of Mt. Rainer's Emmons Glacier. Alpine Ascent's home is at *www.alpineascents.com/guides.asp*.

Resistance-Training Terms

Before we describe certain routines, we're going to get some basic resistance-training terms out of the way.

Reps 'n' Sets

The *repetitions*, or reps, are the number of times you lift a weight before you take a rest. For example, 10 reps of a bench press at a certain weight involves executing the bench press 10 times in a row without racking the bar/weight and 15 reps of Hindu pushups simply means doing this type of pushup 15 times. A set is a group of reps that you do before resting or moving on to a set of another activity, as in "one set of 10 reps." Imagine an egg carton as a set and the eggs as reps. A typical egg carton is one set of 12 reps (unless it's a baker's dozen, then it would be 13 reps).

Of course, there are many more notations for sets and reps, including forms of shorthand. Although many people (including me) just keep track in their heads, others like to write down what they've accomplished in the gym, or check notes describing their workouts. In order to reduce writing or typing, you can write "3 x 10 x 150# or kg," meaning "three sets of 10 reps each at 150 pounds or kilograms"—kg—a kilogram is 2.2 pounds. Or you can use something slightly more verbose, such as "150 lb x 3 reps x 3 sets."

Sessions and Volume

A *session* is one workout, as in a weightlifting session. A session usually contains more than one exercise and more than one set, but it doesn't have to. Your training routine will include a certain number of sessions per week, from one to up to four or more if you're an experienced weight trainer.

You can also keep track of the *total volume* lifted in the session, day, or week, or even within a time period (say, in a set of bench presses with short rests between each rep). *Volume* is the total amount of pounds or kilograms you lifted during an exercise or a session. For example, if you did 10 reps of bench presses at 150 pounds, the volume was 1,500 pounds.

> *Volume is impressive and motivating—as in, "Hey, I lifted three tons of weight during that session!" But it may not be as relevant as the incremental gains you are making in strength for the different exercises. Volume is a statistical or aggregate figure that has anecdotal value at best (as in, "During my lifetime, I've run the equivalent of once around the equator").*

The RMs: Repetition Maximum

Repetition maximum, or RM, is a term that's bandied about a great deal in weightlifting circles. RM is a way to express the relative intensity of an exercise, so one repetition maximum, or "1RM," for the squat would be the most weight you could squat one rep. As another example, if you can bench press 200 pounds once, your 1RM for the bench press is, you guessed it, 200 pounds.

Higher RMs reflect the weight that you can lift for multiple reps, not just one. For example, 5RM for the military press is the weight that you can presently do five repetitions of for that exercise (it will, of course, change as you get stronger).

Similarly, 10RM for the leg press is the weight that you can push on the leg press for 10 reps. The higher the RM, the lower the weight; your 1RM for the bench press might be 200 pounds, but your 10RM might be 150 pounds.

Your RMs can also, of course, be specified in kilograms—1 kilogram (kg) equals 2.2 pounds (lb).

As you might have guessed, the "protocol" or the plan for your weight routine might not change as rapidly as your increase in strength. For example, midway through your routine, Tuesday's schedule might call for 5RM of the deadlift. When you first started lifting weights, this might have been 100 pounds. Now you can do 155 pounds five times, or more, but the exercise is still referred to as "5RM deadlift."

Percentages of RM

A weight for a particular exercise is often referred to as a percentage of RM. Let's say you wanted to start off an exercise with a set of weights that was not quite as difficult as 10RM (the weight you can only do 10 reps of before you're maxed out). The level of intensity could be referred to as "80 percent of 10RM." If your 10RM is 150 pounds, 80 percent of your 10RM is 120 pounds. Or you could be doing a high-intensity session that falls just short of an all-out effort, such as "85 to 90 percent 1RM."

How do you know what your 1RM is? You could perform a 1RM test with spotters, say, on the bench press (a certain safety technique by which one or two spotters can steady or lift up the bar if you fail to complete the rep—*very important* with exercises like the bench press). That can be kind of risky, though, particularly for beginners. At least one equation exists for estimating the 1RM based on lifting multiple reps with a lighter weight.

The formula goes like this: 1RM = ((# of reps) / 30 + 1) x weight lifted

The higher the RM, the lower the weight; your 1RM for the bench press might be 200 pounds, but your 10RM might be 150 pounds.

For example, say you lifted 150 pounds 11 times, or for 11 reps. The equation will look like: $(11/30 + 1) \times 150 = 205$. This equation estimates that your 1RM for that exercise is 205 pounds.[4]

The "predictions [based on estimations] are more accurate when the equations are based on loads equal to or less than a 10RM," and they get more accurate the closer you get to 1RM, according to the excellent reference book *Essentials of Strength Training and Conditioning*.[5] In other words, the amount you can do for 5RM or 3RM is a more accurate predictor of your 1RM than your 10RM.

What's Your Plan? How Many Sets and Reps

Alright, enough of the RMs. Exactly how many sets and reps do you perform for each exercise?

So you've decided that you are going to initiate a resistance-training routine involving the bench press, the deadlift, and the bicep curl in one session. How many sets are you going to do for one session? In instances when you are using a trainer, this plan will be handed to you, for better or worse (you can tell I like to design my own training sessions).

This issue is another area of great debate among resistance trainers. The protocol or scheme, a kind of recipe for what combination of sets and reps will make you stronger for each exercise, will often be different for each trainer or expert you consult. There are numerous different protocols for weightlifting, which just means that you have a lot of room for variety and experimentation.

> *The rule of thumb is that "lower reps, higher weights," closer to your 1RM for each exercise, will help build power and muscle. Higher reps, lower weights will help increase muscular endurance.*

The protocal should take into account whether you are a beginner, when you're probably starting off with higher reps and lower weights, or an experienced personal weight trainer.

Everyone is different, in terms of factors such as baseline fitness, strength, and age, when they begin weight-training programs. Another major consideration is the goal of your resistance-training program. Someone who's a competitive power lifter has a different goal than a geek who is just trying to get fitter. One strategy is to try different protocols and see what makes you stronger and what works for *you*.

There are actually three components to a protocal: the actual weight you'll be lifting, the number of sets in one session, and the number of reps per set (not to mention the different exercises that will comprise one session and the number of days during the week you will work out).

The 1-Set Method

I know a good athlete who prefers doing one set of 10 reps to "failure," or 10RM, for each exercise. This is easy to remember, but it can be a little difficult at first for inexperienced lifters to determine how much weight to use. 10RM is about 75 percent of your 1RM, so if you have already determined that in the leg press machine, say, your 1RM is 160 pounds, then your 10RM should be about 120 pounds.

What if you don't know what your 1RM is? How do you know what failure is? In this case, you can just make a subjective determination that "I can't do another rep" (but never do this unspotted with exercises that could be risky, such as the bench press!). The more experience you gain as a resistance trainer the easier it will be to tell when you're reaching your "failure" point. Similar to that feeling of "I don't have one more sprint interval left," the muscles are quivering and you're building up a lot of tightness or lactic acid, which is a byproduct of the muscle's energy output.

An old chestnut for track workouts or intervals is to finish your interval session when you feel that you can only do one more sprint.

Pre-Exhaustion

Another scheme for determining sets and reps is to use a lighter weight and multiple reps to "pre-exhaust" the muscle group first, before you hit it with a heavier set, such as 85% of 1RM. This method also offers the advantage of warming up the muscle group and lets you smooth out your technique first without the pressure of having to tackle the heaviest weight. The first set might be considered aerobic, while the second set is *anaerobic*, roughly similar to sprinting at 75 percent of max speed for 100 yards prior to going all-out for 100 yards.

Still another variation is the inverse of pre-exhaustion, where you follow up a hard set with a high-rep, lighter-weight set. The idea is that the first set fatigues the powerful, fast-fatiguing Type II muscle fibers, while the second set takes care of the less powerful, slower-fatiguing Type I fibers.

Vary your routine; do both methods. Mix things up. Combine a body-weight exercise with a hard barbell exercise. For example, I will follow up a hard set of bench presses with a set of inverted pushups (feet on the bench), to failure.

GAIN and WODs

The two tools we discuss in Chapter 9, GAIN Fitness (*www.gainfitness.com*) and a "workout of the day" generator, also offer some insight into sets and reps. GAIN Fitness recommends two sets of 12–13 reps for each exercise, with a 40-second rest between sets. They include body-weight-type exercises, barbells, and kettlebells (these are basically cannonballs with handles, a popular new tool in CrossFit circles).

Here's what The WOD Shop (*www.wodshop-service.org/getWod.do*) generated for me when I requested a workout involving lifting weights:

> *Rest 1 minute between rounds, add 10# per round, continue until failure: 2x Back squat (185#/95#)*

Unless I'm misinterpreting these instructions, what they are specifying here is, "Do one rep of back squats with 185 pounds, then one rep with 95 pounds; rest one minute; add 10 pounds to each exercise and do the same thing." The exercise calls for unlimited rounds "to failure," meaning you keep doing these sets, two reps each, until you can't any more. There's always a minute between the "rounds" (which in this case encompasses one set and two reps).

Low-Rep Methods

You've probably concluded by now that there are countless variations or schemes for sets and reps. I've seen schemes where lifters have done 10 or more sets of 3 reps for the same exercise, over and over again with a heavy weight, or 5 sets of 5 reps at 5RM.

My wife's training facility uses four sets for each exercise, but they don't count reps, they have the athletes perform reps for 45 seconds, with short rests between sets.

The bottom line with resistance training when choosing these schemes is that heavier weights with exercises that recruit more muscle groups, and lower RMs, produce the best results. Hormones send signals to the cells to synthesize new protein, and thus new muscle. Hormones rule! You can eat as much protein and take as many supplements as you want, but the signal to make new muscle is delivered by a hormone—and involves the mTOR pathway.

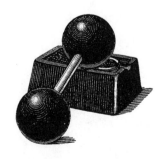

To make more lean mass for your body, you have to use the routines that best cultivate muscle-building or anabolic hormones such as testosterone and growth hormone.

Here's another quote on this matter from *Essentials of Strength Training and Conditioning*:

> When the intensity used was 10RM (heavy resistance) with three sets of each exercise (high total work, approximately 60,000 J) and short (1-minute) rest periods, large increases were observed in serum [growth hormone] GH concentrations. The most dramatic increases occurred in response to a 1-minute rest period when the duration of exercise was longer (10RM vs. 5RM).[6]

SAMPLE ROUTINE FROM A BBS GUY

It is instructive to examine a brief rundown on what other dedicated athletes do for exercise. Bob Watson is a Spanish teacher and cross-country coach (his teams do far more variety than run training—I've trained with them). I asked him what kind of weight routine he does.

"I try to do all of my workouts fasted, and I am just starting a Doug McGuff–style protocol," he told me. Dr. Doug McGuff wrote the excellent book *Body by Science*, which, in a nutshell, recommends a high-intensity routine about once per week, or even once every 10 days or more. He argues, using good scientific data, that it takes that long for the muscles to legitimately heal and rebuild after the workout, which is to failure. Dr. McGuff writes convincingly about the futility of overtraining. Read the book (its method is referred to as *BBS*) if you want to learn something about exercise physiology.

"I lift 2x/week: day 1 is pull-downs and overhead press," Bob said. "Day two is chest press, seated row, and leg press.

All exercises are one set to failure. I like fasted workouts because I go all out and don't worry about any food in my stomach. I feel sharp physically when I am fasting—energy level is good, and I feel ready to go."

"Also, "he continued," I work hard looking forward to that big meal after the workout (more *leangains.com* influence here). Maybe some would caution against this if one is trying to lose weight, but I'm trying to gain, so it works for me. It's a bit too early to track strength gains. Energy levels are good throughout the day. I used to lean on a cup of coffee after lunch every day to get through afternoon classes, but now find I can take it or leave it—I don't feel fatigued in the afternoon. So if I want a warm drink, I'll have a cup of decaf, maybe with some heavy cream (especially if I'm looking to add calories on a workout day)."

Split Routines and Compound Sets

A *split routine* involves using resistance training for the upper body one day and the lower body another, allowing each muscle group to rest. This is very common, and allows you to train on multiple days without overtraining, if you do it right.

A *compound set*, on the other hand, includes two exercises in the same set. The exercises target the same muscle group, as in performing hammer curls for the biceps followed by some biceps curls.

With all that said, it's about time that we started describing particular routines and weightlifting exercises.

Grand Entry, Time to Warm Up

Now you've made your grand entry to the gym, and you've avoided using the juice bar as a cop-out refuge. You probably want to do some kind of warm-up, and if it's a cardio-related warm-up you are comfortable with, such as sitting on a bike and pedaling for 10 minutes, then have at it.

Personally, I feel that this is a waste of time, and a bit tedious. Why do they provide modern treadmills and stationary cycles with TV monitors, so that you can watch *Real New Jersey Housewives* during your warm-up (or is it *Real Desperate Dallas Housewives*—I don't know, some combination of "real" and "desperate")? Because everyone assumes that spinning or treadmilling is boring, and people require auxiliary entertainment just to get through it.

What I do for warm-ups is a set of dips, and sometimes some push-ups or pull-ups. It only takes a minute, and it gets my blood pumping and my heart rate going. I usually feel the need to stretch out my lower back, so I assume a yoga position called the "child's pose" (see Figure 8-1). Then I take a long wooden staff (most gyms keep these around) and I limber up my back and legs with the staff on my shoulders, sort of like a yoke. This is all over in minutes, and I'm on to my first routine.

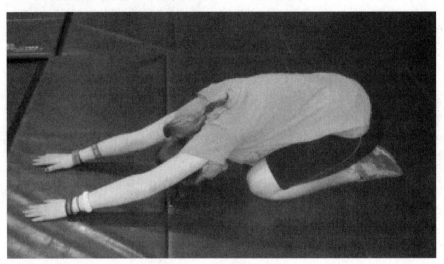

Figure 8-1. *This yoga move can figure into your warm-up*

You can also add or use a first set of lightweight resistance training, as described in "Pre-Exhaustion," as a warm-up, or do a more conventional warm-up, like swimming, which is an excellent loosening activity for the muscles.

Now I'm going to introduce several resistance-training exercises. I'll accompany them with pictures, and, whenever available, link them to a video clip or some other explanatory site. I'm going to start with five go-to routines that use some of the body's larger muscle groups and are proven strength-builders: the bench press, the military press, the deadlift, the leg press, and the back squat. These are tried-and-true resistance-training exercises, and while some have fallen into disfavor on the Internet among hardcore weightlifters (e.g., the bench press), putting these five exercises together will doubtlessly help you increase all-body strength and fitness.

Along the way, you can check out the sidebars, which are examples of routines and interviews with workout mavens. Even if you had a resistance-training program that involved only these five routines, you could still expect to get good results (provided you lifted enough weight, that is).

THE SPARTACUS WORKOUT: 10 MINUTES OF HEALTHY TURMOIL

I love 10-minute workouts, like the "10-minute pull-up marathon" (do as many chin-ups or pull-ups as you can in 10 minutes). A good 10-minute routine is a marvel of efficiency and intensity (and you're not working out, showering, dressing, etc. for two and a half hours…), and will make longer, less intense workouts seem easy. A tough 10-minuter is the *Men's Health* Spartacus Workout. You gals can do it, too, by the way! Find it here: *www.menshealth.com/mhlists/high-intensity-circuit-routine/index.php*.

You can initiate this workout recipe using the *Men's Health* smartphone app that I describe elsewhere in this chapter. The routine involves 10 exercises, mostly using handheld weights or dumbbells, during which you do the reps for 60 seconds. You perform as many reps as you can for a minute, with 15 seconds of rest between sets. Considering that the workout involves nine rest periods of 15 seconds before the last Spartan exercise (if you make it that far!), the entire workout lasts more like 12 minutes 15 seconds.

The exercises include goblet squats (holding a dumbbell in your hands while doing the equivalent of air squats), mountain climbers, single-arm dumbbell swings, jumping drills, and fancy (read: harder than usual) push-ups. This is considered a circuit-training workout, meaning a resistance-training session that moves from one exercise to another very quickly, testing (and building) your muscular strength and cardiovascular fitness.

Like everything else, work up to it using common sense. The first time around with the Spartacus Workout, use lighter weights and/or slightly longer rest periods. Perhaps practice the separate routines involved in the workout before you put it all together. This one seems to be tailor-made for the goal-oriented among us.

The Bench Press

You probably recall this exercise from high school—I do. The "200-pound bench press club," the stocky dudes who used to hang out in the corner of the gym after school. With the bench press, you lie on your back on a bench under the bar, with both feet flat on the floor. You place both hands on the bar, slightly wider than shoulder width (see Figure 8-2), with your palms facing outward, or away from you. Move the bar off the rack, let the bar down toward your chest (but not all the way, obviously!), and push the bar back up, as many reps as you can do. In most cases with the bench press, you will have a spotter.

A warm-up that a beginner can do, with a spotter, is to bench press the bar as many times as he can. In most gyms, the bar weighs 45 pounds, but check with the people who work there first. Another variation on a bench press workout, a kind of compound exercise or superset, is to follow the bench press with inverted pushups off the bench. *You can also do the bench press with dumbbells* of varying weights, which increases the range of motion used for this exercise.

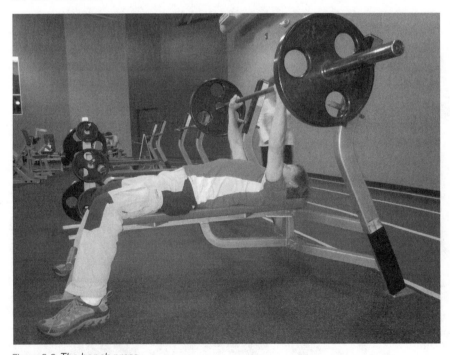

Figure 8-2. *The bench press*

The Military Press

There are a number of different ways to do the military press (such as beginning with the bar on the floor, or a seated military press), but we're going to show a standing variation of the military press, with the bar placed on a rack at about chest height (the equipment is sometimes called a squat rack; it has two hooks placed at different heights for racking the bar). Here's a video link showing the general technique for this exercise from *Bodybuilder.com*: *www.bodybuilding.com/exercises/detail/view/name/standing-military-press*.

With the military press, you grasp the bar with palms facing outward, carefully move it off the rack, then bring the bar down to your chest, and push it all the way over your head. Unlike many other exercises, where you do not lock the joints such as the elbows or knees, the military press pushes the bar in a straight-up-arms position. Figure 8-3 shows the beginning of the rep before the big push.

The military press can also use dumbbells, such as in a seated position, as shown in Figure 8-4. This exercise is also called the shoulder press.

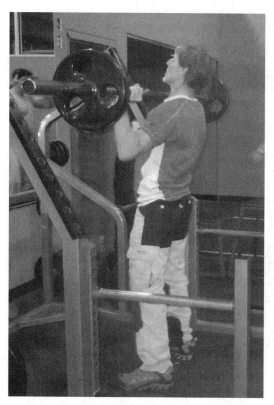

Figure 8-3. *The standing military press*

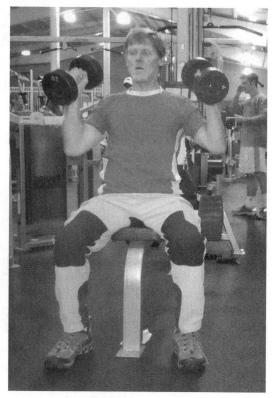

Figure 8-4. *The military or shoulder press, seated*

The Deadlift

For the deadlift, the barbell starts on the floor, or you can take the bar off the rack while standing. You crouch down with your legs bent, and grasp the bar at about shoulder width with your palms down (but there are variations on the grip), shins almost touching the bar. A common instruction for the deadlift is to "drive through your heels" as you pick up the bar, pushing your hips toward the bar at the end of the movement. An excellent demo video from *Bodybuilding.com* is here: *www.bodybuilding.com/exercises/detail/view/ name/barbell-deadlift*.

You should watch this video before you perform the exercise, because you can hurt your back doing the deadlift if it is not executed correctly. Begin with lower weights first as you grow accustomed to the movement. Figure 8-5 shows the finish of the deadlift.

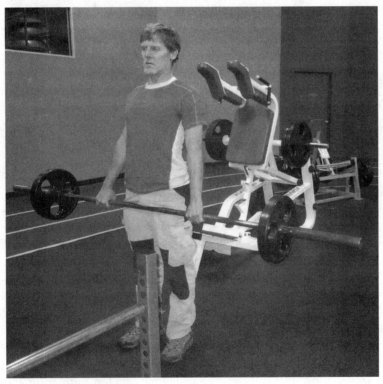

Figure 8-5. *Completing the deadlift*

The Leg Press

The leg press is designed to strengthen the big upper-leg muscles. It is a very effective strengthener for the glutes (your fanny muscles), the hamstrings (the skeletal muscles along the back of your legs), the quadriceps (your thighs), and even your calves. Unlike the other exercises we've described so far, the leg press, in this variation, involves a machine, not a barbell. It's a pushing exercise, rather than a pulling one like the deadlift. You sit in a seat and place both of your feet on a plate or platform about shoulder width apart, as shown in Figure 8-6.

As with many machines, it's a good idea to use the leg press with low weight the first time around, focusing on a smooth, slow motion and proper technique (inhale when the weight comes back toward you; exhale when you push).

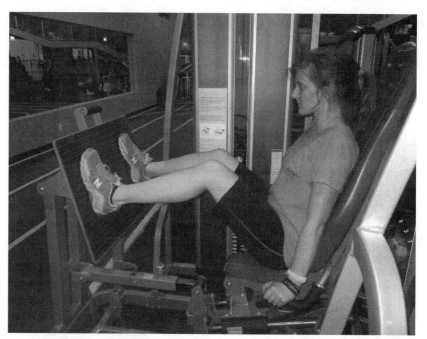

Figure 8-6. *The leg press*

As with many machines, it's a good idea to use the leg press with low weight the first time around, focusing on a smooth, slow motion and proper technique (inhale when the weight comes back toward you; exhale when you push). Do not lock your knee joints during this exercise; keep your legs slightly bent at the end of your push motion. Keep your feet flat on the plate. (A variation of this technique uses only one leg, with comparatively light weights, in order to help strengthen the weaker leg when you have a strength imbalance between your two limbs.)

This is a good conditioning exercise for jumping, sprinting, skiing, and other sports. Here's an excellent demonstration video from *Bodybuilding.com*: *www.bodybuilding.com/exercises/detail/view/name/leg-press*.

The Back Squat

The back squat is another strengthening exercise for your upper leg muscles: the quads and the hamstrings. The bar touches your shoulders behind your head, as shown in Figure 8-7. You place the bar on your back by "stepping into it," when the bar is already positioned with its weights on a squat rack, which is a tool that most gyms will have in their resistance-training areas. The rack allows you to position the bar at different heights. This prevents you from straining yourself trying to get the bar off the floor and onto your back.

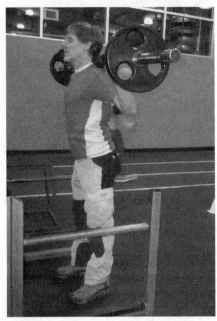

Figure 8-7. *The back squat: tried-and-true, but watch the lower back*

When you're finished with a set, you can just step toward the rack again (not that you're very far away from it in the first place!) and place the bar on the two hooks that are about at your shoulder height. You should probably use a barbell pad as well, as the bar can create some discomfort on the shoulders.

Practice with a wooden staff or a bar alone with no weight before you begin a back squat (or any type of squat) with weighted plates on the bar. You have to be careful with this technique, because the improper usage of it can potentially hurt your knees or lower back (that's why I prefer the leg press for a challenging thigh exercise—there's less of a risk of back injury). The following video provides a demonstration: *www.youtube.com/watch?v=Hyjpz4jkjSQ*.

Figure 8-8 shows a front squat, which is another variation. Figure 8-9 shows a power squat, which is a machine that, in my personal experience, allows you to safely use much more weight than a back squat, without putting potentially excessive pressure on your lower back, for example.

Since it doesn't involve free weights, the power squat can safely substitute for free-weight squats, if you're not quite ready for those.

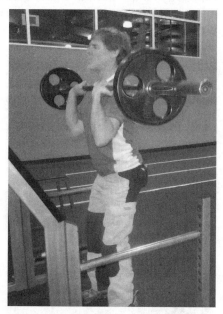

Figure 8-8. *The front squat technique*

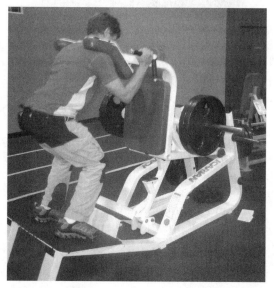

Figure 8-9. *The power squat machine*

Dumbbells

You can use dumbbells to initiate both squats and deadlifts. This is fine; one technique isn't necessarily better than the other, and you're still working hard. For squats, hold a dumbbell in each hand at shoulder height, then perform the squat as you would with a bar. For deadlifts, carefully move a couple of dumbbells to the floor next to your feet: one to your left, one to your right. Bend down and pick them up, drive through your heels and stand straight, as shown in Figure 8-10.

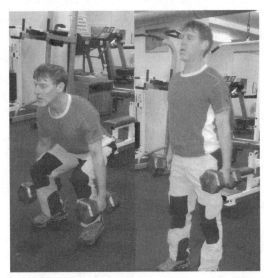

Figure 8-10. *Performing a type of deadlift with dumbbells*

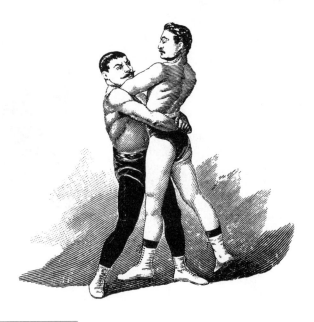

Bicep Curls and Hammer Curls

Bicep curls and hammer curls are two exercises you can do with dumbbells that strengthen your upper arms. The latter are for triceps and the former for biceps muscles. You can do curls standing up or sitting down, but I've found that when standing up, the routine requires more effort (we're not trying to make these workouts easier!).

For hammer curls, for the triceps or the back of the upper arm, the dumbbells are parallel to your body and the grip used is similar to a handshake, as shown in Figure 8-11. This exercise can be combined in a compound set with bicep curls for a complete arm-strengthening exercise.

Figure 8-12 shows the well-known bicep curl with dumbbells. This uses a palms-up grip, similar to a chin-up. One option for your routine is to perform a set of hammer curls, take a short rest or do an upper-body set of another exercise, then complete the troika with a set of bicep curls. Rinse and repeat.

Bicep curls and hammer curls focus on fairly small muscle groups of the arm, so make sure you're not spending too much time on them at the expense of hitting the big muscle groups with your weight training—the hamstrings, quads (thigh muscles), glutes (butt muscles), and lower, middle, and upper back, as well as the trapezoid or shoulder muscles.

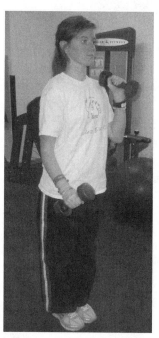

Figure 8-11. *Hammer curls use a different grip than bicep curls*

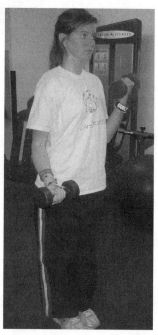

Figure 8-12. *The venerable bicep curl with dumbbells*

Leg Extensions and Cable Pulldowns

The leg extension machine is a machine that you sit down in for exercising the quadriceps muscles. Leg extensions can be performed with either one or both legs (the one-legged exercise to help correct a strength imbalance between the two legs, for example). Use only light to moderate weight at the beginning for this exercise, because you could otherwise hurt your knee joints. I use leg extensions, mostly of the one-legged variety, as a complementary routine following more effective lower-body techniques, such as the leg press or back or power squat. Figure 8-13 shows a leg extension machine.

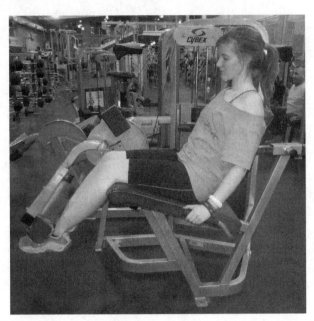

Figure 8-13. *The leg extension machine for the quads*

The cable pulldown is an excellent exercise for the upper back (traps) and arms (seemingly more of an exercise for the triceps, in terms of the arm). There are numerous variations of this exercise, both standing and sitting, as well as with wide or narrow grips. The one I have chosen to show in Figure 8-14 involves sitting down at a cable machine, using a narrow grip, and pulling down on a weighted stack.

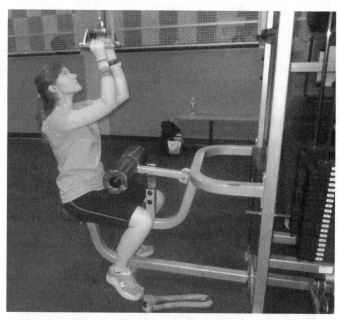

Figure 8-14. *The cable pulldown strengthens the upper back*

You can add strength and lean mass with a small, well-defined set of free weights and machines.

This brief introduction is sufficient, to say the least, to get you started on an all-body resistance-training regimen at the gym. There are nevertheless *hundreds* of exercises that can be performed with free weights and barbells, machines, dumbbells, kettlebells, weighted balls—you name it. To come right down to it, you don't need the endless flood of "new and improved" fitness tools, wherein it is difficult to separate slick marketing from an actual tool or device that has a practical, beneficial effect. You can add strength and lean mass with a small, well-defined set of free weights and machines, for instance.

FIGURING OUT PROGRESSION IN WEIGHT TRAINING

When you're lifting weights, how do you know by how much to increase the weight when you are progressing to a higher level of resistance?

This is another "art versus science" issue. An experienced weightlifter knows when a particular weight, say with the bench press, is getting too easy: you obviously can do multiple repetitions with the weight with a lower level of exertion.

We recommended 10RM (10 repetition maximum) as a pretty good level of resistance to use for one set of repetitions. This is the highest weight that you can do 10 repetitions of. For example, if you're performing the leg extension, and by the 10th rep your thighs are really burning to the point where you cannot wait to let the weight down and conclude the set, then you have probably used a 10RM

weight for that exercise. If it seems really easy (you have plenty of reps still in your legs), you need to increase the weight, up to your "true 10RM."

The excellent book *Essentials of Strength Training and Conditioning* offers a few rules of thumb that you can use for increasing the weight: when you can do two more reps than usual (say, 12 reps) for an exercise, during two consecutive sessions, try increasing the weight. For beginning weightlifters, increase it by 2.5 to 5 pounds (or about twice that for lower-body exercises). For the experienced, add 5 to 10 pounds additional weight (10 to 15 pounds for lower body). Or, use your best judgment and increase the weight by anywhere from 2.5 percent to 10 percent of the current weight.[7]

Instructional Video Sources

It helps to watch technique-oriented videos before you start a new resistance-training routine. The Mayo Clinic website has an extensive collection of "how-to" videos: *www.mayoclinic.com/health/strength-training/MY00033*. They are mostly designed for beginners and include coverage of machines, free weights, and body-weight exercises.

Bodybuilding.com also has a huge library of instructional videos and other resources: *www.bodybuilding.com/exercises/*. If that's not enough, a Google search on "resistance training videos," for example, produces more than 10 million hits.

The next section describes a couple of apps that you can use to track your sets and reps. Then we conclude the chapter with a segment that introduces CrossFit, a variation on the local gym that you might be interested in trying out at some point. CrossFit offers a few useful routines that you cannot find at a typical fitness facility, like climbing ropes!

Using an App, or Not, to Record Sets

Remember that "what gets measured gets managed" paradigm we mentioned in the preface—the measure first mantra? It's often a good idea to keep track of your sets and reps over time, as well as the subjective aspects of weightlifting (e.g., "I was maxed out by that last set, even though last week I got through it no problem."). The data is not only motivational, but it shows you what you're doing right, what you're doing wrong, when you need to rest, and what type of rest works best.

> *Consider recording sets, reps, and the weight used for various exercises, as well as the effect of sleep and nutrition on your energy levels.*

The purpose of resistance training is to increase muscular strength by gradually increasing the resistance or weight you are lifting. This action stimulates the muscles and other physical systems to adapt to an ever-increasing load or level of weight. If you want to be scientific about your weightlifting, it can be difficult to remember the weight that you used for various exercises, and thus to manage the sequential incrementing of that weight as you develop strength, if you don't keep records.

Traditionally, people bring lists they've written down or printed out of their exercises, sets, reps, and weight used, as well as their goals for the day or session. It's a tried-and-true method, and it might be useful if you have a particularly complicated session planned for that day—say, half a dozen or more exercises. Or, you may be able to keep your set-and-rep scheme in your head. Either "low-tech" option works fine; I don't use any recording apps for my typically short and efficient workouts.

If something more high-tech appeals, though, you can use a smartphone app to set up and record your weightlifting, and there are some good ones out there.

Men's Health Workouts

Men's Health Workouts is a comprehensive app (for both Android and the iPhone) that includes numerous recipes and descriptions of resistance-training techniques, as well as methods for recording them. Before you get into the description of this app, be advised that it is not designed to record exercise routines you have invented. You have to perform the Men's Health routines (there are dozens to choose from), and it provides you with a feature to save the sets and reps. This app also does not have a web-connected dashboard and graphics, at least at the time I checked it out, for viewing your workouts.

Figure 8-15 shows the main screen, which gives you the choice between exercise descriptions, workout recipes, and logging (inputting reps and sets).

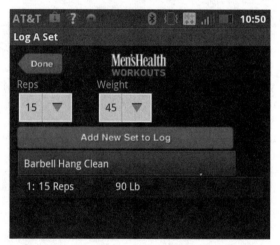

Figure 8-15. *Get some good ideas for workouts from the Men's Health Workouts app for smartphones*

Choose Workouts and Build New Muscle from the resulting screen, and you get a little description of the recommended program. Specifically, this routine involves four weeks of training using eight exercises, of the "3 sets, 8 to 10 reps" variety. The routines are of the "do this, do that" prescriptive variety, but you can obviously adapt them to your own program. Perhaps run through the whole routine once to determine if you want to adopt parts of it or the whole thing. The app does a pretty good job of briefly describing and illustrating the exercises, as shown in Figure 8-16.

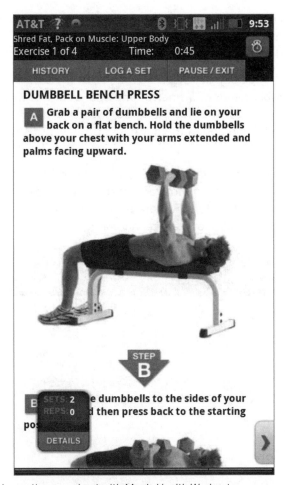

Figure 8-16. *Implementing a workout with Men's Health Workout*

Run through the whole routine once to determine if you want to adopt parts of it or the whole thing.

The app times your sets, with an option to pause or exit a workout. It can be inconvenient and awkward to carry around a smartphone (thus all the armbands and similar accessories they're willing to sell you!) and push buttons during your workout. Some athletes respond better to using devices in the weight room than others. When it's time to log the workout, select "Add New Set to Log" and the app saves it on your device's storage medium, as shown in Figure 8-17.

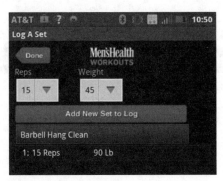

Figure 8-17. *Log a set and save it on your phone*

Hello, Gym! Finding Your Way Around the Fitness Facility

The big missing element—the elephant in the room, so to speak—is the absence of an accompanying website with all your workout data uploaded and displayed with charts and graphics.

We described Fitocracy in Chapter 2. If you're a Fitocracy member, you can use its mobile site (not a smartphone app, as of this writing) to record weight-training sessions. Go to the site at *www.fitocracy.com/m/play/*. The sets will be saved and added to your data at the website, on the cloud, so to speak.

This site has an intuitive design for entering weightlifting data. Given that your own data is stored on Fitocracy's servers (for viewing/manipulating once you log onto the site), the data is accessible on your phone via the mobile app. Figure 8-18 shows a screen for logging a set.

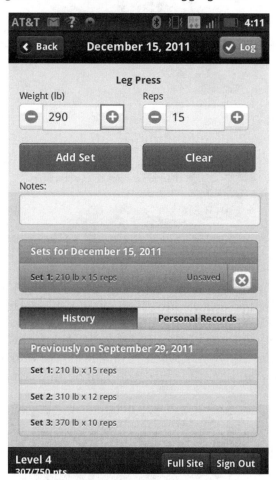

Figure 8-18. *Fitocracy's mobile app for logging sets*

Given that your own data is stored on Fitocracy's servers (for viewing/manipulating once you log onto the site), the data is accessible on your phone via the mobile app.

Tracking on Bodybuilder.com

Bodybuilder.com has a pretty good website for tracking sets and reps—it's called the BodySpace Workout Tracker. It has the nice feature of creating a template from a previous workout, and you can use that template to enter data for a current session. Figure 8-19 shows the screen for creating a workout involving inverted pushups.

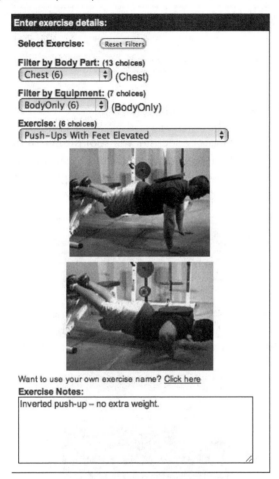

Figure 8-19. *Bodybuilder.com's screen for creating a workout and entering exercise data*

Using the template, you enter a new workout into the tool using a calendar and an intuitive screen, and the tool saves the data for you, as shown in Figure 8-20.

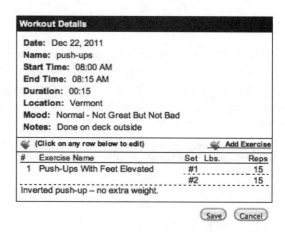

Figure 8-20. *Entering workout data for a couple of sets of inverted pushups*

In the site's View/Edit History section, the tool proffers a nice set of charts and aggregate statistics for previous workouts, as shown in Figure 8-21. The app compiles statistics such as volume (total weight lifted) and calculates your 1RM (highest total you can lift one rep) for the workout's exercise.

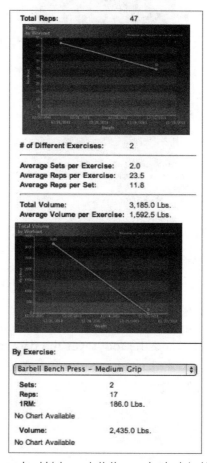

Figure 8-21. *Viewng your workout history, statistics, and calculated RMs*

Chapter 8

CrossFit

We include an introduction to CrossFit here, but not because it is one of the loudest recent buzzwords of the exercise world (although that noise may well lead you to wonder, "What is CrossFit?"). As a cross-training regimen, it seems to be a very good fit with the other regimens we covered in Chapter 7 and earlier in this chapter, such as sprinting, body-weight exercises, and weightlifting. CrossFit involves all of these activities, and more. We'll let the developers speak for themselves, from the introductory page at: *www.crossfit.com/cf-info/what-crossfit.html*:

> *CrossFit is the principal strength and conditioning program for many police academies and tactical operations teams, military special operations units, champion martial artists, and hundreds of other elite and professional athletes worldwide. Our program delivers a fitness that is, by design, broad, general, and inclusive. Our specialty is not specializing. Combat, survival, many sports, and life reward this kind of fitness and, on average, punish the specialist.*

We'll talk about CrossFit again in Chapter 9, when we discuss using a WOD (or workout of the day) generator. The CrossFit gang also pay more than lip service to additional health-related aspects such as nutrition and fasting, which are widely discussed in this book.

Cross-training

CrossFit might be thought of as cross-training on steroids. Cross-training is the traditional term for using exercises that promote variety and focus on both cardiovascular strength and power, for example, combining running, sprinting, and weightlifting. Cross-training was an outgrowth of people finally burning out on "just running" or "just cycling," as well as the proliferation of extensive year-round training programs for one team sport (promoting more burnout), leading many to realize that they needed some variety throughout the year.

CrossFit is basically offered at gyms that are specially designed for those purposes, and you can find them in the Yellow Pages and advertised on the Web. They have introductory courses on the huge variety of techniques they use, and the Web also offers a ton of descriptions and videos. Just go to the CrossFit Frequently Asked Questions (FAQ page), for instance, at *www.crossfit.com/cf-info/faq.html#General0*.

The list of CrossFit videos is here: www.crossfit.com/cf-info/excercise. html.

CrossFit involves a smorgasbord of weightlifting, gymnastics, body-weight exercises (all kinds of pushups), newish techniques (such as hoisting kettlebells around), and the kind of climbing maneuvers you might see at a military boot camp or "muddy gladiator"–type weekend race, like climbing ropes. The CrossFitters pride themselves on being all-rounders and "functional," meaning their techniques are meant to make you strong in a practical way, instead of just making a particular muscle group bulge out or giving you six-pack abs.

The six-pack ab mentality is so pervasive that my 7-year-old blurted out one day that he "only had a two-pack."

With CrossFit, you can work out alone or in a class full of sweaty people doing mountain climbers and hoisting barbells, which a lot of people apparently like to do. Class-style fitness has never appealed to me, but I suppose that depends on your personality and experience. I've found that some CrossFit facilities are particularly rigorous about making you take classes and/or move about the facility with an instructor, so you may have to shop around if that's not your style.

With all the information available on the Web you are certainly capable of buying the equipment or just using your local gym to initiate your own CrossFit routine. CrossFit proponents often recommend that you learn the different techniques, then use the various WOD generators.

CrossFit also has competitive tournaments, and the various techniques involved in the competitions are a reflection of just how versatile and strenuous CrossFit can be. The tournament might require its entrants to do as many pull-ups as they can, run a 5k, run a 400-meter dash, squat as much weight as they can, do a timed weightlifting contest for total volume, and so on. Just looking at the results will knock you out. It is the Everyman's Olympic decathlon.

Randomizing Fitness and the Importance of R & R

9

Consider an imaginary world where your job is to move the cream puffs off the assembly line. I seem to dimly recall an *I Love Lucy* episode along those lines. Anyways, the crux of your tasks could be reduced to "cream puff… cream puff… cream puff." What do you think your brain would be like at the end of the week, or the month, without any other stimulation? You might be wearing one of those T-shirts that reads "My brain on cream puffs." Do you think your brain would grow and thrive? Obviously not—our nervous systems and neural networks need constant stimulation of a *varying* nature to sustain themselves and grow more robust. A little math here, some programming, a new language; finally, you get to a complete reading of Herman Melville's *Moby Dick*.

The brain needs to be surprised and challenged, along the lines of a Lumosity test.

You can access this "exercise your brain" online site at www.lumosity.com.

Shock the Monkey

Your body and physique require constant shocks and challenges, too, in the form of surprises and new techniques to learn. The idea that surprising your body with good stress, as in a hard and/or explosive movement that you're not accustomed to, has gained a lot of traction lately in the fitness world. Art De Vany, an impressively fit economist in his seventies, the "grandfather of Paleo," and one of the first to apply Chaos Theory to health and fitness, is a big proponent of shocking or surprising your own metabolism with a fast (the no-food kind) or a high-intensity workout. The idea is that we seem to benefit from brief, acute stresses that excite adaptive processes and help make us stronger. We're designed for variety and the adaptation of our physiques to multiple skills.

De Vany has written an interesting book called The New Evolution Diet; *check it out at http://amzn.to/newevolutiondiet.*

We'll discuss good stress, or *hormesis*, more in Chapter 11.

Shake It Up in the Morning

Imagine that when you wake up in the morning you know you're going to do *some* kind of exercise, but you don't know exactly what it will be. It will be randomly chosen for you. Randomizing exercise is one of the new frontiers of fitness you can explore.

We're talking about exercise within certain parameters, not injury-prone surprises, such as, "This morning you'll pull a truck up the driveway with a cable and your teeth."

We're going to start off this chapter with a discussion of randomness and variability in the workout realm, and tools you can use to take part in that. These include the new website GAIN Fitness, and a random CrossFit-workout picker called The WOD Shop.

I'm Only Sleeping

The rest of the chapter covers sleep, rest, and sleep/rest tools mixed together. Why bother to even write about sleep or to use sleep analysis tools?

Sleep is a deeply underappreciated aspect of fitness and health, particularly among geeks. Most geeks would rather write code and hack and eat pizza than sleep at night, whereas if they want to gain fitness and stay healthy, the inverse would be better: writing code and hacking standing up during the day, and taking naps and sleeping at night.

A friend of mine summed up the state of sleep among modern techies when he said, "Society shouldn't call it 'sleep'—it should be renamed along the lines of 'human cell-rejuvenation time' or the like." We usually view sleep as optional, and something kind of cool to skip. We like to be up when others are snoozing, as if we are going to experience some intriguing life revelation that others will not, such as watching intoxicated people say awful things and do face-plants in front of nightclubs.

Sleep is a deeply underappreciated aspect of fitness and health, particularly among geeks.

Better to get a good night's sleep so you can wake up refreshed and have a gratifying, perhaps randomly assigned bit of exercise under the sun. We'll check out some apps for analyzing the quality of sleep, such as the Zeo sleep manager tool.

RESTful Programmers

We're also going to discuss the importance of rest for athletes, as in taking days off from the fun stress your body undergoes. You need the rest to rebuild and recharge. People tend to not rest enough, particularly when they get excited about a new routine, start seeing some results, or compete in the endurance world. Exercise can also be physically addictive, as in something you crave each day.

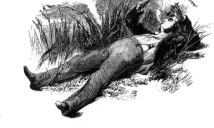

> Overtraining, at least amongst sports-medicine geeks, is considered a kind of disease, complete with a set of physical and mental symptoms, like a racing heart rate, irritability, and not sleeping well.

Two concepts—"less is more," along with another old expression that is still useful to us fitness geeks, "quality not quantity"—are important for staying rested, strong, and infection-free.

We're going to discuss an interesting tool called RestWise that serious athletes and daily fitness hackers alike can use to analyze their current state or level of rest.

Randomize It

Ever programmed a random() function in your code? The typical setup is to have an array of items that the program has to display or use, but it doesn't matter which item the code plucks out of the array. I did a JavaScript program that had to display a book cover whenever a web page was displayed in the browser, but not the same book cover every time. I had an array of "book image" objects representing the different book covers, and when the page was loaded, the JavaScript shuffled the array and chose the first member to display. Parts of the code are shown below:

```
var bookCoverJava = new BookImage(…);
var bookCoverGWT = new BookImage(…);
var bookCoverAjax = new BookImage(…);
var imgArray = new Array(bookCoverJava, bookCoverGWT, bookCoverAjax);
// randomly shuffle the book covers using a custom function
imgArray.shuffle();
//choose the book cover to display
var bookObject = imgArray[0];
```

What if you could choose your exercise workout this way? Well, you can. You can create your own array of workout objects, shuffle them up, and write a program that chooses one for you each morning. That would be fun, but labor-intensive. Also, *you* would be writing the workout routines, so a certain amount of bias would be baked into the workouts. You wouldn't *truly* be surprised or shocked by the routines, since you would be making them up.

The WOD Shop

We don't always have to reinvent the wheel. At least one site will do this for you. The WOD Shop is a website that lets you choose from a category of workout types (e.g., weightlifting, endurance, body weight, or kettlebells), and it will generate a workout for you. You can access it at *www.wodshop.org*.

In CrossFit circles (see Chapter 8) a WOD means "workout of the day"; however, for our purposes, it could also mean "workout on demand." Figure 9-1 shows what The WOD Shop's menu page looks like.

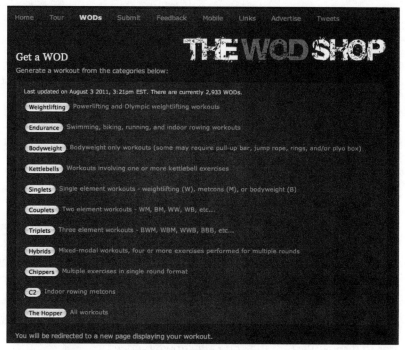

Figure 9-1. *The WOD Shop for dynamically generated workouts*

You are presented with the choices of Weightlifting, Endurance, Bodyweight, Kettlebells, and more. I'm going to choose Bodyweight for today, and we'll see what it comes up with.

A list of videos describing many kinds of CrossFit exercises can be found at www.crossfit.com/cf-info/excercise.html#Exer.

Figure 9-2 shows the result: a tough series of different forms of pushups, squats, and other exercises, like "mountain climbers" (see Chapter 8 for more details on some of these CrossFit variations).

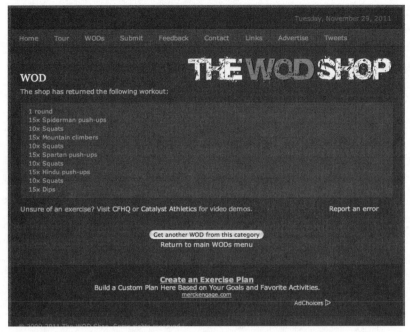

Figure 9-2. *Spartan push-ups, Hindu push-ups, Spidermans, and more*

This workout specifies:

- 1 round (so you only do this once)

- 15x Spiderman push-ups

- 10x squats

- 15x mountain climbers

- 10x squats

- 15x Spartan push-ups

- 10x squats

- 15x Hindu push-ups

- 10x squats

- 15x dips

Chapter 8 describes some of these different types of exercises. You shouldn't use any weight on your back for the squats (it's not specified). They're more like "air squats." A Spartan pushup, for example, is a normal pushup, except that your hand positions are staggered; one is in a normal position while the other is behind that position, closer to your chest. With each pushup, you exchange the hand positions.

The whole workout should take about 10 minutes (believe me, it's a very efficient and intense 10 minutes!), unless you take longer rests in between sets.

You could do this workout anywhere: in a hotel room, your mother-in-law's living room, or, if you were really brazen, an airport terminal lounge. You can also adapt the workout to your own body and needs; you don't have to perform it exactly as specified (for example, you'd probably have to practice Spartan pushups and do fewer reps).

You can also access this site from your mobile phone at *www.wodshop.org/mobile/index.html*. Figure 9-3 shows a dynamically generated weightlifting workout on my mobile phone.

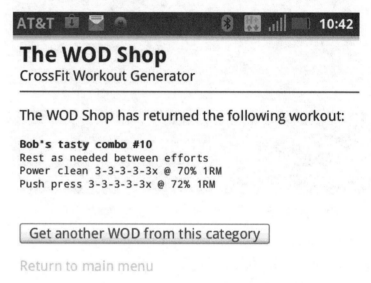

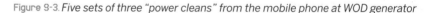

Figure 9-3. *Five sets of three "power cleans" from the mobile phone at WOD generator*

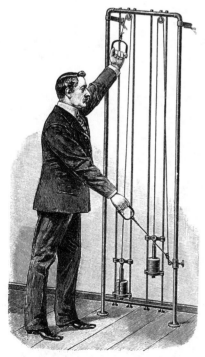

These instructions mean two upper-body barbell exercises (power clean and pushup press), five sets of three reps, at about 70 percent of "one rep max" (1RM). What's 1RM? This is a relative way to gauge how much each individual lifts for a certain exercise. One RM is the most weight you can do for one repetition with a specific exercise, such as 150 pounds for the bench press. So, 70 percent of 1RM for this bench press would be about 105 pounds.

See Chapter 8 for more details on repetition maximums and weightlifting in the gym.

> It can be hazardous to try to find out an unknown 1RM for a certain exercise. You can try to estimate your 1RM by how many reps you've done with a lighter weight. A number of equations have been proposed to calculate a maximum load lifted—a 1RM—from performing the same exercise with less weight on the bar. Here's one: 1RM = ((# of reps) / 30 + 1) x weight. So, if you bench pressed 145 pounds 10 times (and that was all you could do), the equation would be (10/30 + 1) x 145 = 193. This equation suggests that you could bench press 193 pounds once.

GAIN Fitness

Another workout generator I like comes via GAIN Fitness at *http://gainfitness.com*. It was in an alpha stage at the time I was using it in early winter 2011/12. To build a "quick workout," as GAIN Fitness describes it, you use the screen shown in Figure 9-4. I like the various "tuning options" you're given for determining a workout that includes equipment like kettlebells and barbells, or not.

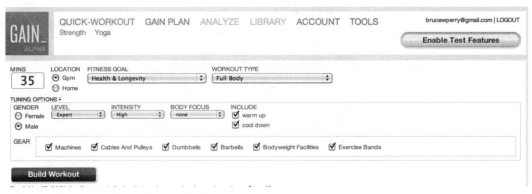

Figure 9-4. *Tuning a workout at* www.gainfitness.com

You can even configure the number of minutes that you want to devote to the exercise, and set the gender, level of fitness experience, and which part of the body you want to focus on. Then you just click the Build Workout button.

The results are quite impressive and intuitive. The app displays a series of exercises with videos (for some of them) and descriptions, as well as a timer and some stats to start with (such as how long it should take you and the total number of reps). Figure 9-5 shows the top segment of the results. I liked the ability to choose a menu item for a text description or a video.

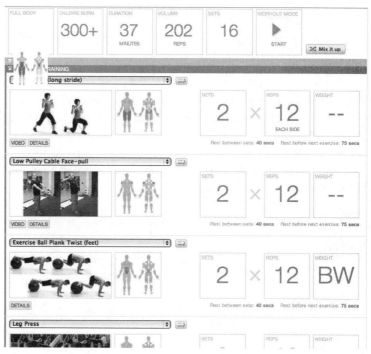

Figure 9-5. *The GAIN Fitness site generates a workout for you, with some instruction videos*

The tool also will also generate a fitness *plan* or routine for you, although this doesn't have anything to do with randomizing fitness. You might just get some more good ideas for additional fitness or strength-building methods. Figure 9-6 shows the different components you can configure for the plan, such as muscle groups targeted, whether you're in gym or home settings, the time devoted to each workout, how many days per week you want to train, and so on.

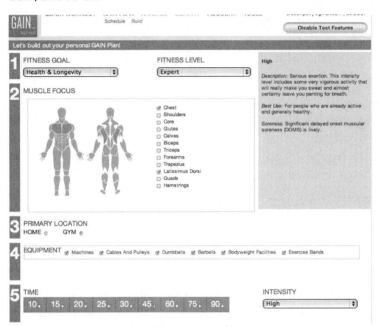

Figure 9-6. *Use a GAIN Fitness template for an autogenerated fitness plan or routine*

Once you generate the plan, the tool displays a calendar view, as Figure 9-7 shows. This view rotates through a couple of routines that are similar to the ones that can be dynamically generated for you in the quick workouts mode. For example, you do one kind of workout on Monday, a different one for Thursday, and the tool configures the routines for you.

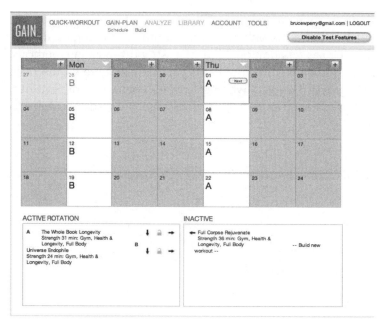

Figure 9-7. *The GAIN Fitness app creates a calendar for your workout plan*

Whether or not the recommended workouts are hard enough to make a difference is for you to test, but its clean design and usability make GAIN Fitness a promising site for generating workouts in the future.

The important thing is to find a tool to make up the "surprise" workouts for you. Otherwise, you'll fall prey to the tendency to hit your comfort zone with the same set of static exercises that you've done for months, a sure prescription for the plateauing of your fitness level. In general, with a randomizer, who needs a personal trainer?

If you like to work out with other people, get together with friends and randomize, then treat yourself to a pizza (but with Paleo crust and plenty of veggies for a topping!).

Mashing Up Your Sports Devices

One of the ways you can add variety to your routine, and to make sure all your fitness databases (such as Endomondo, the Fitbit Tracker, and Garmin Connect) are up to date with your latest workouts, is to mash up the various devices and tools you use. All of these tools include internal databases that store your workouts historically. If you go from one device to another—from a Garmin device to a smartphone, for instance—various databases will get out of sync with your training and exercise data. Horrors!

The important thing is to find a tool to make up the "surprise" workouts for you. Otherwise, you'll fall prey to the tendency to hit the comfort zone with the same set of static exercises…

You could bring two devices along—a watch and a smartphone, for example—to determine if there are significant differences in the way they collect data. How close are the mileage calculators, and which device has the most accurate GPS? Thankfully, the devices do tend to play well with each other in terms of being able to export GPX files that can be imported into another tracker's database.

> *GPS can be notoriously imprecise in terms of measuring up to the tenth of a mile. Different devices tend to disagree with each other in measuring the exact length of runs, for instance. This drives runners crazy. Most of the time, however, the GPS-enabled devices serve our purposes fine.*

During this interlude, we're going to take a look at combining Garmin with Endomondo. My Forerunner 301, an older GPS-enabled watch that records workouts, provided the data for Garmin. As described in Chapter 2, the watch plugs into the USB port of your computer, then uploads its data to Garmin Connect, a nifty web-based dashboard sporting all kinds of features. It's located at *http://connect.garmin.com*.

The Endomondo smartphone app, another GPS device that connects with an elaborate training website, is discussed at length in Chapters 2 and 7.

Figure 9-8 shows the Garmin Connect window displaying various features of a mountain-bike ride.

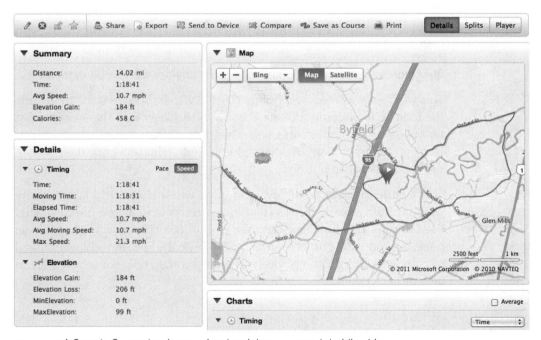

Figure 9-8. *A Garmin Connect web page showing data on a mountain-bike ride*

One of the nice features of Garmin Connect is that it includes a Player (an embedded Adobe Flash program) that allows you to replay the entire workout and check out the sequential data along the way, such as your speed and elevation. Nifty! Figure 9-9 shows the Player in a Garmin Connect window.

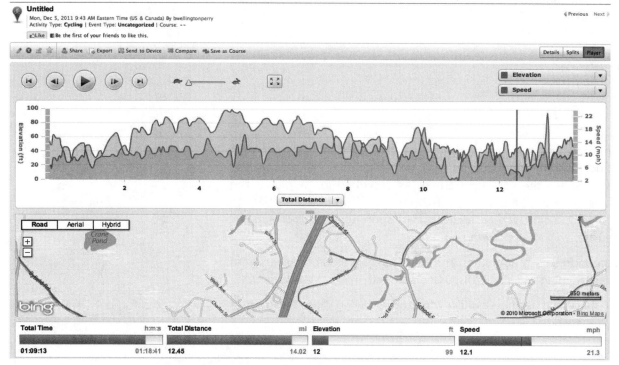

Figure 9-9. *Replay your workout using Garmin Connect's Player*

But I digress; let's return to mashing up the devices' associated databases.

This workout was recorded on my Garmin watch, but we want to include the training in Endomondo's database as well. Never fear. There are at least two ways to accomplish this task. One is to go to *www.endomondo.com/ workouts/* with the Garmin device plugged into your USB port, then choose the Import Workout button.

This feature displays a window that gives you a choice of importing the workout from a file or from a Garmin device. As long as you have installed the Garmin Communicator browser plug-in (which you *have* if you have been playing with one of Garmin's GPS devices), Endomondo will pull all of your workouts off the device and give you the choice of which ones to include in its database.

You can also export a file from Garmin Connect, then import the same file into Endomondo. This is easy to do. In the activities segment of your Garmin dashboard in the browser, select an activity or workout. The selection will bring you to a detailed page on that activity. This page has an Export button, which allows you to generate a GPX file, for example, representing that activity.

Save that file on your computer. Then, once again, go to *www.endomondo. com/workouts/* and choose Import Workout. This time, select the file you downloaded to your computer. Figure 9-10 shows the same mountain-bike ride at Endomondo, so now you've synced your databases at both sites.

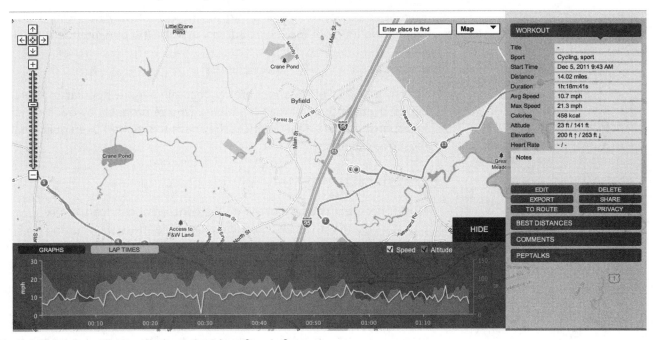

Figure 9-10. *Presto, you've imported a workout from Garmin Connect*

With your Garmin watch plugged into the USB port (and using the Garmin Communicator plug-in), you can import your workouts en masse into Endomondo.

Rest and Taper

Resting is the part of fitness that few people are particularly good at. Just about all of us are good at being a couch potato, but not working out at all during the day? "Gotta get my fix!"

Tapering is also an important concept for people who like to do races. Tapering means gradually cutting back during the days and weeks leading up to a race or competition—in a way, like taking an "active holiday." Tapering is almost more art than science. You have to listen to your body, and that goes for resting as well.

Exercise is addictive, and it's hard to know intuitively how much rest is neither too little nor too much. But rest assured (no pun intended), *you will fail to get stronger with either resistance or endurance training if you don't rest enough*.

In fact, the idea of "less is more" is becoming more popular in exercise circles, even among Ironman triathletes, who've probably by tradition (and in response to the brutal distances they have to train for) been guilty of the most overtraining.

Decelerate, Strategically

Most fitness regimens are based on the concept of overload, or taxing your physical system with an intense but manageable stress, then cutting back, or completely stopping any hard exercise (short of a walk), to allow your body and mind to recover and initiate the adaptations that will make you stronger.

As you can probably imagine, you could fill books—and authors have—with the varying strategies for how to spread exercise and rest periods throughout a week or month. Runners and triathletes have their *periodization* plans for an entire season, dictating when their training will peak, ebb, and flow leading up to their events, with complicated calendars and designated rest days. Traditionally, these athletes use Sunday as a rest day, but they're usually doing *something* out at the gym or on the road on all of the other days.

Tapering means gradually cutting back during the days and weeks leading up to a race or competition, in a way, like taking an 'active holiday.' Tapering is almost more art than science. You have to listen to your body, and that goes for resting as well.

The Wound Healing School

CrossFitters also tend to have a schedule that keeps them working out hard four, five, or six days out of the week (see Chapter 8 for the skinny on CrossFit). On the other hand, the popular high-intensity training (HIT) school of weightlifting recommends training very hard just once every 7 or 10 days, for example.

This "wound healing" school of iron pumpers bases its strategy on the notion that it takes a week or more to heal from a very hard weight-training session and to rebuild the targeted muscles, and it has good physiological evidence to back it up.

It's essential to introduce variety into your routine, and this built-in variability usually includes rest as a side effect. For example, you might work out really hard with weights or a CrossFit routine once per week, and let walks, romps in the park with dogs and/or kids, and bike commutes take care of your remaining desire and need to get outdoors. You have to see what works for you; everyone is different.

> *I devised my own strategy in the old days for preparing and tapering for races, like a 10k or a triathlon. About 7–10 days out I would do a short, intense race (such as a 5k) as a "tune-up," and then I'd cut back my daily training significantly, by about half. Every other day I would take a complete day off, especially the day before a race. I focused on getting good sleeps every night. About 48 hours out I would get a sports massage (see Chapter 10). This usually worked for me; I was almost always very fresh for races.*

As you may have predicted, there's a software tool (at least one!) for gauging your rest levels and patterns.

RestWise

RestWise is an online tool for calculating the restfulness levels of athletes. Its literature describes the tool as a "non-invasive fatigue monitoring system" (meaning, needles aren't involved). It's basically a way to "hack your rest levels." RestWise is designed for pro or amateur superstars, their coaches, and regular Janes and Joes like you and me. While it's a for-pay service, you can try it out for free for two weeks at *restwise.com*.

Resting is the part of fitness that few people are particularly good at.

The way it works is that you sign in at the website, then go to the page for submitting your physical or biological data (nothing too complicated). Figure 9-11 shows this page. You enter values for several parameters, including resting heart rate, oxygen saturation (more on that in a moment), your weight, the hours you slept, as well as several subjective categories, such as your mood, energy level, and whether you have muscle soreness. You even enter an estimate on a sliding color scale of your pee color, as this is a very good barometer of your level of dehydration (*really* yellow is bad; clear is good).

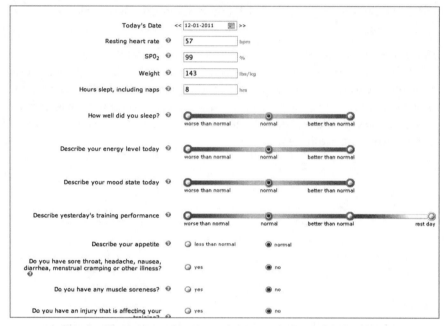

Figure 9-11. *Entering the various subjective and objective biological stuff at RestWise*

Oxygen saturation is a measure of how well oxygen is being diffused throughout your body. If you've ever been in a hospital intensive care unit (ICU), they are always sticking this device that looks like a clothespin on the patient's finger. This is measuring the oxygen saturation. For healthy values, they look for a result in the high 90s, such as between 96 and 99.

A pulse oximeter is the hardware tool that comes with the RestWise software service (and *it* looks like a fancy electronic clothespin): you use this device as you are entering data. It captures both your resting heart rate (how many times your heart beats per minute) and your oxygen saturation.

Once you enter the data, you click a button for the results, which Figure 9-12 shows.

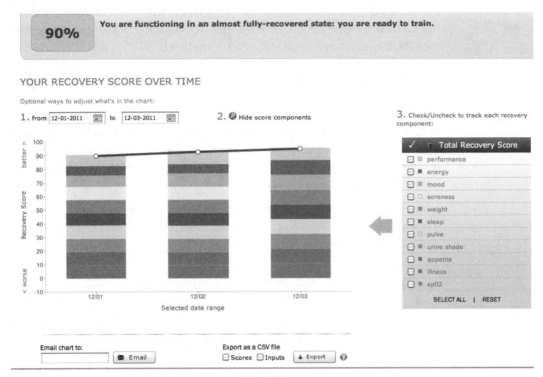

Figure 9-12. *Checking out your recovery score with RestWise*

The results give you a "recovery score" of up to 100 percent, which means "all systems go," and you're ready to train again. If you get a lower percent value in the red zone, that means take it easy on training today, or take the day off. You can email the resulting chart and download it in comma-separated-value (CSV) format (for Excel and other applications).

The FAQ at the site (*restwise.com/contactus/askus/*) discusses the proprietary algorithm it uses to produce recovery scores, without completely letting the cat out of the bag. Here's the answer to the question about whether all the values you enter are weighted the same (they're not):

> *The weighting varies for each marker and is dependent on the strength of the empirical and anecdotal evidence of each. Keep in mind also that the algorithm is specific to the individual by intelligently referencing to an individual's baseline data and also intelligently responding to the degree by which specific markers change over a few days; for example, the weight of last night's sleep score (a proprietary algorithm for duration and quality) is dependent on the previous two night's scores, with the understanding that the effect of poor sleep is cumulative.*

What if fitness chiefly revolved around how well you slept and handled stress…

It also points out that the recovery scores will probably be low if you are in an overload or *supercompensation* mode of training (in which you have actually stressed or broken the body on purpose). If you're just day-to-day training for health, however, only the complete cessation of training will help you recover. You just have to take days off sometimes.

The All-Important Zees

Maybe we're all wrong about nutrition and exercise as the primary touchstones of fitness. What if fitness chiefly revolved around how well you slept and handled stress, and that food and muscle-work represented the icing on the cake and were comparatively incidental to sleeping well and putting life's stressful interludes into perspective?

In my own experience, sleep seems to be at the top of my agenda just when it is least attainable. With few exceptions, I feel awful without it—the bottom line for me is, sleep is wicked important!

And it should be for you, too (see the "Melatonin: The Darkness Hormone" sidebar). Medical researchers have associated long-term sleep deprivation with all kinds of serious medical issues,[2] as well as inflammation in general.[3] Enough said on the dark side of going withovut sleep; let's discuss the benefits, basics, and tracking considerations of getting a good conk-out.

This chunk of the chapter covers some of the basics of sleeping, followed by a rundown of a few tools and apps you can use to monitor and track your entrance into the luxurious realm of dozing—hacking your sleep, in other words, with a tool called Zeo or the Fitbit.

We also discuss an app that helps with *meditation*, which is a tool you might consider including in your own stress-reducing repertoire.

Sleep Basics

Most of us require anywhere from seven and a half to nine hours of sleep per night. Sleep is essential for the repair and growth of cells, and it's a crucial stage of the circadian rhythm or "biological clock" by which your body times and controls its various physiological states. For example, when life intercedes and whacks out our normal sleep patterns, the timing for the secretion of certain hormones, such as growth hormone, which is used to repair and build tissue, and a stress hormone called cortisol, is disrupted. A lousy sleep once in a while is natural, but the deprivation isn't usually a good thing over a long time.

It's just a theory, but sleep studies indicate that proper sleep is essential for creating cognitive order out of neural chaos; during sleep's deepest stages, our minds sift through and process the fog of data the daytime has immersed us in, filtering out the dross from the information that can be committed to memory and learned.[4]

> *There's probably good evidence for this, considering the cognitively disorienting effects of just a few bad nights of sleep.*

Sleep Stages: NREM and REM

There are two principal stages of sleep that cycle off and on, distinguished by brain waves of differing types, throughout the night. Non–rapid eye movement (NREM) sleep is composed of four different stages, from "just drifting off" to deep, restorative sleep. You spend about 75 percent of sleeping time in NREM sleep.[5] The muscles relax, blood pressure and body temperature drop, growth hormone is released, and the repair and restoration mechanics of sleep take place.

You typically traverse each stage of NREM, one through four, before you reach the rapid eye movement (REM) stage of deep dreaming.

> *The sleep graph produced by the Zeo Sleep Manager indicates that, at the very least, the stages can get "mixed up," so that you may not have a latter-stage NREM sleep segment before you drop off into REM. The sleep stages are linear, but not strictly linear.*

The entire cycle of four-stage NREM to REM is repeated roughly every 90 minutes; yet, you can experience situations where you undergo hours of stage 3 and 4 NREM sleep without falling into REM. Imagine that you're ascending the floors of a building, and each floor is more comprehensive and dream-filled.

Befitting the REM stage's name, the eyes dance around behind the eyelids during this cycle, as the theory goes, following the actions and imagery of our dreams.[6] The first drift into REM lasts only up to 10 minutes, but the duration of the final REM cycle(s) can be from 20 minutes to more than an hour.[7] It seems that if you have a full eight hours of sleep, you undergo at least four or five of these 90–120 minute NREM-to-REM cycles. This is yet further evidence that you shouldn't eschew the various components of a full night's sleep, say, by constantly going to bed too late and getting up too early (if it fits your schedule, that is). You could be missing out on one or more of these essential REM and NREM components.

Disrupted or habitually deprived sleep will reduce the growth hormone releases that take place during normal NREM cycles—what the Zeo tool calls "deep sleep." At the very least, this state will result in less cellular repair and less new tissue growth. If you want to build more lean mass or muscle, sleep a lot!

Most dreaming takes place during REM, although you can experience nightmares and "night terrors" during NREM (it seems that sticking to REM dreaming is the way to go!). The brain uses more oxygen during REM sleep than it does during normal wakeful activities, belying the myth that everything "just shuts down" during sleep.[8]

MELATONIN: THE DARKNESS HORMONE

Melatonin is a hormone or signaling chemical that the pineal gland synthesizes and secretes (tryptophan, an essential amino acid, is an ingredient for melatonin). The pineal gland, a pinecone-shaped gland about the size of a pea positioned alongside the brain, is sometimes called the "third eye," because it can convert environmental-lighting signals about the time of day and season and send those signals to the rest of the body.

While melatonin makes us sleepy, this hormone lies at the center of an intricate biological clock by which our bodies synchronize all types of crucial activities. When we expose ourselves to bright lights at night, instead of sleeping away in our pitch-black man- or girl-caves, we disrupt these rhythms to an extent that could make us susceptible to cancer, according to an article by David E. Blask, Ph.D., M.D. at Tulane University called "Melatonin, Sleep Disturbance, and Cancer Risk." The article appeared in a 2009 issue of *Sleep Medicine Reviews*. Here are some highlights:

- For all but the last 120 years or so, humanity and her distant ancestors lived by the solar clock, and there's physiological evidence of this. Sunlight enters the eyes and stimulates photoreceptors in the retina—these receptors send neural signals to a part of the brain's hypothalamus called the suprachiasmatic nuclei (SCN). The SCN synchronizes the internal 24-hour rhythms, including the melatonin surges at night. Very little melatonin is secreted during the day.

- "The nocturnal melatonin signal provides time of day information to all the cells, tissues, and organs of the body."

- Numerous bodily sites contain melatonin receptors; the hormone is involved in no less than "the control of sleep, circadian rhythms, retinal physiology, seasonal reproductive cycles, cancer development, immune activity, antioxidants and free-radical scavenging," as well as mitochondrial respiration, bone metabolism, and other processes.

- While sleep deprivation suppresses the immune system, a problem in and of itself, it's the exposure to light at night that messes with melatonin messaging. If you're not sleeping, but in darkness, the melatonin secretions *still* continue (one consolation of tossing and turning). "Darkness at night is an absolute requirement" for melatonin production.

- "It has been postulated that light exposure at night may represent a unique risk factor for breast cancer… via its ability to suppress [melatonin production]… while male night-shift workers are at a significantly increased risk of developing prostate cancer."

The bottom line? It helps to feel the warmth of the sun on your face in the morning, thus sending a natural signal to the hypothalamus/SCN and the pineal gland, as well as to turn the lights off at night. Try to follow the sun.

What are those twitches you experience just before nodding off to sleep? Scientists call them hypnagogic myoclonus, or sleep-related muscle spasms. It appears to be just an occasional motor response to entering the first stage of NREM sleep. I pumped the term into Google Scholar, and one of the results I got was "Exploding head syndrome and idiopathic stabbing headache…" so I decided not to explore that subject any further!

Low-Tech Sleep Tracking

Not everyone wants to know exactly what's happening while they're asleep, or is comfortable being connected to some device that's monitoring them at night, à la Malcolm McDowell in *A Clockwork Orange*. Others are thrilled or at least intrigued by that notion and keen to look at the data afterward (if that's you, see just ahead for a description of the Zeo Sleep Manager).

If you're looking for clues to inconsistent sleeps, you might find them in your own wave patterns, or how NREM or REM stages relate to certain days, scheduling changes, and what you eat or drink before going to bed.

If you don't want to be hooked up to a monitor, you can track sleep quality and quantity with a remarkably simple regimen. For example, for years, all I've done is recorded my sleep hours in a "fit log" that usually encompasses no more than one line of text (sometimes it turns into a kind of pithy diary; such as when a child is born, which is nice, considering that it's more than 12 years old).

Record your sleeping hours, including the all-important naps, for a month or longer. Compare the data to your resting heart rate and even your blood pressure at times. You'll probably learn that there is a strong relationship between sleep and other fitness parameters.

Oddly, sleep quality (or lack thereof) has seldom affected the ability of myself and other people to competently get through big athletic or physical events (just don't make them do math!), such as a triathlon, or summiting a mountain in the middle of the night. I think there's evidence that we are capable of tremendous physical achievements on little sleep—as certainly required on an evolutionary basis—but we can't count on "the borrowed time" lasting very long.

Hacking Your Sleep with the Zeo Sleep Manager

The Zeo Sleep Manager is one of the power tools that you can use to analyze and improve your sleep. Zeo is a combination of hardware and software: a clock, a headband with an attached tracking device, an SD card for storing your sleep data, and a USB connector for uploading the data. Figure 9-13 shows the equipment setup, which costs $100 or more depending on the options you choose (*www.myzeo.com/sleep/*).

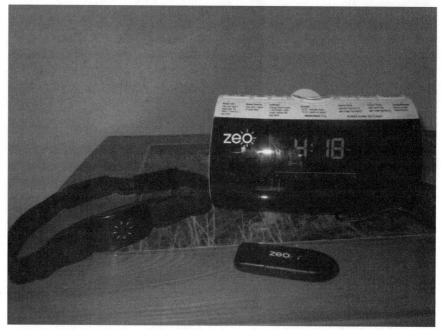

Figure 9-13. *The Zeo Sleep Manager hardware setup, with headband and USB connector*

Zeo also offers a smartphone version that doesn't require the bedside clock; it just has the headband, docking station, and smartphone app.

The way it works is that the headband rests in a cradle that is attached to the clock for recharging. When you go to sleep, you wear the headband, which connects wirelessly to the clock, recording your sleep data or biofeedback on an SD card. The card is easily inserted into and subsequently removed from a slot on the side of the clock. The clock does provide a way of turning down its glowing luminescence so you don't violate the darkness of your man- or girl-cave.

The device that Figure 9-13 shows sitting in front of the clock is the USB connection to your computer. When you're ready to upload the sleep data or feedback, you remove the SD card and hitch it to this device, which you attach to a USB connection, as Figure 9-14 shows. Then you connect with Zeo and click Upload Your Sleep Data. This action is similar to uploading the data from a Garmin watch to Garmin Connect.

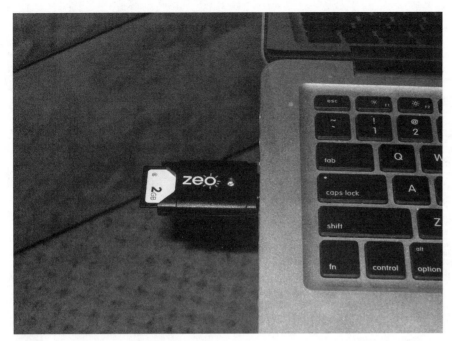

Figure 9-14. *Upload your Zeo sleep data with an SD card attached to a USB connection*

On a Mac, the USB device is mounted on the desktop and the data is stored in a zeo/zeosleep.dat *file.*

The upload widget at *http://mysleep.myzeo.com* asks you to choose the *zeo-sleep.dat* file. The website software then gobbles up your data and displays it with fancy graphics, as shown in Figure 9-15. The chart shows the color-coded patterns of your sleep stages for the night, if you were lucky enough to produce a lot of NREM and REM sleep.

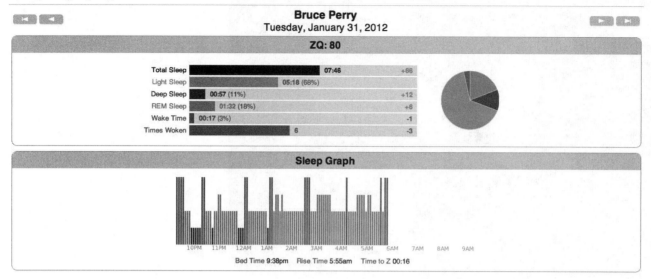

Figure 9-15. *The MyZeo charts display the sleep stages with colored patterns denoting REM and NREM sleep*

The Zeo FAQs and literature, which are quite extensive on the website, define stage 3 and 4 NREM sleep as deep sleep (the dark green bar) and early stage NREM as light sleep (the gray-colored bar).

Very nifty. This sleep chart actually represents a good snooze recorded by my wife. The lighter green lines on the chart represent REM, a very restorative, dream-filled stage. She chalked up 92 minutes of it, and you can see that she had four progressively longer (in general) stages of it, similar to our earlier description of the basics of sleep.

The ochre or orange lines represent times spent awake.

The MyZeo website, which is set up for you after you have registered with the serial number from the bedside clock, includes all sorts of structured content, blogs, forums, and "hack your sleep" tips that are designed to polish your snoozing skills. They set up a personalized sleep coach for you, for example, and there are graphics that compare your ZQ, or sleep quality, with that of other Zeo users of the same age group.

Figure 9-16 shows how a ZQ for a night's sleep breaks down into different sleep segments, such as time in REM. The ZQ is basically a numerical index of sleep quality.

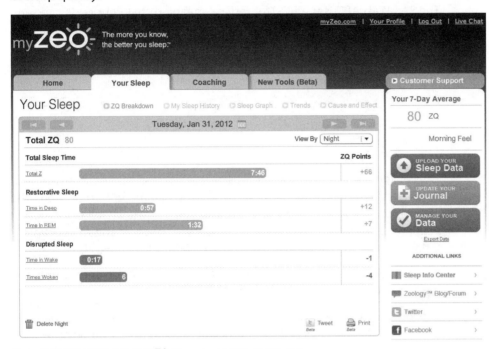

Figure 9-16. *Checking out your ZQ at* www.mysleep.myzeo.com

The Zeo Web API

For really hacking your sleep, Zeo offers a Web API with which you or a third party can use software code to access your sleep data from Zeo's servers.

For example, you might want to display the data in a customized way on your own web page, or another personal tracking outfit can integrate Zeo's data with its own features. The API site with documentation is at *http://mysleep.myzeo.com/api/api.shtml*.

The Web API works with several different programming languages, including Java, PHP, Perl, Python, and Ruby. Before you can use the API, you have to apply for an authentication key, a long string of hexadecimal numbers, which will accompany your programmatic calls for the Zeo sleep information. Zeo sends you this key in an email message.

For really hacking your sleep, Zeo offers a Web API with which you or a third party can use software code to access your sleep data from Zeo's servers.

API nitty-gritty

The API documentation is quite complete, but I'll give you a taste of it here.

The Zeo Web API uses a RESTful service, meaning that your code can send HTTP requests for the sleep data in the form of a URL, such as this example from the instructions (you plug in the various components in square brackets): *https://api.myzeo.com:8443/zeows/api/*[version]/[response_type]/[service_name]/[action_name]*?key=*[key]&[parameters].

> *A real URL looks like this: https://api.myzeo.com:8443/zeows/api/v1/ sleeperService/getOverallAverageZQScore?key=54CAE7B527B0CD8EA D5875A20F214CDD.*

The version is the software version, as in "v1"; the response type (an optional parameter) is "xml" by default (if you leave the parameter out) or "json"; the service name is "sleeperService"; and the action name is whatever method or action you are calling, as in "getOverallAverageZQScore." The API documentation provides the details on the different actions you can use.

You can also use the open source OAUTH protocol for authorizing the requests for data: see *http://oauth.net*.

The key that you receive from Zeo will go right into the URL as the "key" parameter. The key is locked to a particular domain (e.g., your website, as in *www.fitnesskg.com*), which you specify when you register with the Zeo Web API. This means that you won't be able to grab real sleep data unless the code that executes the Zeo request is hosted on the specified domain.

I tested these Web API calls by making requests directly from the Firefox browser, putting the URL containing all the specified parameters, including my key, into the browser location field (even though I didn't have any data on Zeo's website yet). The response gave me an error message telling me that the request did not derive from my specified domain, but at least I was able to test using different parameters in the URL, as well as the API's two response types, XML and JSON.

XML and JSON are two structured languages for displaying data.

Here's the XML version (the key has been changed):
```
//The URL :: https://api.myzeo.com:8443/zeows/api/v1/sleeperService/
//getOverallAverageZQScore?key=54CAE7B527B0CD8EAD5875A20F213CBB
//The XML response
<?xml version="1.0" encoding="UTF-8" standalone="yes"?>
<response versionBuild="1.0.10186" versionApi="v1"
    status="5" rspId="0" reqId="0">
<errMsg>API Key does not match caller domain.</errMsg>
</response>
```

And here's the JSON version:

```
//The URL :: https://api.myzeo.com:8443/zeows/api/v1/json/sleeperService/
//getOverallAverageZQScore?key=54DBE7B527B0CD8EAD5875A20F214CDD
{"response":
{"@versionBuild":"1.0.10186","@versionApi":"v1","@status":"5","@rspId":
"0","@reqId":"0","errMsg":"API Key does not match caller domain."}}
```

Here's an example from the API documentation of XML and JSON responses:

```
XML Output:
<response versionBuild="1.0.0054" versionApi="v1"
status="0" rspId="0" reqId="0">
    <name>
getOverallAverageZQScore
    </name>
    <value>
79
    </value>
</response>
JSON Output:
{
    "response": {
            "@versionBuild": "1.0.0054",
            "@versionApi": "v1",
            "@status": "0",
            "@rspId": "0",
            "@reqId": "0",
            "name": "getOverallAverageZQScore",
            "value": 79
    }
}
```

More Web Tracking

Other tools abound for tracking your sleep in more detail with devices and gear. You can find a list of self-tracking tools for sleep at Quantified Self: see *quantifiedself.com/guide/tag/sleep*.

For example, the Fitbit Tracker discussed at length in Chapter 2, has a feature for these purposes. It includes a whole section on tracking your sleep from the night before and over time, as Figure 9-17 shows.

The Fitbit comes with a wristband or armband that you use to take the tracker along on your snooze fests. You can wear it on your wrist to record your night's sleep. Figure 9-17 indicates that I was awakened 12 times on this night. Ah, reflections of the old days when the kids weren't sleeping!

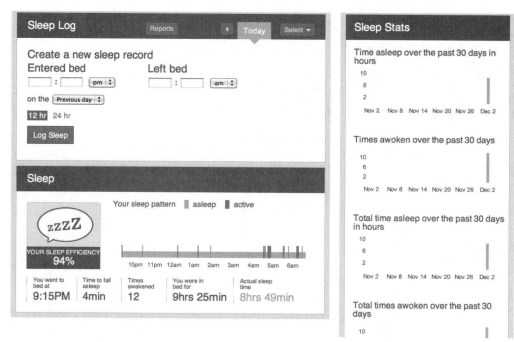

Figure 9-17. *Use Fitbit to record and examine sleep*

Ever hear a comedian say, "I slept like a baby last night—I woke up every two hours and cried"?

In this case, every time my hand moved, the Fitbit flagged that as "He's awake," so there were probably a few times when unconscious rearranging of the pillows or yanking the blanket (sorry, spouse) triggered the device. Actually, I only remember waking up once during a deep night of snoozing on that date. This was otherwise a fairly accurate rendering of what kind of sleep I got that night.

Meditation Tools

Meditation is a useful habit to add to your fitness program. It has the potential to lower your blood pressure and heart rate, at the very least, and to help you dial down the stress and cultivate a sense of peace. If you doubt whether the latter mood aspects have health ramifications, you should rethink or simply meditate on the topic.

Meditation comes in all shapes and sizes, including transcendental meditation and *mindfulness*. A Center for Mindfulness, for example, exists at the UMass Medical School in Massachusetts, and the technique is used extensively to help people with the stress induced by chronic illnesses.

Mindfulness is based on the notion that you can "live in the moment" while meditating and simply let thoughts flow in and out of your consciousness unheeded, without being preoccupied by their meanings or responding stressfully to them. One mindfulness expert used the metaphor of thoughts flowing through your mind heedlessly like clouds moving across the sky.

Here is a more formal definition, from a 2002 journal article called "What Do We Really Know About Mindfulness-Based Stress Reduction?":[9]

> *The meditation techniques are used to develop a perspective on thoughts and feelings so that they are recognized as mental events rather than as aspects of the self or as necessarily accurate reflections of reality.*

Vonnegut Would Have Grokked It

Okay, so it's difficult to precisely pinpoint meditation in plain language. I view the general mindset as similar to that of a Kurt Vonnegut character, shrugging his shoulders and saying something nonsensical like, "Hey ho," no matter what comes along.

To my mind, anytime someone is sitting or lying down in a dark room listening to music and attempting calmness, his behavior is already a whole lot healthier than about 1,000 other things he could be doing, so the techniques are at least an excellent attempt at fitness. This is why I offer up a meditation tool at this point in the chapter. It's called Attunement, and I've tried it a few times myself.

> *What I consider to be meditation happens a lot on the tops of mountains and beside lakes and oceans. Calm sitting and letting the scenic view pour over you, emptying your mind, filling your soul—that counts; it undoubtedly has the same physical and psychic benefits.*

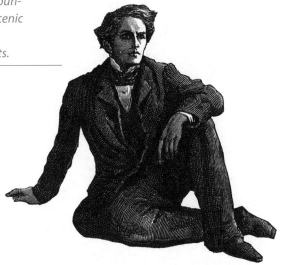

Once you've installed the app on your phone, Attunement works by giving you a choice of several songs, some of which are designed to induce calm meditating, and some of which are designed to accompany yoga. Figure 9-18 shows my choice—"Primordial," of course.

Choose the song length and off you go, into a stress-reduced universe of your own creation. Although it's no different than what you could initiate with your own iPod or other MP3 player, Meditation Oasis, the group who distributes the app, has hand-picked the music as appropriate for meditating. It has a whole site that's devoted to meditation instructions, podcasts, and other tools. It's worth a visit: *www.meditationoasis.com/how-to-meditate/simple-meditations/*.

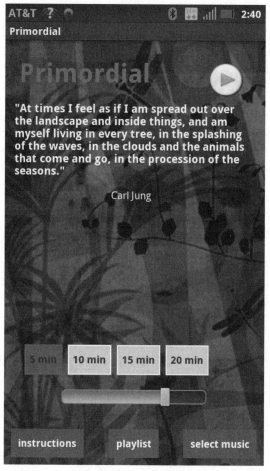

Figure 9-18. *A song on your phone corresponds to mindful meditation*

Code Maintenance:
Human Fueling and Supplements

10

You fancy yourself the human equivalent of a Formula I race car. Or at least, that metaphor reflects how much you value your health. You want your engines to operate on the finest fuel, not the leftover stuff at the bottom of the deep fryer at your cousin's big-box restaurant (although it would be noble if your car ran on that residue). If an important part of fitness is exercise, then the raw ingredients for that regimen—the food you eat before and after (even if you bow out of eating *during* the workout)—are essential as well.

The rules of thumb for eating aren't very different for people who are strenuously active and people who are mainly interested in staying out of the doctor's office but have no desire to train for climbing Kilimanjaro. Eat well; eat nutritiously—and perhaps more copiously, if your adventures burn tons of calories.

Consume real, nutrient-rich food (fruits, veggies, fish, fowl, beef, pastured eggs, nuts, whey protein/berry smoothies, etc.), not just filler that seems sinfully good at the moment but packs a big negative payback later.

This chapter presents a few general guidelines for the best ways to tweak your diet in a quest to fuel your fitness goals.

Fueling Fitness

If you're an athlete or are taking part in fitness activities for the purpose of health and maintenance, you're probably wondering if there is a better way to eat and drink to make you stronger, quicker, faster, and indefatigable.

No magic nutrition bullets exist for fueling fitness, despite the giant industry that has been assembled to sell us supplements that suggest we can be Superman or Superwoman as long as we consume their products (I did find references in the scientific literature that specify *some* supplements that may be of benefit—see the sidebar "Consider These for Supplement Experimentation").

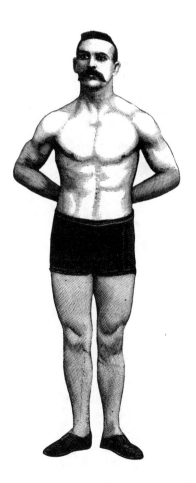

While they may be of help to some athletes, the supplements are unlikely to be a major part of your fueling process. They can give you an extra edge going into a high-intensity training session or a competition, but you can get that from something as simple as having a cup of coffee an hour before a run or a weightlifting session.

Fueling fitness for people who want to remain healthy yet add sport-specific strength is more a matter of small adjustments than radical changes in an otherwise healthy diet. Stick to the "eat for health" strategy and avoid processed foods.

> *One larger adjustment of note, however, could be moving from a high-carb diet, which has been almost universally recommended for athletes, to a Paleo diet for athletes involving a preference for fat and protein. I'll cover this issue a bit in a sidebar at the end of this chapter.*

This chapter covers some of the following aspects of sports-nutrition basics:

* Increasing your protein consumption a bit to provide the raw materials for synthesizing and repairing muscles, as well as maintaining the integrity of all of the protein components of your body that need to have enough amino acids available for their cell- and tissue-building processes.

* Increasing caloric intake in general to accommodate the extra fuel you will need for your activities—you might want to lose a few extra pounds, but you don't want to eat away your hard-earned lean body mass as your physical system reaches out for the extra gas it needs.

* Knowing the signs of dehydration, and drinking plenty of water before, often during, and after hard exercise.

* Using the "magic hour" following exercise, particularly weightlifting, to consume a high-quality protein meal such as one containing branched-chain amino acids (BCAAs) and possibly a protein/carb mixture to produce the best results for muscle growth.

* Making sure you are properly fueled with micronutrients—all the vitamins and essential minerals important for fueling physical activity. Being geeks, we'll also go into some details on these nutrients.

Fueling fitness for people who want to remain healthy yet add sport-specific strength is more a matter of small adjustments than radical changes in an otherwise healthy diet.

Maintaining a Reasonable Protein Intake

For the strength- and power-related activities such as weightlifting, body-weight workouts, and sprinting, it's essential to absorb enough grams of protein on a daily basis to keep you *net positive* for that nutrient (i.e., so you're making more protein tissues than you are breaking down for energy during the course of training).

For most people, it's easy to derive enough protein from a Western-style diet, unless you're a vegetarian or vegan. In the former case, you have to be more conscientious to aim for protein sources that don't involve meat or fish (eggs, milk, cheese, yogurt, avocados, nuts, whey protein shakes, tempeh, etc.), and for vegans, it's just plain tough to maintain an adequate intake of essential amino acids on an active lifestyle (see Chapter 3 for more dietary protein specifics). Lots of nonmeat or nondairy foods, including vegetables and grains, contain protein, just not in a high enough quantity—i.e., these meals don't have enough grams or milligrams of amino acids.

According to the article "Nutrition and Athletic Performance" from the journal *Medecine & Science in Sports & Exercise*, "Protein quality is a potential concern for individuals who avoid all animal proteins such as milk and meat (i.e., vegans). Their diets may be limited in lysine, threonine, tryptophan, or methionine."[1]

For the strength- and power-related activities such as weightlifting, bodyweight workouts, and sprinting, it's essential to absorb enough grams of protein on a daily basis to keep you net positive for that nutrient.

How Much Protein Is Enough?

Of course, a geek is going to want to know exactly how much protein she needs to take in (in grams) on a daily basis, and where it's going to come from. You probably don't have to be obsessive about exact amounts, or too concerned with erring on the high side. But you might recall our discussion in Chapter 3 about the potential negative health ramifications of taking in more than about a third of your calories in protein—that's one of the things you have to keep in mind as you plan meals over the long term.

A 2007 scientific-review article in the *Journal of Sports Science* called "Nutrition for the Sprinter" makes this sound recommendation:

> *Habitually high intakes, often greater than 2 g per kg per day, appear to be unnecessary for muscle hypertrophy and increased strength and power. It is likely that protein intake in excess of 1.7 g per kg per day is simply oxidized.*[2]

I can tell you that the upper limit the article discusses (two grams per kilogram per day) is easy to obtain if, for instance, you eat a nutritious diet that includes a big omelet (with real eggs) for breakfast and have meat, fish, potatoes or rice, and salad (with cheese) for dinner. The limit would only be 130 grams for someone my size (65 kilograms); one decent-sized filet of salmon would get you about a third of the way there.

Tools

You can use a simple web-based protein calculator, and the Web is full of them. Here's one: *www.healthcalculators.org/calculators/protein.asp*. You enter some criteria, such as your size, age, and activity level, and it spits out a number, such as 107 grams for me.

NutritionData (*www.nutritiondata.com*) is a very good tool for determining the protein content of individual foods (see Chapter 2 on tools). FitDay (*www.fitday.com*) provides you with a more comprehensive picture of how much protein is contained in an entire meal, or your food intake for the day or week. Figure 10-1, for example, shows the protein content of an omelet with tomato, broccoli, and Swiss cheese, and a kiwi on the side. That chow contained about 29 grams of protein.

Food Log	Total Nutrition	Custom Nutrition Goals					
NAME	**AMOUNT**	**UNIT**	**CALS**	**FAT(G)**	**CARBS(G)**	**PROT(G)**	
Tomatoes, raw	3	medium slice (1/4	11	0	2	1	
Broccoli, cooked	4	floweret	22	1	3	1	
Kiwi fruit, raw	1	fruit	46	0	11	1	
Butter	1	pat	36	4	0	0	
Cheese, Swiss	2	cracker-size slice	53	4	1	4	
Egg, whole, cooked	2	medium	147	11	1	11	
egg beater	2	serving	60	0	2	12	
		Totals	375	20.3	20.2	28.9	

Figure 10-1. *Figuring out your protein with FitDay*

Make Sure the Tank Is Full

It might seem counter to the prevailing wisdom to recommend taking in more calories. If your goal, however, is to put on additional muscle and prevent the degradation of your lean mass, you'll probably have to ingest more calories than you were prior to beginning your training program. The journal article "Nutrition for the Sprinter" points out that:

> As early as 1907, Chittenden demonstrated that as long as energy intake is sufficient, athletes will gain muscle mass and increase strength even during periods of low protein intake. More recently, positive energy balance has been demonstrated to be more important than the amount of protein ingested for gains in lean body mass during resistance training.[3]

By "positive energy balance," the journal quote means taking in more calories than you expend. Go to FitDay or use your Fitbit dashboard, for example, to determine if you're in a positive or negative calorie balance (Fitbit is covered in Chapter 2).

If your total energy expenditure exceeds the calories you consume, you won't be able to add lean mass (the exception being when you are making big gains at the very beginning of a new exercise regimen by losing that extra fat you've been carrying around, while adding a bit of muscle).

This balancing act might be a little more nuanced than you think, because you don't want to add food to your plate and end up putting on a lot of extra fat. Rather than viewing this strategy as a license to eat, drink, and be merry, you might want to analyze the number of calories you are *burning* with the extra exercise. For this analysis, you can use Endomondo, the Fitbit Tracker, or any of the other tools we discuss in Chapter 2 and throughout the book.

Basal Metabolic Rate and Activity Calculator

You can also estimate the number of calories you're expending using a formula called the Harris-Benedict equation (*http://en.wikipedia.org/wiki/Harris-Benedict_equation*). The first part of the equation estimates your basal metabolic rate (BMR), or the amount of calories you expend in a day just keeping your internal organs and overall system functioning, but not including the energy costs of exercise or general movement.

The key: w = weight in kilograms; h = height in centimeters; a = age in years.

For men: (13.75 x w) + (5.003 x h) - (6.7775 x a) + 66.5

For women: (9.563 x w) + (1.85 x h) - (4.676 x a) + 655.1

Next, take the total of your BMR and multiply it by the appropriate "activity variable" in Table 10-1 (e.g., 1.9 for extremely active).

Table 10-1. Activity variables for determining calorie requirements

Activity variable	Activity level	Description
1.2	Sedentary	Little or no exercise and desk job
1.375	Lightly active	Light exercise or sports 1–3 days a week
1.55	Moderately active	Moderate exercise or sports 3–5 days a week
1.725	Very active	Hard exercise or sports 6–7 days a week
1.9	Extremely active	Hard daily exercise or sports and physical job

Let's say you get a BMR of 1,668 (for a 5' 9" 35-year-old male who weighs 70 kilograms, or 154 pounds). You are very active, so your total calorie expenditure comes to an estimated total of about 2,877 calories.

Add a few hundred *high-quality calories* (e.g., lean meats, energy-packed veggies) per day above that amount, boosting it to 3,077, or about 3,000 calories. This is the amount of calories you will need to consume per day if you're working out very hard with resistance training, and want to add some extra pounds of muscle. Make sure to drink plenty of water as well.

If the estimated figure seems low (as it does to me), experiment. If you cannot add any weight after a few weeks, add another hundred good calories per day. And make sure you are eating well in the hour following training, as we'll discuss later in the chapter.

The *timing* of when you take in these extra calories is important, as the article "Nutrition for the Sprinter" points out:

> *Training adaptations may depend less on the amount of protein ingested, and more on the type of proteins ingested, timing of ingestion, and other nutrients ingested in the same meal.*[4]

For example, eating within an hour after training will improve the likelihood of building lean mass for someone like a sprinter or team-sports person who desires to add strength and muscle.

Pre-Exercise Eating

In terms of timing, however, consuming *carbs* before, for instance, a typical gym workout actually inhibits your ability to burn fats during the exercise. Again, from "Nutrition for the Sprinter":

> *Carbohydrate ingestion has a very strong inhibiting effect on fat oxidation. The ingestion of 50–100 grams [or 200 to 400 calories' worth] of carbohydrate in the hour before exercise will inhibit lipolysis and will also reduce fat oxidation [during the exercise] by about 30–40%.*[5]

Lipolysis means the release of triglycerides from your fat stores so that they can be broken down into free fatty acids (FFAs) and used as muscle fuel. Eating carbs before exercising restricts this mechanism. However, endurance athletes who are entering a fast-paced workout have to make sure that their glycogen stores are topped up, so they have a different priority *vis à vis* the carb meals. See the sidebar titled "A Paleo Diet for Athletes" for a related discussion.

All Protein Is Not Created Equal

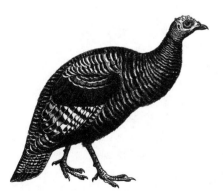

As Chapter 3 discusses, proteins are made up of chains of amino acids. A subset of these amino acids, the branched-chain amino acids (BCAAs), are growth-promoting and therefore of particular interest among certain kinds of athletes.

The BCAAs, a subset of the *essential amino acids* (see Chapter 3), are leucine, isoleucine, and valine. The amino acids arginine and glutamine, along with leucine, also play a role in stimulating the growth pathway in the body, mTOR. (see the sidebar titled "The mTOR Pathway Is Our Growth Machine").

A recently published study review from the journal *Nutrition & Metabolism* underlines the efficacy of whey protein, which contains the three BCAAs, as a muscle-building and -sparing supplement. The amino acid leucine, which whey contains, seems to be a key constituent for building muscle, according to the review:

> *Leucine, acting as a signaling molecule in the mTOR cascade…, has been shown to be a critical amino acid for increasing skeletal muscle protein synthesis. [...] Leucine may also be involved in suppressing muscle protein degradation.*[6]

Leucine is present in adequate amounts in most of the typical sources of protein you will be eating. The following sources have more than three grams of that amino acid (per 200-calorie serving): eggs, fish (many varieties), chicken, turkey, various game meats such as elk or buffalo, dried seaweed (spirulina), pork, shrimp, duck, etc. See the whole list here: *http://bit.ly/ nutritiondataleucine*.

A whey protein shake with a typical serving (for example, the one I use in smoothies) provides the following amounts of the BCAAs: leucine (2.9 grams), isoleucine (1.6 grams), and valine (1.7 grams).

THE MTOR PATHWAY IS OUR GROWTH MACHINE

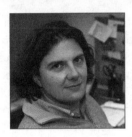

If you frequent any of the muscle-building sites on the Web, looking to pick up some tips, you're going to encounter a lot of articles and references to mTOR. This is a pathway in the human body whose name stands for *mammalian target of rapamycin*. A pathway is a built-in sequence of chemical reactions.

People who want to add lean mass are not only trying to impress their friends with geeky biological acronyms, but they want to stimulate mTOR, which is responsible for anabolism, or cell growth in the body.

I talked with Professor David Sabatini, whose lab studies mTOR at the Whitehead Institute in Cambridge, MA. He's an Associate Professor of Biology at the Massachusetts Institute of Technology (MIT), among many other things.

Why is mTOR important to someone who is trying to build lean mass?

mTOR is a central pathway for anabolism—the regulator in the balance between making or breaking stuff down. It controls if you're in a catabolic or anabolic state. The pathway is on if you have [the presence of] nutrients and growth factors like insulin and IGF.

How do you turn on mTOR?

What's most interesting from a scientific standpoint is that mTOR senses everything; it has antennae out there that detect pretty much anything you can think of. The key nutrients mTOR senses are glucose and amino acids (AA)—leucine is a very important AA [for turning on mTOR]. The other amino acids mTOR cares about are glutamine and arginine.

Where is mTOR centered in the body?

mTOR exists everywhere in the body; that's the simple answer. From a functional point of view, tissues like your muscle, fat, and liver have mTOR and are kind of on the receiving end. When they receive signals that say, "Hey, we're in an anabolic state," then they build mass: muscle will build muscle protein, the liver will build glycogen and protein, fat cells will build fat—there are many tissues that have what I would call the receiving mTOR, waiting for signals to build stuff.

Then there is the MTOR that's in more specialized master-controller tissues, like the hypothalamus and pancreatic beta cells where the role more is to sense that you're in the anabolic state. To tell tissues to grow.

THE MTOR PATHWAY IS OUR GROWTH MACHINE (continued)

So we think always of mTOR as upstream and downstream of itself; it does the sensing of the appropriate state, then it does the work of turning on the machinery to make growth happen. You don't think of your hypothalamus as growing, but mTOR is there saying, "Hey, there's amino acids around [so] let's send signals to tell other big tissues to grow."

So you can turn on mTOR with resistance training?

You can do resistance training and that will turn on mTOR, but it's almost like a computational AND gate. You need the resistance training, but if you don't have the nutrients, nothing's going to happen, because the system is smart. You can't make mass without nutrients or energy. Whether the input is IGF, weight lifting, AMP kinase inhibitor—if you don't have the raw ingredients, the system is built to turn things off.

I've read about, and experienced, good results with fasting and weightlifting. How does this fit in with mTOR and the required nutrients?

Our bodies have strong homeostatic mechanisms. We certainly have plenty of nutrients flowing through our blood, but once your body can no longer keep a homeostatic nutrient level, it's going to be much harder to let growth happen.

[Editorial note: that's why it's important to eat *after* fasting and training.]

David Sabatini's faculty bio page is at *www.wi.mit.edu/research/faculty/sabatini.html*.

Carbs and Protein: Both in the Mix

In terms of eating after exercise to maintain and add lean mass, it seems both protein and carbs play important roles.

"Carbohydrates and proteins may be the best strategy for [the] stimulation of anabolic pathways," according to "Nutrition for the Sprinter." The "utilization of ingested amino acids for [the] synthesis of muscle proteins is greatest when carbohydrates are ingested concurrently with an amino acid source…. The effect of carbohydrates is presumably due to the associated insulin release. Insulin increases net muscle protein balance following resistance exercise primarily by blocking the rise in muscle protein breakdown."[7] So, add some berries and/or banana to your whey protein shake just after working out, or a pile or rice or sweet potato with your fish or steak.

WHERE DID YOU GET ALL THAT ENERGY?

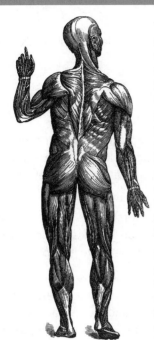

The human body is a smart system that has evolved to offer a number of different energy sources throughout the body to fuel activities of varying intensities. The fuel sources range from creatine phosphate (CP) in muscle cells, to the stored glycogen in the liver and skeletal muscles, to stored fat in muscles and adipose tissue. Different types of exercise rely on these energy sources in varying ways.

CP is an anaerobic energy source in the muscles (meaning it does not require oxygen). It fuels very short duration, high-intensity contractions—such as up to 10 seconds. "The amount of creatine phosphate available in skeletal muscle is approximately four times greater than ATP and, therefore, [CP] is the primary fuel used for high-intensity, short-duration activities such as the clean and jerk in weight lifting or the fast break in basketball."[8]

This mechanism is called the *phosphagen system*.

Glycolysis is a mechanism that the body relies on to fuel longer events, such as a 400-meter sprint. Glycolytic fuel derives from glycogen, as well as any glucose that the body has made available in the bloodstream. Recall that the liver and muscles store relatively small amounts of glycogen—roughly 1,200 or more calories' worth—in the form of animal starch. From the journal article "Nutrition and Athletic Performance":

Approximately 25%–35% of total muscle glycogen stores are used during a single 30-s sprint or resistance exercise bout. Neither the phosphagen nor the glycolytic pathway can sustain the rapid provision of energy to allow muscles to contract at a very high rate for events lasting greater than 2–3 min.[9]

What about all those longer endurance events? The body uses the aerobic, or oxidative, pathway to fuel hours-long exercise—glycogen, fats, and to a lesser extent amino acids (including from the carbs, fats, and protein you consume during the event). "As oxygen becomes more available to the working muscle, the body uses more of the aerobic (oxidative) pathways and less of the anaerobic (phosphagen and glycolytic) pathways."[10]

At "70 percent of maximal oxygen capacity," about 50 to 60 percent of energy comes from carbs, and most of the rest from fats.[11] When exercise intensity drops, you start utilizing more fats for energy, which makes sense, considering that you have so much more available and stored in the body compared with glycogen. In fact, the amount of calories stored as triglycerides in the muscles, not even counting all the other fat depots in the body, *exceeds the storage capacity of glycogen*.

"As a result of aerobic training, the energy derived from fat increases and from carbohydrates decreases. A trained individual uses a greater percentage of fat than an untrained person does at the same workload. Long-chain fatty aids derived from stored muscle triglycerides are the preferred fuel for aerobic exercise for individuals involved in mild- to moderate-intensity exercise."[12] So as you're walking or hiking, for instance, the preferred fuel is fat, just as it is at rest.

These facts suggest that you should replenish your glycogen levels with carbs before short, intense events, and don't shrink from fats as a major source of fuel for long, slow efforts.

Water and Hydration

Remaining properly hydrated when you exercise is important and, most of the time, easy to do. Use common sense and listen to your body. The hydration requirements for weightlifting at room temperature for up to 40 minutes are not that great; drink enough water beforehand so you're not going into the training session thirsty. The requirements for running in a

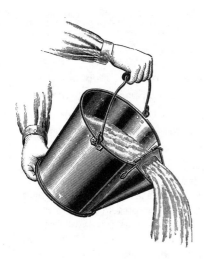

hot road race or summer triathlon are a different ballgame—you have to be well hydrated before the event and have a plan for adequate hydration during the race.

The consequences of dehydration can be very bad, particularly if it's a hot, humid event promoting a lot of sweat loss.

Sweat loss can vary among individuals and weather conditions, from 0.3 to 2.4 liters per hour!

First it's muscle cramps, and you're basically reduced to walking out the course. The cramps probably reflect the significant loss of potassium and sodium in sweat. You can replenish both minerals with a decent electrolyte sports drink such as Accelerade or Heed.

Heat stroke can follow the cramping, in the worse-case scenario, if you haven't properly responded to the dehydration and you're trying to push through the heat. Heat stroke involves a body temperature in excess of 104, and it can be fatal.

I've heard of more cases of *hyponatremia* lately. This malady besetting some marathoners involves drinking *too much* before and during an event (or simply excessive salt loss through sweating), to the level of diluting the salt in your body (a serum sodium concentration of less than 130 mmol·L).[13] It can also be fatal. So, the bottom line is to properly hydrate if you're going to do long, challenging events and, in general, monitor your hydration levels while exercising.

Guidelines

There isn't any more suave way to put it: you can find out how well hydrated you are by observing the color of your pee. If it's clear, you are well hydrated. If it's dark yellow, drink up. Make sure it's clear before any event you are doing, like a weekend bike ride or road race.

The best thing to do is to practice your hydration strategy for weeks in training if you're going to enter something challenging. The article "Nutrition and Athletic Performance" contains other hydration reminders:

The goal of drinking is to prevent dehydration from occurring during exercise and individuals should not drink in excess of sweating rate. After exercise, drink approximately 16–24 oz. (450–675 mL.) of fluid for every pound (0.5 kg) of body weight lost during exercise.[14]

Another guideline is to drink water and/or sports drinks up to four hours before an event. "At least 4 hours before exercise, individuals should drink approximately 5–7 milliliters (mL) per kilogram (kg) body weight (2–3 mL per pound) of water or a sport beverage."[15] This means if a person weighs 140 pounds, she should drink about 14 ounces; or, if she weighs 60 kilograms, she should sip up to half a liter four hours before the event.

These levels seem a bit low to me, especially four hours before an event. Heat, nervousness, and the warm-up can dehydrate you prior to an event or big exercise bout. Hours before you start, monitor your pee color and respond to your body's thirst reflex, and drink accordingly.

This protocol is more difficult to meet if the event starts at seven in the morning (unless you're tossing and turning). You could make sure your pee was clear before you went to bed.

PRE-EVENT JITTERS AND COFFEE: IT'S ALL IN YOUR HEAD

So much of health and physical preparation is psychic and spiritual. *Belief* is very powerful; never underestimate it. It's actually reassuring to know that there are elements of your body and mind that no scientist may ever put his finger on, and thus reduce them to a pill, for instance. I have one funny story that in its own small way illustrates this notion.

I was signed up for a triathlon once in Vermont, and I had a small motel room facing the woods. I kept the window open all night because the room was stifling. The motel had a swamp or wetlands behind it, and all night it emitted an incessant cacophony of frog croaks. I don't remember falling asleep at all. I finally rolled out of bed in the morning, somewhat in a panic (I used to really obsess over pre-event sleeps; now I don't, knowing I'll focus on a good sleep afterward).

"At least I've got strong coffee with me!" I thought. I made a big pot of strong dark roast, and started quaffing it down. I had a banana, a bagel with peanut butter, and a Powerbar. Feeling the caffeine kick in, I headed off to do all the little things you have to do before a triathlon starts. I ended up having a great swim-bike-run for me, feeling strong throughout, and shattered my course record.

I headed back to my motel afterward to pack my stuff, my little finisher's medal dangling around my neck, and happened to pick up the bag of coffee I'd used that morning. It was decaf! My brain had actually tricked me into thinking that I was stoked on strong coffee, and that phenomenon had suitably prepared me for the two-hour-plus event.

Cold and Altitude Also Affect Hydration

Just because it's not hot doesn't mean you don't have to hydrate. People often get dehydrated in cold environments because the tendency to drink falls off. You spend so much time preoccupied with staying warm that you don't bother to guzzle water or tea. Use the pee test in these environments as well.

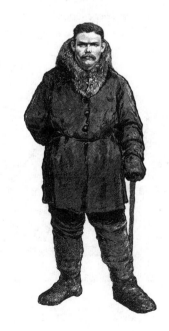

You pee more at altitude (sorry for all the pee references—this increased urination at altitude is called *diuresis*), so you have to be conscientious about hydrating during hikes and climbs, especially above 8,000 feet, or 2,438 meters, of elevation. According to "Nutrition and Athletic Performance":

Respiratory water losses may be as high as 1900 milliliters (mL) [per] day (1.9 L [per] day) in men and 850 mL [per] day (0.85 L [per] day) in women. Total fluid intake at high altitude approaches 3–4 liters (L) [per] day to promote optimal kidney function and maintain urine output of ~1.4 L in adults.[16]

You begin to lose your appetite at altitude as well, which can mean fewer opportunities to reach for the fluids, as you're not gobbling food.

Proper hydration is absolutely key to staving off Acute Mountain Sickness (AMS), which will definitely ruin your summit attempt.

A FEW SUPPLEMENTS FOR ATHLETES TO CONSIDER

Carnosine may be a useful supplement for sprinters and other fast-running athletes (e.g., soccer players), according to the *Medicine & Science in Sports & Exercise* article "Nutrition for the Sprinter."

Carnosine is a protein involving the amino acids alanine and histidine. "Carnosine is found primarily in type IIa and type IIx fibers in skeletal muscle."[17] It is not difficult, however, to locate a supplement company that will be happy to sell you carnosine products, so try to be sensible and selective in your considerations (it's not to be confused with creatine, another supplement).

Carnosine is a primary substance the body uses for buffering, which means compensating for the rising acidity levels in muscles and blood when you're exercising strenuously. The increase in lactic acid is what causes the "exercise burn" at the end of a sprint or a tough series of weightlifting reps, for instance. Sodium bicarbonate is also a buffering agent.

Carnosine may show some promise in other health areas, according to this article and its concluding references.

In theory, increasing skeletal muscle carnosine levels (via beta-alanine supplementation or intense training) should increase buffering capacity, delay fatigue, and increase exercise performance. Higher carnosine concentration in muscle was associated with higher mean power from a 30-[second] maximal sprint on a cycle ergometer.[18]

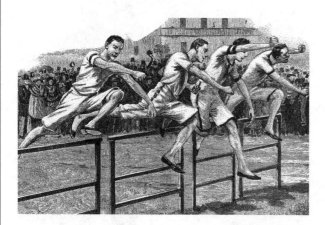

Caffeine, such as that found in a strong cup of coffee or tea, is a suitable supplement before a sprint, a weightlifting session, or even a longer event. Caffeine mobilizes free fatty acids and acts as a central nervous system stimulant.[19]

Sodium bicarbonate, or baking soda, is also a well-documented supplement for sprinters (e.g., track and field, cycling, rowing), but you should only experiment with it in small doses because it can cause gastrointenstinal distress such as diarrhea:

Reviews of the available literature suggest a dose–response relationship between the amount of bicarbonate ingested and the observed performance effect (Horswill, 1995). A dose of 200 milligram (mg) per kilogram (kg) body mass ingested 1–2 hours before exercise seems to improve performance in most studies, but 300 mg per kg body mass appears to be the optimum dose (with tolerable side-effects for most athletes). Doses of less than 100 mg per kg body mass do not affect performance.

Intakes of more than 300 mg per kg body mass tend to result in gastrointestinal problems. Most of these studies, however, used exercise lasting longer than 1 min and in most the exercise intensity and duration were comparable to middle-distance running not sprints.

No studies have shown an effect on performance in high-intensity exercise lasting less than 1 min. Therefore, a window for efficacy of bicarbonate has been identified between approximately 1 and 7 min and sprint events are not likely to be affected. Nevertheless, the use of bicarbonate is common in 400-m running, with anecdotal support for its efficacy.[20]

Creatine is manufactured in the human body out of amino acids, and most of it is found in skeletal muscle.[21] Creatine increases energy or ATP for the muscles, which has obviously sparked interest in its use as an energy-boosting supplement.

A FEW SUPPLEMENTS FOR ATHLETES TO CONSIDER (continued)

Whereas the creatine studies do not show sprinters running faster[22], it could help them gain lean mass and power, and certainly the latter benefit would be of interest to resistance trainers:

> …It is important to emphasize that results from well-controlled laboratory studies consistently indicate that creatine supplementation can enhance power output during short maximal exercise…, in particular during intermittent series (10–30 s) of maximal muscle contractions… interspersed by 1–2 min rest intervals[…]

Heavy resistance training accounts for an important fraction of the total training volume in elite sprinters. It has been well documented that creatine supplementation can potentiate the gains in fat-free mass and muscle force and power output that accompany resistance training…. Thus, creatine supplementation conceivably could contribute to improving sprint performance by enhancing the efficacy of resistance training.[23]

Micronutrient Replenishment

Vitamins and minerals are obviously of paramount importance. An athlete who's training harder needs more food, and thus increased amounts of vitamins and minerals, to make up for greater "metabolic turnover"—i.e., using up the micronutrients at a higher rate than average, because she is generating more energy and ramping up her metabolism.

The bulk of this extra nutrition can come from all those nutritious extra foods you are eating. A multivitamin/mineral (MVM) supplement or individual supplements (e.g., vitamin D3 or magnesium) might be necessary, however, if your training load is particularly high or you are a vegetarian/vegan, if you're not consuming enough fat and thus fat-soluble vitamins (A, D, E, and K).

RDA Levels May Not Be Enough

The Recommended Dietary Allowances (RDAs) for these vitamins and minerals are really minimum levels for the average person. If you have a very high activity rate, you may focus on getting higher levels than the RDAs for micronutrients. According to "Nutrition and Athletic Performance": "The most common vitamins and minerals found to be of concern in athletes' diets are calcium and vitamin D, the B vitamins; iron, zinc, magnesium, as well as some antioxidants such as vitamins C and E, β-carotene, and selenium."[24] In other words, with increased levels of exercising come the risks of deficiencies in most of the major micronutrients.

If you're exercising moderately most days and have been conscientious about taking in larger amounts of nutritious foods (a big *if*), *and* if you don't have a nagging fatigue or difficulty healing from injuries, you're probably getting adequate vitamins and minerals.

Here are some highlights of how important vitamins are for the training/ competing athlete, as well as for anyone who has ramped up their exercise levels significantly:

- "The B-complex vitamins have two major functions directly related to exercise. Thiamin, riboflavin, niacin, pyridoxine (B6), pantothenic acid, and biotin are involved in energy production during exercise…whereas folate and vitamin B12 are required for the production of red blood cells, for protein synthesis, and in tissue repair and maintenance including the CNS [central nervous system]."[25]

- We wrote a lot about vitamin D in Chapter 4; it may be advantageous for athletes to supplement vitamin D at greater than the RDA level.

- "Athletes at [the] greatest risk for poor antioxidant intakes are those following a low-fat diet, restricting energy intakes, or limiting dietary intakes of fruits, vegetables, and whole grains."[26] This means that you have to make sure to get enough vitamin C and E, and the mineral selenium. See Chapter 4 for more information on antioxidants.

- "The high incidence of iron depletion among athletes is usually attributed to inadequate energy intake. Other factors that can impact iron status include vegetarian diets that have poor iron availability, periods of rapid growth, training at high altitudes, increased iron losses in sweat, feces, urine, menstrual blood, intravascular hemolysis, foot-strike hemolysis, regular blood donation, or injury…. Athletes, especially women, long-distance runners, adolescents, and vegetarians should be screened periodically to assess and monitor iron status…. Because reversing iron-deficiency anemia can require 3–6 months, it is advantageous to begin nutrition intervention before iron deficiency anemia develops."[27]

A PALEO DIET FOR ATHLETES

Some active people are experimenting with a so-called Paleolithic, or Paleo, diet for fueling sports, feeling that the answer doesn't always lie in the prototypical high-carbohydrate diet for athletes. The adaptation to the diet may be difficult at first, as there is little to no carbo-loading—the spaghetti, pizza, and bread that have been a part of so many preparations for marathons and triathlons.

Paleo certainly doesn't mean that you give up salads or potatoes, by the way; it simply means that you move to a lower percentage of carbs in your dietary ratio—a change that may be metabolically healthier.

Athletes who adopt a higher-fat diet experience some beneficial adaptations: they increase the oxidation or usage of fats while exercising, and become more efficient at burning the fats that the muscles store for energy. [28]

High-carb diets appear to still be necessary for endurance athletes who are competing at long distances and cruising along at very high rates, such as triathletes, middle-distance runners, and cyclists doing time trials. Combining a high-fat diet with a two- to three-day carbo-loading period (to top off the glycogen) appears to have some promise. [29]

Another study discussed the notion of taking more energy-dense foods such as fats on ultra-endurance events where athletes are largely responsible for providing all of their food. [30] High-fat diets like a Paleo approach might be optimal for these ultra distances, where the athlete motors along at a slow but persistent rate.

There is at least one book devoted to this topic that you might want to check out, called *The Paleo Diet for Athletes*. [31]

The athletes who go Paleo often point to feeling less sore post-exercise and the day after hard efforts, after removing the bulk of the grains from their diet. It provides plenty of energy too, but more from fats and protein than from the extra carbs.

The personal evidence is empirical, but hey, I have a lengthy experience with both approaches, so I might as well throw in my own two cents. I used to eat a lot of spaghetti, rice, salad, and meat before my long races, and most of the time I got good race results. For various reasons, such as less inflammation and the probability that we are not evolved for a heavy-carb diet, I now lean toward an approach that involves the consumption of a more moderate amount of these macronutrients.

Back in the day, I found a really good carb-rich sports drink that worked well to sustain energy levels during a two-hour+ event (it will go unnamed as I'm not interested in using a brand-name beverage as a whipping boy), but unfortunately it also ended up giving me the only cavity I've gotten since childhood, due to its sugar content and how much I was taking in.)

Jump ahead to a long, difficult mountain climb I did in my fifties, similar to an ultra-endurance event. Slow, with lots of pauses. Suffice it to say, the effort required thousands of calories per day; especially the last day, which was cold, at altitude, and lasted the better part of 17 hours. I did bring carbs along in the form of energy bars, but far better than half of my calories were fat and protein (nuts, high-cacao chocolate, and chunks of my favorite raw cheddar).

While that's not orthodox Paleo, because it includes dairy, it is more of a high-fat and -protein approach, and the mountaineer's mess tent cooked up plenty of protein and fat too, like cheesy eggs and bacon, as well as avocado and tomato burritos.

The feeding strategy worked very well; I climbed well and never had altitude or energy problems. I consumed very little simple sugars. My preparations were rushed and, as a result, I'd probably do it differently next time, bringing a greater variety of snack foods for climbing.

In a nutshell, a Paleo diet for athletes involves eating more meat, fish, plenty of veggies and fruit, nuts such as almonds and macadamias, pastured eggs, coconut milk/whey protein shakes for a good protein/healthy fat supplement—a macronutrient ratio that generally emphasizes fat (no trans fat and ease up on the Omega 6s) and protein over carbs. Tubers and starchy vegetables such as sweet potatoes and plantains are also a part of Paleo mealtimes. It's becoming easier for Paleo athletes to find foods these days as the diet eases into the mainstream, such as Paleo energy-bar recipes.

Lifestyle Hacks for Fitness 11

Little things matter when it comes to fitness, particularly when multiplied over a lifetime. That's why I don't think it's superficial to consider various "hacks" or health-related habits and borderline-kooky angles (e.g., diving into freezing water) that do not necessarily fall under the rubric of the "fitness big three" of nutrition, proper exercise, and sleep/stress management. I know of a Brooklyn, New York man, a famous Coney Island strongman, who was known to take frequent, not just annual, winter swims. He swore by the health benefits of cold-water immersion; he lived to be 105, and the only reason he didn't live longer was that he was struck by a minivan a few years ago while taking a five-mile walk in the city. It appeared that but for this tragic accident, he was well on his way to being perhaps the oldest, strongest-for-his-age American male in history. It doesn't seem a stretch to view his cold-water swims as one healthy component of this extraordinary example of a long "health-span."

This chapter discusses other little hacks, such as the concept of *hormesis*, or good stress, sports massage, and the aforementioned cold-water immersion, that can make a difference in the pursuit of fitness.

Hormesis

What doesn't kill you makes you stronger, or so goes a saying. Ernest Hemingway wrote a memorable line in *A Farewell to Arms*: "The world breaks everyone and afterward many are strong at the broken places."

Scientists actually have a word for a stimulus or good stress that has an adaptive effect on the body—hormesis. The word is derived from the Greek *hórmēsis*, meaning "rapid motion, eagerness" (even though that definition does not seem to fit with our discussion here—see *http://en.wikipedia.org/wiki/Hormesis*). A number of activities, some widely familiar and some not, fall under hormesis, and they've been the subject of numerous laboratory studies and published hypotheses. Here's how a scientific journal article called "Dose Response" described the hormetic phenomenon:

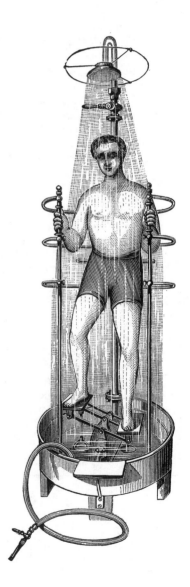

Low doses of otherwise harmful agents are beneficial at threshold low levels. The beneficial hormetic response involves the adaptive stress response to the low dose toxic challenge as multiple conserved protective enzymatic and signaling systems are activated by stress…. These fundamental survival pathways, when activated, confer plasticity [or better fitness and adaptability to changes in the environment] to species longevity.[1]

USING ANTI-PATTERNS FOR FITNESS

Anti-patterns are a concept that is popular in the programming or geek world. The idea is that you learn efficient methods of designing code by studying lousy code. It really makes sense, when you think about it. You don't know what good code is until you've seen bad code, which, unfortunately, many of us in the software world have encountered many times. For example, a basic anti-pattern in the object-oriented programming world of Java and C Sharp is a piece of code that does something complicated, but only uses three or fewer classes (units of code), thus failing to adhere to the basics of object-oriented design by separating the program's various responsibilities into a cluster of uncoupled, logical classes. The classic unreadable blob of "spaghetti code" is another typical anti-pattern.

Chapter 1 actually begins with an anti-pattern for fitness—sitting all day in the dark, hardly ever moving, and living off of vending machines. That's kind of an obvious anti-pattern for living, and one we Westerners at least have been advised to avoid since the get-go (unfortunately, the advice hasn't affected our behavior very much; we still "cheat" too much). Anti-patterns, however, can represent small subtleties and nuances. For example, here's a "do's and don't's" site for Java programmers: *http://javaantipatterns.wordpress. com.*

One example is if you have a method in your program that returns an array or Java `List` object (a collection of things like numbers, as in `[1,2,3,4,5]`, an array of numbers), never return `null` from the method; always just return an empty `List` or array (one of the ideas being that you could cause the caller of that method to crash by trying to invoke a method on the returned null object, which raises an exception in Java).

Fitness abounds with potential anti-patterns, or wrong ways of doing things, and examining them can be instructive. A classic anti-pattern is overtraining, and what immediately comes to mind is an anecdote from the excellent book by Dr. Doug McGuff called *Body by Science*. In this book, he discusses training some hockey players during the preseason. The young players gained several pounds of muscle weight, or lean mass, and had excellent body composition after leaving his gym. They then entered traditional hockey training at the rink, and their coaches overtrained them, apparently to a high degree. The end result was that even though they were working much harder at the rink, they had actually lost the hard-earned new muscle and had poorer body composition.

Whether or not you think they are useful, the popular sleep-analysis devices like Zeo are fertile sources for anti-patterns for presleep nutrition and behavior. Just eat at the wrong time and drink too much wine or caffeine before sleep, and view the literal sleep patterns that the device produces, showing the poor-quality REM sleep and disrupted patterns. The data represents an anti-pattern we can study to determine better ways to eat or drink to produce higher-quality sleeps.

Another anti-pattern that comes to mind is taking a single-dose megavitamin. You might have a good reason to take a large dose of vitamin C, for example, but the dose is better absorbed if the supplement is taken throughout the day in smaller units (of, say, 200 mg) than in one massive hit. Another fitness anti-pattern is doing the exact same workout all the time. A lot of people do that; we're creatures of habit. You're likely to plateau fairly quickly, however, in terms of strength or cardiovascular fitness, unless you vary your routine.

Translation: our bodies have built-in metabolic pathways that are "switched on" by various environmental stresses (cold, heat, exercise, etc.). Good things happen physically as a result of the activation of these signaling pathways, such as a potential for improved immunity against diseases, the upregulation of machinery for repairing damaged DNA and proteins (a damage that can lead to cancer), and improved antioxidant defenses.

A vaccine is an example of hormesis, in that we inject ourselves with a weakened pathogen, and this action "tricks" the body or educates the immune system to defend itself against that germ. This is a disease-prevention measure, however, and not really a fitness tweak.

The dose matters, however. And that makes sense. Low doses of nutritious substances can be hazardous at high doses, even in regard to drinking water (*hyponatremia*, the dilution of your body's salt content, can be caused by excessive hydration). With hormesis, a concept you should keep in mind while rebooting your lifestyle is that discrete small doses of the following foods or activities can have beneficial effects over the long run:

- Cold and heat stress, such as through cold showers or saunas, and particularly the combination of the two.

- High-intensity exercise—we'll discuss "exercise stress" later in this chapter.

- Caloric restriction and fasting, discussed at length in Chapter 6.

- Assorted other things, such as having one drink at night (without driving, of course), consuming substances such as curcumin or turmeric, and other activities that I cannot prove but suspect may have a hormetic effect, such as wilderness treks that involve potential (but seldom realized) hazards that temporarily scare the crap out of you, in a good way. I explain this theory in more detail later in this chapter.

Cold and Heat Stress

Experiments have shown that cold and heat stress increase cellular defenses against these conditions, and various published hypotheses have pointed to cold-water exposure as a potential treatment for depression,[2] as well as a possible boost for the immune system.[3] So, for practical purposes, what is heat and cold stress?

An example of heat stress is a sauna. The combination of a sauna and a cold shower is popular in countries such as Finland, and a number of northern European cultures and others throughout the world have adopted variations of these practices. A sauna that is not too hot, and where you sit or lie for a reasonable amount of time, provides enough heat stress to possibly have a hormetic effect.

Our bodies have built-in metabolic pathways that are "switched on" by various environmental stresses (cold, heat, exercise, etc.).

A rule of thumb in saunas, for adults, is that if your hair becomes hot to the touch, you've been in there long enough. Very hot dry air can be bad for the lungs. As a result, many saunas include some water to splash over the hot coals or rocks, thus moistening the air. Children should not spend much longer than a minute in a sauna; in my experience, they're usually smart and instinctive enough to leave a sauna right away anyway. A typical heated-up sauna can be 130 degrees Fahrenheit (F) or thereabouts. Combine a sauna with a cold shower or pool.

Heat stress such as running a marathon in 90+ degrees F is not a good example of hormesis—the heat-stress dosage is way too high and can damage the body, or even kill you with heat stroke (or hyponatremia, if you guzzle too much water).

An example of cold stress is a cool shower or the classic polar plunge in 40- to 68-degree F water for a short period of time (particularly at those freezing temperatures).

One study found that cold-water immersion elevated several immune-system factors by small but significant margins, but only after six weeks of pretty regular immersions at 57 degrees F, 14 Celsius (C).[4] The study also found that the cold-water swimming, predictably, increased the subjects' metabolic rate.

When you shiver in the cold, this is the body's natural reaction to generate its own heat with automatic muscle contractions in order to keep your body temperature warm and stable. Non-shivering thermogenesis can also occur in the cold. The net effect is that you burn more calories via thermogenesis, particularly if you are outside in the cold most of the day, as in the case of outdoor workers, ski patrollers, or just someone winter hiking or Nordic or alpine skiing.

Another study, titled "Improved Antioxidative Protection in Winter Swimmers," suggested that winter swimming increases the body's utilization of its major antioxidant biochemical, glutathione.[5] Glutathione is a key biochemical in mopping up oxidative damage, or "bodily rust," which is at the center of aging and some diseases such as cancer.

I think we can more or less conclude that exposing yourself to a cold shower or swim once in a while is healthy, and it feels really good, once you get over the initial discomfort. See the sidebar on the mammalian dive reflex for information on what happens to us physiologically when we dive into cold water, and obviously, take care not to do anything dangerous like hurl yourself into 38-degree rapids, unless that's your job (like Bear Grylls of *Man vs. Wild* fame).

BEFORE YOU TAKE THE DIVE, CONSIDER THE MAMMALIAN DIVE REFLEX

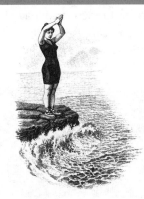

One way to take advantage of the benefits of cold-water immersion is to take the plunge in a cold river or ocean. But take some precautions first, such as making sure you can get out quickly if it's very cold, as in 55 degrees F or colder. You also probably shouldn't take a very cold water plunge if you have a preexisting heart condition.

You have only about five minutes when the water is 50 degrees F or cooler before you lose dexterity in your arms and legs, and if it's colder than 60 F, you have about 10 to 15 minutes without protective clothing.[6]

As mammals, humans have a built-in physical response, an oxygen-conserving mechanism, to diving into cold water. It's called the *mammalian dive reflex*. This is an anatomical response we share with other mammals that have a superior dive reflex to ours, such as whales and seals. At least three things happen to your body when you are submerged in water that is less than 68 degrees F, or 21 degrees C. The purpose appears to be the body's conservation of oxygen for the brain and heart, which are more sensitive to a sudden anaerobic environment than the skeletal muscles controlling your arms and legs, for instance. The three things that occur are:

- *Bradycardia*, or a slow-beating heart. Your heart rate slows by up to 25 percent, so if you have a resting heart rate of 60, it drops to 45 beats per minute. Before you panic, coffee or caffeine also slows the heart rate, while increasing blood pressure.

- *Vasoconstriction* of capillaries. Blood flow to the extremities begins to shut down in order to reserve blood and oxygen for the internal organs such as the brain and heart. First the fingers and toes go numb, then hands and feet, and gradually the arms and legs become pretty useless in extreme cold water. This vasoconstriction can also raise the blood pressure dangerously in people who have heart issues.

- A *blood shift* occurs, but only during deep dives. Blood plasma fills the lungs' alveoli, returning to normal upon the diver's reemergence at the water surface and within dry-land air pressure.[7]

In humans, the dive reflex is thought to be the reason some people have survived for extraordinary periods of time (especially children) when accidentally submerged in cold water (particularly compared with trying to hold your breath for a similar period of time on land).

Tools

The most obvious tool for swimming in cold water is a triathlon wetsuit, although this might actually be too efficient (because you don't get cold enough to enjoy the benefits of hormesis). Buying a wetsuit without the arm coverings might decrease your body temperature a little more during a cold swim, but that's a consideration only for the purpose of this chapter's discussion of cold-water benefits. Obviously, the typical function of a good wetsuit is to keep you *warmer* in most other circumstances.

> *I did a one-mile triathlon swim in New Hampshire once, when the water was 62 degrees F (and the air was 59 degrees F). My wetsuit was cut off at the shoulders, so my arms weren't covered, and I was never cold except for the first minute or so. I was also wearing a swim hat and goggles.*

I use a *pool thermometer* before I decide to jump into a cold river in the early or late spring. Figure 11-1 shows the thermometer—just dip the blue part into the water, tie it off to something like a stick or branch, and leave it in there for a minute or two. As a safety precaution, you can use the list of tips from this website on the effects of different temperatures on your ability to survive in cold water: *http://www.shipwrite.bc.ca/Chilling_truth.htm*.

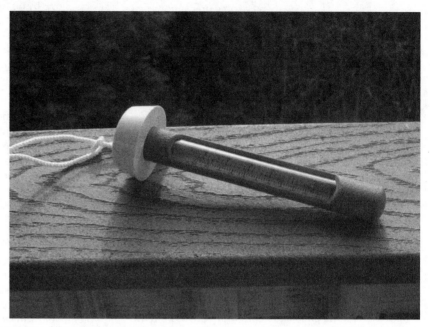

Figure 11-1. *Use a pool thermometer to test the temperature of a water body before swimming*

More tips for cold-water immersion:

- If you're doing winter or early-spring swimming, you might find a club of people with like interests. This means you have people around when you're doing a swim, especially the first time, just in case.

- Make sure your swimming spot doesn't include any other potential difficulties like tricky currents or unknown depths (this isn't the time for cliff jumping!). It should be very easy swimming so you can focus on adapting to the water temperature.

- Have a goal in mind, such as a rock a few meters away. If the water's really cold, swim in sprint form for a few strokes as you warm up in the chill environment. It also helps to swim in cold shallow water, like in a river or stream without much depth, so you can stand up whenever you want and warm up.

Chapter 11

- Have a place and clothes to get warm quickly after a cold-weather or winter swim. It's not necessarily the swim that will cause hypothermia (a potentially fatal drop in body temperature); it's the inability to get warm after emerging from the water, for the next 15 to 30 minutes. Make sure you have a towel and plenty of clothing layers for after the swim, and that shelter, your car, or the like is nearby.

- By far the easiest way to take advantage of hormesis and cold water, and one that is also effective, if less adventurous and gratifying, is a *cold shower*. The shower is more convenient than going to a swimming hole and allows you to gradually adapt to cooler temperatures. The *shower/sauna combination*, and going back and forth between the two in a single session, is the simplest way to expose yourself to cold and heat stress. Stay in the sauna until you're hot, then take a cold shower (at this point, it's less of a shock than relief), then get back into the sauna again. It feels great!

A number of websites can provide up-to-date water temperatures so you can determine whether the water is too cold or just right for a bit of hormetic swimming. This site provides maps showing the water temperature in the ocean throughout the east and west coasts of the United States: *www.nodc.noaa.gov/dsdt/cwtg/natl_tmap.html*.

Simply walking in the cold is healthy. I can't prove it or cite studies, but hey, perhaps cold-weather hiking or *Nordic walking* provides a hormetic effect. You're exposing yourself to a cold stress, but a manageable one if you've dressed appropriately (in layers, using wind-resistant materials and fibers that are designed to retain warmth, such as SmartWool). You may also burn more calories than usual, as your body seeks to keep its internal temperature stable. When you generate heat internally, but are not yet shivering, this state is called *non-shivering thermogenesis* (NST). The liberation of fats from your storage depots (lipolysis) is one of the sources of energy for NST.[8]

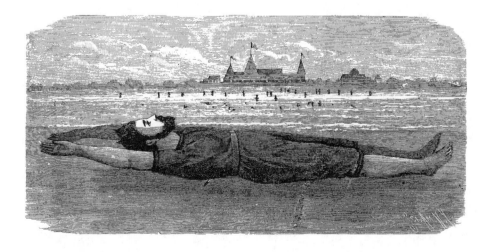

Sometimes things happen coincidentally, and at other times they have a cause-and-effect relationship. Keep your eyes open concerning what works, fitness-wise. My son recently had an upper-respiratory infection (URI), a "hack" that wouldn't go away, for weeks. Then he went skiing in Vermont for more than two weeks. He skied 14 out of 16 days. By around the beginning of the second week, the infection had gone away completely. Did the cold-weather exposure have a hormetic effect, strengthening his immune system? What gives? I thought cold, dry air was bad for the lungs. Continuous exposure to the cold and being outside, often in the sun, seems a healthy way to deal with cold-weather climates, and better than shrinking from the outdoors in artificially warmed environments all day.

Bring a pair of trekking poles on winter walks if you live in the northern climes to help deal with the snow and ice, as in Nordic walking.

Cryotherapy

Cryotherapy is a recent term for using extreme cold for medical purposes, but people have been icing their aches and pains for what seems like generations now. Beyond hormesis, cold-water immersion and swimming are very effective at reducing inflammation. The inflammation could be caused by arthritis or simply overexertion.

I have swum in the Walensee, a large lake about 70 kilometers from Zurich in Switzerland, a number of different times after hard hiking in the steep Alps. I'd be pretty banged up after the hikes, but I would always feel great, all inflammation having subsided, after these swims. I presumed the lake contained some magic mixture of minerals, when it was probably the water's cool temperatures that took care of the inflammation. Even in June through August, the lake water would often be only in the high 50s to 60s F, or 14 to 20 C.

ADAPTIVE THERMOGENESIS IN THE COLD MIGHVT AFFECT YOUR BODY-FAT LEVELS

We've discussed in this book how little things matter with fitness. For example, if you move around a lot to the tune of six miles per day compared with someone else's three (even if that doesn't equate to more formal exercise, just informal movement throughout a day), you're burning roughly 200 more calories per day than that person. That's 73,000 calories in a year, or about 21 pounds of stored calories, or fat.

A 2010 study in the *Obesity* journal found that the way people responded to a cold environment tended to differ depending on whether they were overweight or not (*www.nature.com/oby/journal/v18/n6/full/oby201074a.html*).

In the study, titled "Cold-Induced Adaptive Thermogenesis in Lean and Obese," researchers took a group of people and had them live in a temperature-controlled chamber for a few days. During the first part of the stay, the chamber was kept at 72 degrees F, or 22 C, and they cooled the chamber to 61 degrees F, or 16 degrees C, during the second part of this sequestered study. That's actually not very cold; my house during the winter is barely kept at 60 degrees F. I don't like paying utility bills, and when in Vermont, which is a lot of the time, I sleep at 50 degrees F).

During the study, researchers tested various parameters like total daily energy expenditure (TDEE), skin temperature, and hormone levels.

They found that the lean subjects tended to increase their activity levels to maintain warmth in the cooled environment, but the obese did not. This is called *adaptive thermogenesis*, representing the combination of behaviors and physiological effects that take place to keep one warm when a room is cold.

The study pointed out that "Energy Expenditure (EE) in the cold increased significantly in the lean subjects, but did not in the obese subjects. In both groups, interindividual differences in EE changes were large…." Some people just move around more in the cold, and they tend to be leaner to begin with.

The study also pointed out that the obese subjects had more insulation (their body fat, obviously). They therefore required less physical activity to deal with the cooler room temperatures. The authors speculated that modern life involves too little variability in room temperatures (we keep office and house temperatures too warm and static despite what's going on outside, in most cases). The baking room temperatures where we work and live probably contribute to people falling out of shape, because there is little motivation to move around and develop adaptations to the temperature. In other words, blasting the heat all the time inside is not only expensive from an energy standpoint, but it doesn't contribute to health in the long run.

Sports recovery and the use of cryotherapy has gone high tech, as an article about soccer players in England describes. The players enter special chambers in which the temperature can drop below −200 F (*www.dailymail.co.uk/sport/football/article-1335496/How-hot-Spurs-stay-cool-Rafael-van-der-Vaart-finds-ice-easy-way-recover-hamstring-injury.html*).

This kind of therapy is called *whole-body cryotherapy* (WBC), and it's used to relieve pain and improve the healing of injuries. A number of studies have been implemented to determine the effects of very short-term exposure to extreme cold (such as 20-second winter swims versus 2 minutes of WBC).[9]

Exercise Stress

Exercise itself is a form of stress—particularly short-term, high-intensity exercise, which Chapters 7 and 8 cover in depth. Exercise is hormesis; the body will respond to the short-term intensity or the gradual demands of moderate endurance exercise with positive adaptations, such as a stronger musculature (as with weightlifting) and even improvements in the way your hormonal or endocrine systems function.

According to our originally quoted scientific article ("Mimetics of Hormetic Agents: Stress-Resistance Triggers"), exercise is a hormetic agent that triggers positive gene expression.

In other words, exercise will trigger signaling pathways that make you metabolically more efficient, as long as you don't overdo it (the positive adaptations of training are dose-dependent, like other forms of hormesis, which are toxic when they involve excessive doses).

For example, one study that reviewed the evidence for hormesis and exercise pointed out that moderate running had benefits at the muscular and skeletal levels. These included increased antioxidant capacity in the muscles and improved bone strength, whereas higher-intensity running for long periods catabolized, or broke down, muscles and led to reduced bone-mineral density (these studies were performed on rodents).[10]

This review also pointed out a number of dose-dependent effects (meaning too much treadmill running had a bad rather than beneficial effect) with several internal organ systems.

For example: "Moderate exercise increases pancreatic volume and β-cell mass… and reduces circulating insulin levels, indicative of enhanced insulin sensitivity" (which is a good thing).[11]

The bottom line is, if you've never heard of hormesis before and you are training strategically, as in aiming for resistance training and/or moderate endurance exercise, then you've already been doing it!

Caloric Restriction and Fasting

Intermittent fasting (IF) is itself a stress to the system and hormetic. Chapter 6 includes a detailed discussion of the existing research on the benefits of IF. Caloric restriction (CR) is different than fasting—it involves a chronic, not just temporary or intermittent, reduction of calories consumed per day, by up to 40 percent. In other words, a typical diet for a male American involving 3,200 calories per day would drop to 1,920, and a female's intake of 2,000 calories per day would be reduced to 1,200 calories.

Exercise is hormesis; the body will respond to the short-term intensity or the gradual demands of moderate endurance exercise with positive adaptations, such as a stronger musculature (as with weightlifting) and even improvements in the way your hormonal or endocrine systems function.

CR is one of the few proven life-extension strategies for laboratory animals such as rats (lab experiments using CR have significantly increased lifespan, in the realm of 25 percent).[12]

IF is quite easy to integrate into your lifestyle. Chapter 6 includes several recommendations for making short-term fasts (up to 16 hours) a part of your routine.

CR, however, despite the positive lab results and hormetic effects (in studies), is difficult and enervating for most people. In a word, it's like starvation. This eating (or noneating) strategy provides very little energy for making athletic gains or putting some additional lean mass on your body.

Assorted Hormetic Activities

Having one drink periodically may have a hormetic effect, according to the journal article "Mimetics of Hormetic Agents: Stress-Resistance Triggers":

> *The cardio-protective advantage of moderate consumption of ethanol in popular beverages [the so-called "French Paradox"] may result from ethanol-induced favorable changes in lipid metabolism, antioxidant effects, changes in homeostasis and platelet aggregation, arterial vasodilatation mediated by NO release, expression of cardio-protective proteins, insulin sensitization and lower levels of inflammatory markers.*

> *In humans, a beneficial induction of plasma antioxidants is achieved with one drink (5% v/v alcohol) while an increased prooxidant state occurs after three drinks from volunteers averaged over 360 minutes. One drink of red wine, beer, or stout provided equivalent increases in plasma antioxidant activity without induction of pro-oxidative stress…. Thus, at different doses, different physiological responses occur from benefit to harmful response.* [13]

Translation: one drink, such as a glass of wine or beer, might be good for you, but no more than that can really be called hormesis.

Is *being scared or at a heightened level of alert for a short period of time* hormesis? You could make an argument for it. The short-term fear elicited by, for example, a bungee jump or a trek or hunt in grizzly-bear country (Montana or Wyoming) seems to provide the same "rush" as similar high-intensity physical states. The resulting sensation is one of a heightened sense of connection with your surroundings (like the discussion in Chapter 7 of the Scandinavian concept of *friluftsliv*), and of all your senses acquiring a greater level of acuity.

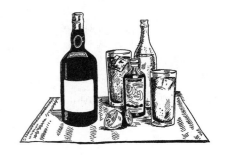

One drink, such as a glass of wine or beer, might be good for you.

Could this short-lived stress be good for you, as opposed to the chronic, thousand little stresses of a typical day lived in the Digital Age (e.g., you're late for the school pickup, you're behind on deadlines, you don't get along with your boss, someone's posted something sociopathic on your Facebook wall, and you're getting subtle slights from the nearby cubicle guy…)? Yeah, I know, this brief discussion is unscientific and unproven, but it's nonetheless worth exploring. Maybe one way we stay fitter is by never ceasing to pursue the natural, ultimate high. Go ahead, challenge yourself. Never stop.

Sports Massage

I included sports massage in this chapter as a legitimate health tweak for people who lift weights, hikes, climbs, skis, bikes, or takes part in a team sport that leaves you stiff, banged up, and with possible overuse issues. There is some controversy about whether sports massage is more art than science, and you can delve into that discussion by searching Google Scholar for "sports massage."

I think there is a good physiological basis for using an experienced sports massage therapist to increase blood flow and help repair damaged muscle fibers, and I can personally attest to its benefits after getting numerous pre- and after-race massages from Sports Massage Pro (*www.sportsmassagepro.com*). Another important consideration is who is doing the massage. Neurosurgery is a highly technical procedure with a scientific basis, but the more subjective consideration of who is actually performing the surgery is critical too.

Check out this rather lengthy review of some of the science on sports massage in the *British Journal of Sports Medicine*: *http://msscentershop.info/content/28/3/153.full.pdf+html/*.

Maybe one way we stay fitter is by never ceasing to pursue the natural, ultimate high.
Go ahead, challenge yourself.

Even if sports massage is more art than science (and I don't think it is, but for the sake of argument)…*so what,* if it works? I once had what I thought was a painful calf tear that lasted more than a week, and was with me for the entire second half of a long duathlon (a race that is a run-bike-run sandwich). I went into Christine's office (see the sidebar on sports massage), she "untied" the knotted calf muscle, and it was completely gone when I walked out of the room.

After that encounter with the sports-massage technique, I was hooked. It seemed so practical. A massage for specific (a muscle or joint problem) or nonspecific purposes will help you recover from hard physical efforts, as well as prepare you for the same kind of activities.

I usually get a deep tissue massage if I don't have any issues, such as niggling soreness or injuries, because the latter technique can kind of hurt in spots (hormesis?). There are numerous kinds of sports massage, from deep tissue to Swedish to Shiatsu. *Many insurance programs will cover massage*, so check with your own provider.

INSIGHTS FROM A SPORTS MASSAGE EXPERT

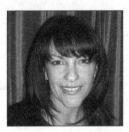

I interviewed Christine Misiano, a wonderful lady who has several decades' worth of sports-massage expertise, mostly in the Newburyport, Massachusetts area. She runs Sports Massage Pro (*www.sportsmassagepro. com*).

What originally inspired your interest in becoming a sports-massage expert?

After being in the massage field for many years I began to realize an affinity toward solving the muscular problems among athletes. I love working with this group of people, because of their proactive attitude when it comes to health and fitness. Working with the body and its repair is also like a puzzle—challenging and rewarding at the same time. To have my clients leave my office feeling calmer and more confident is an amazing job perk!

What are the physical benefits of sports massage?

Sports massage is derived from Swedish massage. From a physical basis, it is designed to stimulate the flow of lymphatic fluid, improve blood circulation overall, improve flexibility by stretching and broadening shortened muscles and breaking up scar tissue, as well as in general prevent injuries and help heal injured muscles and tendons.

What's the typical feedback from your athletes?

The typical result of the massage is that the athlete feels relief, has a considerably better range of motion, and [has] less pain, stress, and tightness. My job is awesome—everyone is happy when they leave!

What do you like most about sports massage yourself, if you're the recipient?

I work out and use my body constantly. After a sports massage, I feel lighter, more flexible, and euphoric—my blood feels like it is flowing more freely. It's a welcome release. Luckily I have never been issued a "Driving While Intoxicated from Massage." That's a joke, by the way!

Conclusion

Here the book comes to an end. I've covered many aspects of fitness—literally as many as I could think of. I haven't flinched from offering technical or scientific information, along with a little homespun wisdom cloaked in a veneer of empirical observation. I hope that you have found the information provocative. I also hope you've found kernels of ideas you have not found in other places and that they make a contribution to your own fitness. After all, what's the use of a book with "fitness" in its title, if not to help make you more fit?

Now it's your turn. Take the information and run with it, and share it judiciously (meaning, don't make a copyright violation!) with friends and loved ones. If you have come across something interesting that you haven't tried before, experiment. If this new technique involves physical activity, especially outdoors, it can never be thought of as a waste of time.

A little analysis often helps and can lead to useful insights. I love recording and digitally mapping my modest outdoor adventures with the best of them. But somehow I think we are living in the age of "hyperanalyzing everything," particularly health and fitness. If somehow you could ask the elegant lynx here in the snowy northern Vermont woods how long it would like to live (it would probably give you an inscrutable look, make a minute fleeting connection, and dash off into the evergreen), it might reply "forever."

Wild animals spend their days simply trying to survive. In a way, their brief, uncataloged lives are dedicated to optimizing survival, and they fit into their niches with a quiet perfection that we have failed to achieve. We don't know how humans spend their days, because the "jury is still out." There are no definitive answers. We've spent eons pondering the meanings of our existence, when maybe a sliver of the answer lies in the gleam of a lynx's eyes before he vanishes into the snow.

I wish you all the best in your pursuit of health. Be strong, help other people, and I hope you find contentment in your fitness efforts.

Chapter 11

Notes

Chapter 1

1. "The Omega-6/Omega-3 Fatty Acid Ratio, Genetic Variation, and Cardiovascular Disease"; *http://apjcn.nhri.org.tw/server/apjcn/volume17/vol17suppl.1/131-134S6-6.pdf*

2. A greatly simplified diagram of human evolution over two million years. See Brian Fagan. *Cro-Magnon: How the Ice Age Gave Birth to the First Modern Humans* (Bloomsbury Press, Kindle Edition), Kindle Locations 567–568.

3. Standing Tall: Plains Indians Enjoyed Height, Health Advantage; *http://researchnews.osu.edu/archive/tallind.htm*

4. Cochran, Gregory; Henry Harpending (2009-01-27). The 10,000 Year Explosion: How Civilization Accelerated Human Evolution (p. 77).

5. Cochran, Gregory; Henry Harpending (2009-01-27). The 10,000 Year Explosion: How Civilization Accelerated Human Evolution (p. 71)

6. Cochran, Gregory; Henry Harpending (2009-01-27). The 10,000 Year Explosion: How Civilization Accelerated Human Evolution (p. 79)

7. Gregory Cochran and Henry Harpending, *The 10,000 Year Explosion: How Civilization Accelerated Human Evolution (Basic Books),* pp. 69-70.

8. ibid, p. 76

9. ibid

10. "Nestle, Glaxo Lobby UN Over Biggest 'Epidemic' Battle Since AIDS"; *www.bloomberg.com/news/2011-09-16/biggest-un-epidemic-battle-since-aids-pits-nestle-glaxo-vs-health-lobby.html*

11. *A* "Origins and Evolution of the Western Diet: Health Implications for the 21st Century"; *www.ajcn.org/content/81/2/341.long*

12. *B* "Eating, Exercise, and 'Thrifty' Genotypes"; *jap.physiology.org/content/96/1/3.long*

13. *C www.thyroid8.com/brooklyn-eagle-bay-ridge-eagle-brooklyn-ny-daily-paper-in-brooklyn.html*

14. "Health-Chair Reform – Your Chair: Comfortable but Deadly"; *http://diabetes.diabetesjournals.org/content/59/11/2715.full*

15. The Engineering Toolbox; *www.engineeringtoolbox.com/met-metabolic-rate-d_733.html*

Chapter 2

1. "The Engineering Toolbox"; *www.engineeringtoolbox.com/met-metabolic-rate-d_733.html*

2. "Screen-Based Entertainment Time, All-Cause Mortality, and Cardiovascular Events,"; *http://content.onlinejacc.org/cgi/content/abstract/57/3/292*

Chapter 3

1. "Alternatives for Macronutrient Intake and Chronic Disease: A comparison of the OmniHeart Diets with Popular Diets and with Dietary Recommendations"; *www.ajcn.org/content/88/1/1.full.pdf+html*

2. *www.iom.edu/Global/News%20Announcements/~/media/C5CD2D-D7840544979A549EC47E56A02B.ashx*

3. *http://nutritiondata.self.com/facts/sweets/5465/2*

4. "Hypothesis: Could Excessive Fructose Intake and Uric Acid Cause Type 2 Diabetes?"; *http://edrv.endojournals.org/content/30/1/96.full*

5. ibid

6. "Is the Fructose Index More Relevant with Regards to Cardiovascular Disease Than the Glycemic Index?"; *www.ncbi.nlm.nih.gov/pubmed/17763967*

7. ibid

8. "Fructose: Metabolic, Hedonic, and Societal Parallels with Ethanol"; *www.ncbi.nlm.nih.gov/pubmed/20800122*

9. ibid

10. "Maltose – Virtual Chembook"; *www.elmhurst.edu/~chm/vchembook/546maltose.html*

11. "Review of Food Chemistry"; *www.vivo.colostate.edu/hbooks/pathphys/digestion/basics/foodchem.html*

12. Shabne, Bilsborough and Neil Mann, "A Review of Issues of Dietary Protein Intake in Humans," *International Journal of Sport Nutrition and Exercise Metabolism*, 2006, pp. 1, 129

13. Patricia Gadsby, "The Inuit Paradox," *Discover Magazine*, Vol. 25 No. 10, October 2004

14. Elaine Marieb and Katja Hoehn, *Human Anatomy & Physiology*, Seventh Edition (Benjamin Cummings), p. 971

15. ibid, p. 49

16. ibid, p. 929

17. ibid, p. 973

18. Bilsborough and Mann, 2006; *International Journal of Sport Nutrition and Exercise Metabolism* "A Review of Issues of Dietary Protein Intake in Humans," Bilsborough and Mann.

19. Source: *http://nutritiondata.self.com/facts/legumes-and-legume-products/4415/2*

20. Source: *http://nutritiondata.self.com/facts/legumes-and-legume-products/4380/2*

21. Bilsborough and Mann, 2006: *International Journal of Sport Nutrition and Exercise Metabolism*, "A Review of Issues of Dietary Protein Intake in Humans"

22. Source: *http://en.wikipedia.org/wiki/Fatty_acid_metabolism#Fatty_acids_as_an_energy_source*

23. Source: *http://nutritiondata.self.com/facts/fats-and-oils/509/2*

24. "Fats and Fatty Acids"; *www.chemistryexplained.com/Di-Fa/Fats-and-Fatty-Acids.html*

25. Gerard Mullin, M.D., "Search tor the Optimal Diet"; *http://ncp.sagepub.com/content/25/6/581.full*

26. *http://lpi.oregonstate.edu/infocenter/othernuts/Omega3fa/*

27. *http://nutritiondata.self.com/facts/fast-foods-generic/9277/2*

28. *http://lpi.oregonstate.edu/infocenter/othernuts/Omega3fa/#metabolism*

29. See: *http://nutritiondata.self.com/facts/finfish-and-shellfish-products/4038/2*

30. *http://nutritiondata.self.com/facts/baked-products/5003/2*

31. Marieb and Hoehn, p. 969

32. George Cahill; *Annual Review of Nutrition*, 2006; *www.annualreviews.org/doi/full/10.1146/annurev.nutr.26.061505.111258*

33. *www.biomedcentral.com/content/pdf/1476-511x-5-13.pdf*

34. *www.proteinpower.com/drmike/ketones-and-ketosis/metabolism-and-ketosis/*

Chapter 4

1. Frances R. Frankenburg, *Vitamin Discoveries and Disasters*, (Praeger, Kindle Edition), Chapters 2 & 3

2. "Dietary Reference Intakes (DRIs): Estimated Average Requirements; *www.iom.edu/Activities/Nutrition/SummaryDRIs/~/media/Files/Activity%20Files/Nutrition/DRIs/5_Summary%20Table%20Tables%201-4.pdf*

3. "Serum Vitamin C and the Prevalence of Vitamin C Deficiency in the United States: 2003-2004 National Health and Nutrition Examination Survey (NHANES)"; *www.ncbi.nlm.nih.gov/pubmed/19675106*. "More than 20% of adults showed marginal vitamin C status, placing them at risk of vitamin C deficiency, similar to the 20–23% estimates in NHANES III." The study showed about 7 percent of people to be deficient, with serum C levels at <11 uM.

4. "Multivitamin/mineral Suppliments and Prevention of Chronic Disease: Executive Summary"; www.ajcn.org/content/85/1/265S.full

5. "Multivitamin/Mineral Supplements and Prevention of Chronic Disease: Executive Summary"; *www.ajcn.org/content/85/1/265S.short*

6. NutritionData; *http://nutritiondata.self.com/topics/processing*

7. "Radical-Scavenging Activity of Vegetables and the Effect of Cooking on Their Activity"; *www.jstage.jst.go.jp/article/fstr/7/3/250/_pdf*

8. Office of Dietary Supplements; Vitamin A; *http://ods.od.nih.gov/factsheets/VitaminA-HealthProfessional/*

9. University of Minnesota, Nutrition Coordinating Center; *www.ncc.umn. edu/products/databaseNUTvitamins.html*

10. Retinoic acid; *www.sabiosciences.com/pathway.php?sn=Retinoic_Acid_ Mediated_Apoptosis*

11. Linus Pauling Institute: Micronutrient Information Center; Vitamin A; *http://lpi.oregonstate.edu/infocenter/vitamins/vitaminA/index. html#function*

12. Office of Dietary Supplements; Vitamin A; *http://ods.od.nih.gov/fact-sheets/VitaminA-HealthProfessional/#h3*

13. Office of Dietary Supplements; Vitamin A; *http://ods.od.nih.gov/fact-sheets/vitamina/#h7*

14. ibid

15. Vitamin D Council; *www.vitamindcouncil.org/about-vitamin-d/what-is-vitamin-d/what-is-vitamin-d/*

16. page 108 "Hypovitaminosis D in Medical Inpatients"; www.nejm.org/ doi/full/10.1056/NEJM199803193381201#t=article

17. "Vitamin D and Elderly Health"; *www.massgeneral.org/about/pressrelease.aspx?id=1170*

18. Elaine Marieb and Katja Hoehn, *Human Anatomy & Physiology*, Seventh Edition (Benjamin Cummings), p. 638

19. Linus Pauling Institute: Micronutrient Information Center; Vitamin D; *http://lpi.oregonstate.edu/infocenter/vitamins/vitaminD/*

20. Office of Dietary Supplements; Vitamin D; *http://ods.od.nih.gov/fact-sheets/vitamind*

21. ibid

22. ibid

23. Office of Dietary Supplements; Vitamin D; *http://ods.od.nih.gov/fact-sheets/vitamind/#h1*

24. "Markedly Higher Vitamin D Intake Needed to Reduce Cancer Risk, Researchers Say"; *www.sciencedaily.com/releases/2011/02/110222140546. htm*

25. Linus Pauling Institute: Micronutrient Information Center; Vitamin E; *http://lpi.oregonstate.edu/infocenter/vitamins/vitaminE/*

26. Office of Dietary Supplements; Vitamin E; *http://ods.od.nih.gov/fact-sheets/vitamine/#h5*

27. ibid

28. according to a 2006 journal article called "Vitamin K Contents of Meat, Dairy, and Fast Food in the U.S. Diet." A PDF version is here: *www.ars.usda.gov/sp2userfiles/place/12354500/articles/jafc54_463-467.pdf.*

29. "Dietary Intake of Menaquinone Is Associated with a Reduced Risk of Coronary Heart Disease: The Rotterdam Study"; *http://jn.nutrition.org/content/134/11/3100.full*

30. Frankenburg, (Kindle Locations 252–253)

31. Linus Pauling Institute: Micronutrient Information Center Thiamin; *http://lpi.oregonstate.edu/infocenter/vitamins/thiamin/*

32. *http://lpi.oregonstate.edu/infocenter/vitamins/riboflavin/*

33. *http://lpi.oregonstate.edu/infocenter/vitamins/niacin/*

34. *http://lpi.oregonstate.edu/infocenter/vitamins/pa/*

35. *http://lpi.oregonstate.edu/infocenter/vitamins/vitaminB6/*

36. *http://lpi.oregonstate.edu/infocenter/vitamins/biotin/*

37. *http://en.wikipedia.org/wiki/Biotin_deficiency*

38. *http://ods.od.nih.gov/factsheets/folate*

39. *http://ods.od.nih.gov/factsheets/vitaminb12#h2*

40. "Toward a new recommended dietary allowance for Vitamin C based on antioxidant and health effects in humans"; *http://www.ajcn.org/content/69/6/1086.full*

41. Max Hastings, Inferno: The World at War, 1939–1945"; (Knopf), p. 168

42. Marieb and Hoehn, p. 952

43. "Understanding Sources of Dietary Phosphorus in the Treatment of Patients with Chronic Kidney Disease"; *http://cjasn.asnjournals.org/content/5/3/519.full#sec-1*

44. *http://lpi.oregonstate.edu/infocenter/minerals/phosphorus/*

45. "High Sodium, Low Potassium Diet Linked to Increased Risk of Death"; *www.cdc.gov/media/releases/2011/p0711_sodiumpotassiumdiet.html*

Chapter 7

46. *http://en.wikipedia.org/wiki/Sulfur#Protein_and_organic_cofactors*

Chapter 5

1. *www.grownyc.org/ourmarkets*

2. *www.livinghistoryfarm.org/farminginthe40s/crops_02.html*

3. *www.economist.com/node/12792420?story_id=12792420*

4. *http://shine.yahoo.com/channel/food/supermarket-strategies-359780*

5. *www.marketstormer.com/supermarket-merchandising.htm*

Chapter 6

1. Herbert Shelton, Fasting for Renewal of Life, Second Edition (American Natural Hygiene Society), p. 314

2. "Pathophysiology of the Endocrine System"; *www.vivo.colostate.edu/hbooks/pathphys/endocrine/hypopit/gh.html*

3. "Fasting: The History, Pathophysiology and Complications;" *www.ncbi.nlm.nih.gov/pmc/articles/PMC1274154/*

4. "Alternate-Day Fasting and Chronic Disease Prevention: A Review of Human and Animal Trials"; *www.ajcn.org/content/86/1/7.full*

5. "Beneficial Effects of Intermittent Fasting and Caloric Restriction on the Cardiovascular and Cerebrovascular Systems"; *www.jnutbio.com/article/S0955-2863(04)00261-X/abstract*

6. "Beneficial Metabolic Adaptations Due to Endurance Exercise Training in the Fasted State"; *www.ncbi.nlm.nih.gov/pubmed/21051570*

7. "Training in the Fasted State Improves Glucose Tolerance During Fat-Rich Diet"; [*www.ncbi.nlm.nih.gov/pubmed/20837645*

8. "Fasting: The History, Pathophysiology and Complications"; *www.ncbi.nlm.nih.gov/pmc/articles/PMC1274154/*

Chapter 7

1. "Why Are Melanoma Survivors Found to be at Increased Risk of Other Cancers?"; *www.drbriffa.com/2010/0318/why-are-melanoma-survivors-found-to-be-at-increased-risk-of-other-cancers/*

2. *www.sleepfoundation.org/article/sleep-topics/melatonin-and-sleep*

3. "Friluftsliv: The Scandinavian Philosophy of Outdoor Life"; *http://jee.lakeheadu.ca/index.php/cjee/article/viewFile/302/222*

4. "Traditionally Living Populations in East Africa Have a Mean Serum 25-Hydroxyvitamin D Concentration of 115 nmol/l"; *http://journals.cambridge.org/action/displayAbstract?fromPage=online&aid=8478473*

5. "Aging, Muscle Fiber Type, and Contractile Function in Sprint-Trained Athletes"; *http://jap.physiology.org/content/101/3/906.full*

6. ibid

7. "Short-Term Sprint Interval Versus Traditional Endurance Training: Similar Initial Adaptations in Human Skeletal Muscle and Exercise Performance"; *www.ncbi.nlm.nih.gov/pmc/articles/PMC1995688/*

8. *www.ritsumei.ac.jp/eng/html/research/areas/feat-researchers/interview/izumi_t.html/*

9. *www.military.com/military-fitness/navy-special-operations/navy-seal-fitness-test*

10. *www.topografix.com/gpx.asp*

Chapter 8

1. National Strength and Conditioning Association, Thomas R. Baechle and Roger W. Earle, eds.; *Essentials of Strength Training and Conditioning* (Human Kinetics, Kindle Edition), (Kindle Locations 2060–2063).

2. "Nonexercise Activity Thermogenesis (NEAT): Environment and Biology"; *ajpendo.physiology.org/content/286/5/E675.full*

3. "An Easy Approach to Calculating Estimated Energy Requirements"; *www.ncbi.nlm.nih.gov/pmc/articles/PMC1784117/*

4. *http://en.wikipedia.org/wiki/One-repetition_maximum*

5. *National Strength and Conditioning Association, Kindle Location 11890*

6. ibid, (Kindle Locations 2216–2223)

7. ibid, (Kindle Locations 12003–12004)

Chapter 9

1. *http://en.wikipedia.org/wiki/One-repetition_maximum*

2. "Scientists Finding Out What Losing Sleep Does to a Body"; *www.washingtonpost.com/wp-dyn/content/article/2005/10/08/AR2005100801405.html*

3. "Sleep Loss and Inflammation"; *www.sciencedirect.com/science/article/pii/S1521690X10001144*

4. Elaine Marieb and Katja Hoehn, *Human Anatomy & Physiology*, Seventh Edition (), p. 460

5. *www.sleepfoundation.org/article/how-sleep-works/what-happens-when-you-sleep*

6. Marieb and Hoehn, p. 458

7. ibid

8. ibid

9. *www.psychosomaticmedicine.org/content/64/1/71.full*

Chapter 10

1. "Nutrition and Athletic Performance": *http://journals.lww.com/acsm-msse/Fulltext/2009/03000/Nutrition_and_Athletic_Performance.27.aspx*

2. "Nutrition for the Sprinter"; *www.ncbi.nlm.nih.gov/pubmed/18049979*

3. ibid

4. ibid "High-Carbohydrate Versus High-Fat Diets in Endurance Sports"; *www.sfsn.ethz.ch/PDF/06_Jeukendrup.pdf*

5. ibid

6. "Effect of Protein/Essential Amino Acids and Resistance Training on Skeletal Muscle Hypertrophy: A Case for Whey Protein"; *www.ncbi.nlm.nih.gov/pmc/articles/PMC2901380/*

7. "Nutrition for the Sprinter"; *www.ncbi.nlm.nih.gov/pubmed/18049979*

8. "Nutrition and Athletic Performance"; *journals.lww.com/acsm-msse/Fulltext/2009/03000/Nutrition_and_Athletic_Performance.27.aspx*

9. ibid

10. ibid

11. ibid

12. ibid

13. "Nutrition and Athletic Performance"; *journals.lww.com/acsm-msse/Full-text/2009/03000/Nutrition_and_Athletic_Performance.27.aspx*

14. ibid

15. ibid

16. ibid

17. "Nutrition for the Sprinter."; *www.ncbi.nlm.nih.gov/pubmed/18049979*

18. ibid

19. "Nutrition and Athletic Performance"; *http://journals.lww.com/acsm-msse/Fulltext/2009/03000/Nutrition_and_Athletic_Performance.27.aspx*

20. "Nutrition for the Sprinter"; *www.ncbi.nlm.nih.gov/pubmed/18049979*

21. *http://en.wikipedia.org/wiki/Creatine*

22. "Nutrition for the Sprinter"; *www.ncbi.nlm.nih.gov/pubmed/18049979*

23. ibid

24. "Nutrition and Athletic Performance"; *http://journals.lww.com/acsm-msse/Fulltext/2009/03000/Nutrition_and_Athletic_Performance.27.aspx*

25. ibid

26. ibid

27. ibid

28. "High-Carbohydrate Versus High-Fat Diets in Endurance Sports"; *http://www.sfsn.ethz.ch/PDF/06_Jeukendrup.pdf*

29. "Nutrition for Optimal Performance During Exercise: Carbohydrate and Fat"; *http://journals.lww.com/acsm-csmr/Abstract/2002/08000/Nutrition_for_Optimal_Performance_During_Exercise_.6.aspx*

30. "'Fat Adaptation' for Athletic Performance: The Nail in the Coffin?"; *http://jap.physiology.org/content/100/1/7.full*

31. www.amazon.com/Paleo-Diet-Athletes-Nutritional-Performance/
    dp/1594860890/ref=sr_1_1?s=books&ie=UTF8&qid=1327069215&sr=1-1

Chapter 11

1. "Mimetics of Hormetic Agents: Stress-Resistance Triggers"; www.ncbi.
    nlm.nih.gov/pmc/articles/PMC2836146/

2. "Adapted Cold Shower as a Potential Treatment for Depression"; www.
    medical-hypotheses.com/article/S0306-9877(07)00566-X/abstract

3. "Possible Stimulation of Anti-Tumor Immunity Using Repeated Cold
    Stress: A Hypothesis"; www.biomedcentral.com/content/pdf/1750-9378-
    2-20.pdf

4. "Immune System of Cold-Exposed and Cold-Adapted Humans"; www.
    ncbi.nlm.nih.gov/pubmed/8925815

5. www.ncbi.nlm.nih.gov/sites/entrez?db=pubmed&cmd=Search&term=QJ
    M[Jour]+AND+92[Volume]+AND+193[page]

6. www.shipwrite.bc.ca/Chilling_truth.htm

7. http://en.wikipedia.org/wiki/Mammalian_diving_reflex#Effect

8. "Alternatively Activated Macrophages Produce Catecholamines to Sus-
    tain Adaptive Thermogenesis"; www.nature.com/nature/journal/v480/
    n7375/full/nature10653.html

9. "Effects of Long-Term Whole-Body Cold Exposures on Plas-
    ma Concentrations of ACTH"; informahealthcare.com/doi/
    abs/10.1080/00365510701516350

10. "Exercise Induced Hormesis"; www.springerlink.com/content/m76211v-
    7704v0w81/

11. ibid

12. "Role of Hormesis in Life Extension by Caloric Restriction"; www.ncbi.
    nlm.nih.gov/pmc/articles/PMC2477693/

13. www.ncbi.nlm.nih.gov/pubmed/20221297

Index

Colophon

The cover and heading font is BentonSans; the body and margin note font is Myriad Pro; the interview heading font is CamoSans.

About the Author

Bruce W. Perry played college soccer in New York, then amidst a varied career in journalism and software engineering finished literally (ask his knees!) hundreds of road races and multisport events. He's since moved on to family life and recreational alpine hiking, skiing, and resistance training. He has also written two recent software books for O'Reilly Media. After an unguided youth, he now hangs out weightlifting in gyms again, and climbs with guides now, recently Piz Palu in the Swiss Alps, Mt. Whitney's Mountaineer's Route, and Mt. Rainier.

Have it your way.

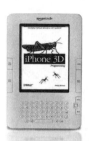 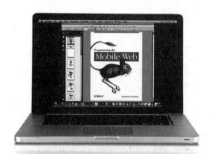 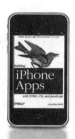 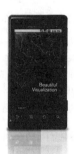
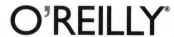
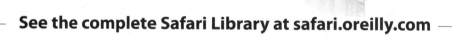

Get even more for your money.

Join the O'Reilly Community, and register the O'Reilly books you own. It's free, and you'll get:

- $4.99 ebook upgrade offer
- 40% upgrade offer on O'Reilly print books
- Membership discounts on books and events
- Free lifetime updates to ebooks and videos
- Multiple ebook formats, DRM FREE
- Participation in the O'Reilly community
- Newsletters
- Account management
- 100% Satisfaction Guarantee

Signing up is easy:

1. **Go to: oreilly.com/go/register**
2. **Create an O'Reilly login.**
3. **Provide your address.**
4. **Register your books.**

Note: English-language books only

To order books online:

oreilly.com/store

For questions about products or an order:

orders@oreilly.com

To sign up to get topic-specific email announcements and/or news about upcoming books, conferences, special offers, and new technologies:

elists@oreilly.com

For technical questions about book content:

booktech@oreilly.com

To submit new book proposals to our editors:

proposals@oreilly.com

O'Reilly books are available in multiple DRM-free ebook formats. For more information:

oreilly.com/ebooks

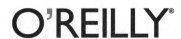

Spreading the knowledge of innovators   oreilly.com